GERIATRIC
SECRETS

GERIATRIC SECRETS

MARY ANN FORCIEA, MD
Assistant Professor of Medicine
University of Pennsylvania School of Medicine
Hospital of the University of Pennsylvania
Presbyterian Medical Center
Philadelphia, Pennsylvania

RISA J. LAVIZZO-MOUREY, MD, MBA
Director, Institute on Aging
Chief of Geriatric Medicine
University of Pennsylvania School of Medicine
Hospital of the University of Pennsylvania
Presbyterian Medical Center
Philadelphia, Pennsylvania

HANLEY & BELFUS, INC./ Philadelphia
MOSBY/ St. Louis • Baltimore • Boston • Carlsbad • Chicago • London
Madrid • Naples • New York • Philadelphia • Sydney • Tokyo • Toronto

Publisher: **HANLEY & BELFUS, INC.**
       Medical Publishers
       210 South 13th Street
       Philadelphia, PA 19107
       (215) 546-7293; 800-962-1892
       FAX (215) 790-9330

North American and worldwide sales and distribution:

       MOSBY
       11830 Westline Industrial Drive
       St. Louis, MO 63146

In Canada: Times Mirror Professional Publishing, Ltd.
       130 Flaska Drive
       Markham, Ontario L6G 1B8
       Canada

Library of Congress Cataloging-in-Publication Data

Geriatric Secrets / [edited by] Mary Ann Forciea, Risa J. Lavizzo-Mourey,
  p. cm. - (Secrets Series®)
 Includes bibliographical references and index.
 ISBN 1-56053-162-2 (paper : alk. paper)
 1. Geriatric-Miscellanea. I. Forciea, Mary Ann, 1949-.
II. Lavizzo-Mourey, Risa. III. Series.
 [DNLM: 1. Geriatrics–examination questions. 2. Aging–
physiology–examination questions. WT 18.2 G369 1996]
RC952.5.G44346 1996
 618.97–dc20
 DNLM/DLC
 for Library of Congress   96-9463
                CIP

GERIATRIC SECRETS   ISBN 1-56053-162-2

Last digit is the print number: 9 8 7 6 5 4 3 2 1

CONTENTS

CONTRIBUTORS

Janet Lee Abrahm, M.D.
Associate Professor of Medicine, University of Pennsylvania School of Medicine, Philadelphia; Chief, Medical Service, Veterans Affairs Medical Center, Philadelphia, Pennsylvania

Elias Abrutyn, M.D.
Professor of Medicine and Associate Dean for Veterans Affairs, Medical College of Pennsylvania and Hahnemann University, Philadelphia; Associate Chief, Medical Service, and Chief, Infectious Diseases, Veterans Affairs Medical Center, Philadelphia, Pennsylvania

Steven E. Arnold, M.D.
Assistant Professor of Psychiatry and Neurology, University of Pennsylvania School of Medicine, Hospital of the University of Pennsylvania, Philadelphia, Pennsylvania

Michelle E. Battistini, M.D.
Assistant Professor, Obstetrics/Gynecology, and Director, Penn Health for Women, University of Pennsylvania School of Medicine, Hospital of the University of Pennsylvania, Philadelphia, Pennsylvania

Marie A. Bernard, M.D.
Associate Professor of Medicine and Associate Chief of Staff, Geriatrics and Extended Care, University of Oklahoma Health Sciences Center, Oklahoma City; Oklahoma University Hospital and Veterans Affairs Medical Center, Oklahoma City, Oklahoma

Elizabeth Capezuti, Ph.D., R.N.
Research Assistant Professor, School of Nursing, University of Pennsylvania, Philadelphia; Nurse Practitioner, Geriatric Nursing Consulting Service, Philadelphia, Pennsylvania

Stephen I. Chavin, M.D.
Professor of Medicine, Medical College of Pennsylvania and Hahnemann University, Philadelphia; Adjunct Associate Professor of Medicine, University of Pennsylvania School of Medicine, Philadelphia; Veterans Affairs Medical Center and Medical College of Pennsylvania—Main Clinical Campus, Philadelphia, Pennsylvania

Grace A. Cordts, M.D., M.S., M.P.H.
Faculty, Internal Medicine, York Health System, York Hospital, York, Pennsylvania

Susan C. Day, M.D., M.P.H.
Adjunct Associate Professor of Internal Medicine, University of Pennsylvania School of Medicine, Philadelphia; Chestnut Hill Hospital, Chestnut Hill, Pennsylvania

William F. Edwards, M.S.N., R.N., C.S., C.R.N.P.
Geriatric Nurse Practitioner, Geriatric Assessment Center, Abington Memorial Hospital, Abington, Pennsylvania

Daniel E. Everitt, M.D.
Assistant Clinical Professor of Medicine, University of Pennsylvania School of Medicine, Philadelphia; Director of Clinical Pharmacology, SmithKline Beecham, Philadelphia, Pennsylvania

Roy S. Feldman, D.D.S., D.M.Sc.
Chief, Dental Service, Veterans Affairs Medical Center; Adjunct Professor of Periodontology/Dental Care Systems, University of Pennsylvania School of Dental Medicine, Philadelphia, Pennsylvania

Mary Ann Forciea, M.D.
Assistant Professor of Medicine, University of Pennsylvania School of Medicine, Philadelphia; Hospital of the University of Pennsylvania and Presbyterian Medical Center, Philadelphia, Pennsylvania

Robert Goldman, M.D.
Assistant Professor, Department of Rehabilitation Medicine, University of Pennsylvania School of Medicine, Hospital of the University of Pennsylvania, Philadelphia, Pennsylvania

Richard Harvey Greenberg, M.D.
Senior Fellow, Hematology and Medical Oncology, Hospital of the University of Pennsylvania, Philadelphia, Pennsylvania

Raquel E. Gur, M.D., Ph.D.
Professor of Psychiatry, University of Pennsylvania School of Medicine, Hospital of the University of Pennsylvania, Philadelphia, Pennsylvania

Ruben C. Gur, Ph.D.
Professor and Director of Neuropsychology, Department of Psychiatry, University of Pennsylvania School of Medicine, Hospital of the University of Pennsylvania, Philadelphia, Pennsylvania

Howard Hurtig, M.D.
Clinical Professor of Neurology, Temple University School of Medicine, Graduate Hospital, Philadelphia, Pennsylvania

Jerry C. Johnson, M.D.
Associate Professor of Medicine, University of Pennsylvania School of Medicine, Hospital of the University of Pennsylvania, Philadelphia, Pennsylvania

Fran E. Kaiser, M.D.
Professor of Medicine and Associate Director, Division of Geriatric Medicine, St. Louis University School of Medicine, St. Louis University Hospital, St. Louis, Missouri

Ira R. Katz, M.D., Ph.D.
Professor of Psychiatry, and Director, Section of Geriatric Psychiatry, University of Pennsylvania School of Medicine, Hospital of the University of Pennsylvania, Philadelphia, Pennsylvania

Glenn W. Knox, M.D.
Assistant Professor of Otorhinolaryngology–Head and Neck Surgery, University of Pennsylvania School of Medicine, Philadelphia, Pennsylvania

Risa Lavizzo-Mourey, M.D., M.B.A.
Director, Institute on Aging, and Chief, Division of Geriatric Medicine, University of Pennsylvania School of Medicine, Hospital of the University of Pennsylvania and Presbyterian Medical Center, Philadelphia, Pennsylvania

Bruce T. Liang, M.D.
Assistant Professor of Medicine and Pharmacology, University of Pennsylvania School of Medicine; Cardiology Staff, Hospital of the University of Pennsylvania, Philadelphia, Pennsylvania

Cheng-An Mao, M.D., M.P.H.
Geriatric Fellow, Division of Geriatric Medicine, University of Pennsylvania School of Medicine, Hospital of the University of Pennsylvania, Philadelphia, Pennsylvania

David J. Margolis, M.D.
Assistant Professor of Dermatology, University of Pennsylvania School of Medicine, Hospital of the University of Pennsylvania, Philadelphia, Pennsylvania

Joseph Robert McClellan, M.D., F.A.C.C., F.A.C.P.
Assistant Professor of Medicine, University of Pennsylvania School of Medicine, Philadelphia; Associate Director, Cardiovascular Medicine Program, Hospital of the University of Pennsylvania; Chief of Cardiovascular Medicine, Presbyterian Medical Center, Philadelphia, Pennsylvania

Harold Mignott, M.D.
Assistant Professor of Medicine, University of Pennsylvania School of Medicine, Hospital of the University of Pennsylvania, Philadelphia, Pennsylvania

David S. Miller, M.D.
Assistant Professor of Psychiatry and Director of Inpatient Geriatric Psychiatry, University of Pennsylvania School of Medicine, Hospital of the University of Pennsylvania, Philadelphia, Pennsylvania

Jeffrey Miller, M.D.
Assistant Instructor, Department of Dermatology, University of Pennsylvania School of Medicine, Philadelphia, Pennsylvania

Paul J. Moberg, Ph.D.
Assistant Professor of Neuropsychology, Department of Psychiatry, University of Pennsylvania School of Medicine, Hospital of the University of Pennsylvania, Philadelphia, Pennsylvania

David W. Oslin, M.D.
Assistant Professor, Department of Psychiatry, University of Pennsylvania School of Medicine, Philadelphia, Pennsylvania

Iris Reyes, M.D.
Assistant Professor of Emergency Medicine, University of Pennsylvania School of Medicine, Hospital of the University of Pennsylvania, Philadelphia, Pennsylvania

Keith M. Robinson, M.D.
Assistant Professor of Rehabilitation Medicine, University of Pennsylvania School of Medicine, Philadelphia, Pennsylvania

Edna P. Schwab, M.D.
Assistant Professor of Medicine, Division of Geriatric Medicine, University of Pennsylvania School of Medicine, Philadelphia, Pennsylvania

Eugenia L. Siegler, M.D.
Department of Medicine, New York University School of Medicine; Chief of Geriatrics, Brooklyn Hospital Center, Brooklyn, New York

Dorothy A. Slavin, M.D.
Fellow, Division of Infectious Diseases, Medical College of Pennsylvania and Hahnemann University, Philadelphia, Pennsylvania

Charles Spencer, M.D., Ph.D.
Clinical Assistant Professor, Division of Geriatric Medicine, University of Pennsylvania School of Medicine, Hospital of the University of Pennsylvania, Philadelphia, Pennsylvania

Joel E. Streim, M.D.
Assistant Professor, Department of Psychiatry, University of Pennsylvania School of Medicine, Veterans Affairs Medical Center, and Hospital of the University of Pennsylvania, Philadelphia, Pennsylvania

Dana L. Suskind, M.D.
Department of Otolaryngology–Head and Neck Surgery, Hospital of the University of Pennsylvania, Philadelphia, Pennsylvania

Raymond R. Townsend, M.D.
Assistant Professor of Medicine, University of Pennsylvania School of Medicine, Hospital of the University of Pennsylvania, Philadelphia, Pennsylvania

David J. Vaughn, M.D.
Assistant Professor of Medicine, Division of Hematology/Oncology, Hospital of the University of Pennsylvania, Philadelphia, Pennsylvania

Margaret E. Yetter-Pritchard, M.S.W., L.S.W.
Division of Geriatric Medicine, University of Pennsylvania School of Medicine, Hospital of the University of Pennsylvania, Philadelphia, Pennsylvania

PREFACE

Geriatric Secrets is designed for medical students and other health care professionals who are learning the principles of geriatric practice. We use a direct approach familiar to students, the question-answer format, because of its ability to cut to the chase. Now more than ever, students must assimilate large amounts of information quickly and effectively. The Socratic method, whether applied on rounds or in board review books, is an effective efficient method of imparting information. We attempted to make the book reader-friendly. Where possible, we encouraged the use of summary tables and bullets rather than long passages of text.

Consider this book a handbook, not a textbook. It provides an overview of the salient issues in the practice of geriatrics, rather than a comprehensive or exhaustive discussion. Within these constraints, we have tried to emphasize the art of geriatrics—the personal touch, the team approach, the clinical challenges, and the tremendous satisfaction of improving the quality of someone's life, however briefly. Chapter 1 focuses on the art of practicing geriatrics and introduces some of the patients who have taught us the real "secrets" of geriatrics.

Next to the satisfaction of practicing geriatrics, our greatest pleasure comes from teaching it. For many reasons, too few students are exposed to geriatric medicine early enough and often enough to experience its rewards. We take pleasure in the fact that the impact of this book will be felt not only by the students who will learn directly from its pages, but also by the clinicians of tomorrow who will benefit from the educational programs of the Institute on Aging at the University of Pennsylvania, to which the royalties from the sale of the book will be donated.

Finally, we gratefully acknowledge those whose contributions helped us turn a concept into a book: the Ralston House for funding the project, the authors for providing content, and the project team, Sandra L. Chaff, Nathan Griffith, and Amy Phillips, for making it happen.

Mary Ann Forciea, M.D.
Risa Lavizzo-Mourey, M.D., M.B.A.

I: Overview

1. THE ART AND PRACTICE OF GERIATRICS

Risa Lavizzo-Mourey, M.D., M.B.A., and Mary Ann Forciea, M.D.

Most of this book focuses on the practice of geriatrics. It strives to impart the basics of geriatric medicine by using a direct approach—questions and answers. However, the art of caring for older patients is as important as the clinical facts, albeit less appreciated. The principles that underlie the art and inherent satisfaction of practicing geriatrics are the "Geriatric Secrets" revealed in this chapter. As with all healthcare, the real secrets reside in the patients. Although every patient is unique, the commonality among them often defines the approach and direction of a specialty or a discipline. Sometimes the commonality is as simple as a particular disease. In the case of geriatrics, the commonalities are more complex, going beyond age, specific diseases, or particular organ systems. This chapter introduces a few of our patients, who, over the years, defined the art and practice of geriatrics for us.

Complex Medicine—Mrs. M

Geriatric patients have multiple chronic diseases, along with all the sequelae and treatments that chronic conditions entail. Chronic disease, coupled with a vulnerability to acute illness and disability, means that geriatric clinical situations are rarely simple. As clinicians, mostly we are taught to make the diagnosis, to find the malady, and to cure it. In geriatrics there is rarely one diagnosis; the average is four. The diagnoses may be related, sharing organ systems or pathophysiology, but just as often coexisting conditions merely fulfill the dictum that common diseases occur commonly together. Whichever the case, multiple chronic diseases interact, adding ambiguity and complications. As a result, geriatric clinical situations are almost always challenging, requiring knowledge, judgment, and good problem-solving skills.

Mrs. M illustrates this point. At 75 years old, Mrs. M has coronary artery disease and a history of two myocardial infarctions despite a series of angioplasties and a coronary artery bypass graft. Mrs. M is a slight woman with limited bone mass and has been on hormonal replacement therapy (HRT) since menopause. We did not question estrogen replacement until she developed stage I breast cancer. The tumor was quickly and effectively treated with lumpectomy and radiation. Then came the complicated question of whether to continue the HRT. Estrogen could stimulate tumor growth, but without it she was at greater risk for another MI and osteoporosis. Moreover, Mrs. M suffered from debilitating hot flushes whenever the HRT was discontinued. Ultimately we continued the HRT, following closely for signs of cancer recurrence. Knowledge, judgment, and active consideration of Mrs. M's preference lead us to the best "solution" for her. Another patient, less compliant or with more advanced cancer, might warrant a different approach.

As challenging as juggling the management of half a dozen chronic diseases—such as diabetes, hypertension, polymyalgia rheumatica, coronary artery disease, nephrosclerosis, and cataracts—can be, it is the superimposed acute disease that often tests one's clinical acumen.

Mr. H

A 92-year-old retired engineer, Mr. H moved in with his son and daughter-in-law after the death of his wife. Mr. H is limited in mobility by coronary artery disease and severe osteoarthritis of both knees. Despite his mobility limitations, Mr. H leads an active intellectual and social life through telephone conversations and visits from neighbors.

One winter, Mr. H developed a severe respiratory tract infection. A chest x-ray revealed multiple smooth pulmonary nodules, which almost certainly represented multiple metastases. His respiratory tract infection resolved. Mr. H and his family discussed diagnostic and therapeutic options with the geriatrics team. Mr. H decided not to pursue further evaluation of the metastases.

Eighteen months later, Mr. H continues to be pain free. He is unable to leave his room due to his dyspnea but still plays a vital role in his family and neighborhood.

In caring for patients with multiple illnesses, patients or their surrogates must determine which symptoms are the most burdensome. The impact of treatment on "critical" symptoms must be evaluated, both in terms of efficacy and potential side effects. To Mr. H, dyspnea was an "old friend." He had adjusted his lifestyle to this limitation and was not frightened by the thought of progression of breathlessness. He was terrified by the prospect of pain or nausea. In his family meetings, he finally concluded that he wished no disruption of his life unless pain intervened. The geriatrics team and Mr. H's family were able to focus on Mr. H's view of his life and to design a program of care that responded to his wishes.

Differentiating Aging from Disease—Mr. I

Shakespeare characterized old age as a second childhood: "sans eyes, sans teeth, sans everything."

The body changes with aging, and many organs and organ systems become more limited in their capacity to carry out prescribed functions. However, the losses conjured by Shakespeare's words generally result from disease, not normal aging. Differentiating the consequences of normal aging from disease so that disease can be treated or managed is a fundamental principle of geriatrics. For example, the ratio of type I to type II muscle fibers changes with age, but does not cause debilitating muscle atrophy. Sleep patterns change—less deep sleep and increased ratios of REM to non-REM sleep. Yet daytime somnolence, insomnia, and early awaking, while common complaints among the elderly, are not a part of normal aging. Part of the art of geriatrics is not only knowing the difference between normal aging and disease, but also being able to convince patients of the difference.

Mr. I could not hear as well as he did as a young man. He saw it as an inevitable consequence of aging and was prepared to accept the attendant inconveniences. It was his wife who insisted that he "look into it." She complained about the blaring television and was growing tired of repeating herself or arguing about what had been said. Mr. I's hearing loss was severe and asymmetric, involving low- as well as high-frequency ranges. Presbycusis, commonly seen in elders (see the chapter entitled "Sensory Changes"), typically involves high frequencies. Mr. I's problem was not normal aging and was treatable with a hearing aid.

Convincing Mr. I that he had a treatable problem meant correcting a lot of misconceptions without creating unrealistically high expectations. After he got a hearing aid, his hearing improved but was not perfect. He admits to being more comfortable in social situations and is amazed at how isolated he had become. In accepting the treatment, he improved his quality of life and taught his physicians the value of pursuing treatable diseases in old age.

Limited Physiologic Reserve—Miss O

Conceptually, older people often tolerate illness and other threats to homeostasis poorly, because they have limited "physiologic reserve." An 80-year-old's minute ventilation may be adequate most of the time, but he or she does not have the reserve necessary to handle two flights of stairs in the setting of a viral upper respiratory infection. Physiologic changes in most organ systems contribute to the diminished reserve observed in the elderly. For example, lean body mass decreases with age, as does muscle strength. Cardiac output with exertion decreases with age. Cognitive functioning, with the exception of executive functions, attenuates. All of these examples can have clinical consequences, particularly when older adults are stressed with an acute illness. Anticipating the consequences of limited physiologic reserves is fundamental to practicing high-quality geriatrics. For example, decreased muscle strength is associated with rapid deconditioning and necessitates attention to ambulation and physical therapy, even during relatively brief illnesses. Miss O was the patient who first peaked our interest in this aspect of geriatrics. She was in her 80s, mildly demented, but still independent in all activities of daily living. Her sister, with whom she shared an apartment, brought her to the emergency department because of her obtunded state. According to the sister, Miss O had been "fine" two days earlier save for a slight fever and foul-smelling urine. Over 48 hours the patient's oral intake progressively worsened, and lethargy developed. On admission to the hospital her serum sodium was 178 mg/dl. That such severe hypernatremia could develop so rapidly seemed improbable at the time, yet we now appreciate that the patient had virtually no reserve and was severely stressed physiologically. Her total body water at baseline was compromised by several factors, including her small size and age-related decreases. Her acute illness, pyelonephritis, exacerbated the dehydration by causing mild diabetes insipidus. Although one cannot be sure that she did not have the infection for longer than two days (but was afebrile), the severity of the dehydration, the devastating effect on her mental status, and the complete reversal of symptoms with hydration left an indelible impression of the need to anticipate the clinical consequences of limited physiologic reserve.

The Interdisciplinary Team Approach—Mrs. W

All too often the uninitiated believe geriatrics to be overwhelming and depressing. Many patients are frail and often have social problems in addition to complex illnesses. To be sure, providing care to such patients in the context of a busy, single-discipline office practice is daunting. Geriatrics is inherently interdisciplinary. To provide comprehensive care across the continuum of potential practice settings (office, hospital, nursing home, and home), a well-functioning, interdisciplinary team is critical.

An interdisciplinary team usually has defined members with defined but fluid roles that, to some degree, frequently overlap. For example, both nurse practitioner and physician may provide primary care, with the nurse taking responsibility for assessment of functional status or other factors, depending on the availability of physical or occupational therapy. Similarly, case management may fall to nursing, social work, or, in complicated situations, medicine. The hallmarks of a well-functioning cooperative team are flexibility, mutual respect, and the ability to stay focused on the patient's needs and goals.

Mrs. W is a 68-year-old woman with insulin-dependent diabetes mellitus of 30 years' duration; complications involve almost every organ system. She requires chronic intermittent bladder catheterization because of autonomic nervous system dysfunction. She cannot perform this task for herself because of peripheral neuropathy involving her fingers. She requires help in drawing up her insulin because of the neuropathy and decreased vision. At a routine office visit, review of her diabetic diary revealed marked deterioration in glucose control. Careful questioning made clear that Mrs. W is no longer certain about guidelines for adjusting her insulin doses to changes in blood sugar level.

A team meeting is followed by a meeting of the team with the patient and her family. The family meeting includes an update of Mrs. W's current complications and their impact on her daily life. The medical team members develop new medication schedules and guidelines. Mrs. W agrees to allow her family to assist in her care and in the adjustment of her insulin doses. Family members volunteer to be trained in insulin administration and in bladder catheterization; team nurses conduct the training sessions. Home health aides are recruited by the team social worker to assist the patient in personal hygiene while the family members are at work.

One month later, the patient and family are much more satisfied with Mrs. W's daily life. Her diary reveals much improved glycemic control. The entire team as well as the patient and her family participated in a series of changes in Mrs. W's daily routine. A crisis that would have required hospitalization for serious hyper- or hypoglycemia was almost certainly averted; the quality of Mrs. W's daily life improved.

Family Involvement—Miss K

Geriatrics is a family-oriented specialty. The geriatrician frequently relies on an older person's family to implement the care plan, to be a surrogate decision maker, and in many ways to function as a member of the team. Yet the family member's unique role and perspective must be preserved. Similarly, geriatricians are faced with the challenge of keeping the patient's interests paramount when day-to-day interactions frequently involve communication only with family members. The rewards of becoming closely involved not only with a patient but also with his or her family are among the most significant in geriatric practice—particularly when the "family" extends beyond the usual definition. While a geriatrician's interactions with family members are complex, four dimensions seem universal: emotional support, decision making, provision of care, and education.

Education is often the foundation on which a sound relationship with the family is built. The willingness to take the time to explain the cause of a clinical event, the next stage of the illness, alternative treatment, and the contents of articles that appear in the newspapers or other lay publications is consistently mentioned by both patients and families as key determinants of their satisfaction or dissatisfaction with physicians. A family that is attempting to cope with a frail elder who may be deteriorating functionally and cognitively is filled with anxiety because they do not know what to expect or when. By educating the family, the clinician not only builds rapport but also gains a critical member of the care team. Family members and other caregivers are the first-line decision makers in any changing clinical situation. The family decides when to call the physician as well as whether to carry out the physician's suggestion, seek an alternative healer, or do nothing at all. Moreover, the geriatrician frequently must make a medical judgment based on the information provided by family members. Confidence in the accuracy and reliability of this information makes decision making easier.

In their roles as caregivers, family members interact with geriatricians in two other ways: as surrogate decision makers and as potential patients. When an elderly person is cognitively impaired, it is often the family who participates in medical decision making rather than the patient. The challenge of keeping the patient's interests paramount while meeting the family's needs can be accomplished only through open communication between the family and geriatric team. When effective, such communication produces gratifying rapport, respect, and closeness. Moreover, it forms the basis for providing ongoing emotional support to the family and offers insight into when more intensive intervention is needed to preserve the caregiver's health and well-being.

The Role of Culture in the Picture of Geriatrics—Mr. M.

Culture is the set of shared beliefs, values, and morals that guide individual behaviors. Culture plays an important role in the way every individual interacts with the health care system. With the elderly, it is often a critical element in the physician-patient relationship. The unprecedented advances in technology and medicine that have shaped much of present-day American culture contrast starkly with the environment that influenced many of our elders' values. Moreover, many of America's present-day elders are immigrants or first-generation descendants of immigrants, making them much closer to a set of values that may be quite different from the dominant values of today. Most elderly patients were teenagers during the late twenties and early thirties, and many immigrated to the United States under political or economic duress. African-American elders endured the humiliation of segregation. While we take antibiotics, chemotherapy, and sophisticated diagnostic procedures, such as MRIs, for granted, rest and good air were the predominant treatment for almost every ailment when most elderly patients were growing up. They were adults when the first antibiotics became available and are all too familiar with the devastation that diseases such as polio can cause. Now most Americans receive more than 13 years of formal education, whereas most elderly people had on average only eight years of formal education. Seventy years ago, health education classes were not a standard part of the curriculum. The basic concepts of biology and human physiology that we take for granted in explaining medical conditions to our patients are not necessarily a part of our older patients' fund of knowledge. An elder's understanding of disease and illness may be rooted in religion rather than biology. Every effort should be made to learn the elderly patient's perspectives and values and to give them careful consideration in explanations, conversations, and care planning.

Mr. M. is an 86-year-old African-American man who grew up in the rural southeastern part of the United States. Despite little formal education, he is articulate and extremely skilled in social interactions. He is quite vocal about his major regrets in life, the most prominent being the missed opportunity to go to college. Mr. M's two clinical problems were hypertension and hearing loss. The hypertension was easily controlled, but over several years the hearing loss became more disabling. Audiometry revealed classic presbycusis, yet Mr. M. adamantly refused a hearing aid. As his disability from the hearing loss progressed and attempts to persuade him to use a hearing aid were repeatedly spurned, an exploration of his health beliefs was initiated. Surprisingly, this worldly gentleman believed that all illness was punishment from God. Once the hearing loss was discussed in the context of a disease caused by God's wrath rather than neuronal loss, we were able to identify the ways in which a hearing aid could be useful. Mr. M illustrates a vital lesson: the sharing of many values, such as love of education, does not necessarily mean that one shares all values, including a belief in the biomedical model.

Bioethics

Unlike clinical situations with younger populations, in which ethical issues arise infrequently, geriatricians often grapple with thorny ethical dilemmas. The difficult decision making surrounding end-of-life choices often gets media attention. However, other decisions—such as the timing of nursing home placement, whether to proceed with a surgical therapy, or whether to place a feeding tube when an elderly person seems unwilling or unable to eat—are equally difficult. The geriatrician's role is complex. The tasks may shift from educator to advisor to sounding board. However, the critical and unwavering role must always be as patient advocate. Older patients can find themselves particularly vulnerable and therefore need the security of knowing that someone will always be their advocate.

Because ethical issues surrounding treatment choices are likely to touch most older people, geriatricians must be comfortable in discussing such issues with their patients. Discussions should occur in the context of the patient's cultural values. Some patients who come from family-centered cultures may prefer to involve family members in the decision-making process, whereas patients from Western cultures are generally comfortable making decisions autonomously. In short, the ethical issues call on all of the other principles of the art and practice of geriatrics. The geriatrician must be knowledgeable about the complexity of medical care in older patients; be able to base prognostications on a clear differentiation between disease and aging; know when to use the other members of an interdisciplinary team; and, above all, discuss such complex issues in the context of the patient's culture and family. Failure to do so can be devastating to the therapeutic relationship and to compliance with recommendations.

II: Symptoms

2. CONFUSION AND AMNESIA

Joel E. Streim, M.D.

1. Are confusion and memory loss part of the normal aging process?

Aging is normally associated with some decline in specific areas of cognitive performance, especially information acquisition, processing, and retrieval, and some language functions. Mild forgetfulness may also be apparent.

Despite this decline in the *speed* of several cognitive functions, older adults normally retain full or nearly-full *capacity* to learn and remember new information, perform problem-solving, and communicate. Confusion and disorientation, or a pattern of memory loss that interferes with the person's ability to function in everyday activities, are *not* normal aging phenomena. They are almost always manifestations of pathologic processes, and some may represent medical emergencies. (See also Chapter 26.)

2. Which conditions are associated with confusion in elderly patients?

Delirium and **dementia** are the two syndromes most often associated with confusional states in older adults. These syndromes, in turn, may each be caused by a wide variety of underlying illnesses and may be exacerbated by environmental factors. Delirium and dementia may also be concurrent.

3. How is delirium distinguished from dementia?

Delirium involves a disturbance of consciousness associated with impaired attention. This may be manifest clinically as waxing and waning lethargy or diminished arousability, with or without intercurrent periods of agitation. By contrast, patients with **dementia** are consistently arousable and able to remain alert without alterations in their level of consciousness, even though they too may have difficulty concentrating on a task or may become agitated at times.

The onset and clinical course of confusion also help to distinguish delirium from dementia. Confusional states with acute onset should always suggest **delirium**. Typically, the syndrome of delirium develops over a short time, becoming clinically apparent over a few minutes, hours, or days—with the level of consciousness and cognitive and perceptual disturbances tending to fluctuate. By contrast, when confusion is due to **dementia**, it usually begins insidiously and becomes apparent over weeks, months, and years. While patients with dementia may exhibit some day-to-day variability in level of confusion, their cognitive and perceptual capacities do not change dramatically over a period of hours or days, and for most patients, the clinical course tends to be stable or gradually progressive, depending on the underlying cause of the dementia syndrome.

4. What causes acute confusional states or delirium?

Almost any medical illness and many medications. The differential diagnosis includes any condition associated with:

- Cerebral hypoperfusion (e.g., hypotension, myocardial infarction, low cardiac output states, arrhythmias)
- Cerebral hypoxia (e.g., pneumonia, COPD, congestive heart failure, pulmonary emboli) or hypercarbia
- Dehydration (mild dehydration as well as intravascular volume depletion)

- Electrolyte disturbances (e.g., hypo- and hypernatremia, hypo- and hypercalcemia, hypo- and hypermagnesemia)
- Hypo- and hyperglycemia and hyperosmolar states
- Infection (e.g., cystitis, urosepsis, pneumonia, peritonitis, and less common CNS infections such as meningitis and encephalitis)
- Fever or hypothermia
- Pain or discomfort (including urinary retention or severe constipation/fecal impaction)
- Intracranial processes (e.g., stroke, subdural hematoma, neoplasm, infection)
- Intoxication or withdrawal states (e.g., alcohol and other drugs)
- Other adverse drug effects (e.g. central anticholinergic, antihistaminic effects)

While this list of potential causes includes conditions that occur commonly in older patients, it is not exhaustive. In many cases of acute confusion or delirium, it is impossible to identify or confirm a single cause. More often, one identifies multiple factors that are suspected to cause, contribute to, or aggravate confusion.

5. Which classes of drugs commonly cause confusion in older adults?

Virtually all drugs that affect CNS function have the potential to cause confusion.

Sedative/hypnotic drugs (e.g., benzodiazepines, barbiturates)
Analgesics (e.g., opiates, NSAIDs?)
Histamine blockers (used for GI disorders, insomnia, pruritus, allergy)
Antisecretory agents (atropinic-like drugs)
Antidiarrheals
Incontinence agents
Tricyclic antidepressants
Antipsychotics (esp. chlorpromazine, thioridazine, mesoridazine)
Antiarrhythmic drugs (e.g., lidocaine, procainamide)
Some antineoplastic agents

6. Who is at risk for developing delirium?

Persons most likely to develop delirium are the very old, those with preexisting brain damage (e.g., from degenerative dementia, cerebrovascular insults, traumatic brain injury), and those with sensory loss (e.g., hearing and visual impairment). Acute confusional states are also more likely to occur in unfamiliar surroundings and environments that cause sensory overload or sensory deprivation.

7. Is sensory deprivation the cause of "sundowning"?

The term "sundowning" usually refers to acute confusional episodes that begin late in the day or at night. The temporal association with the sun's going down has suggested that sensory deprivation may be a cause. However, patients often exhibit a pattern of confusion that has its onset late in the day but before the sun sets. Also, nocturnal confusion has frequently been observed to persist even when adequate lighting and sensory stimulation are maintained after nightfall. Thus "sundowning" may be a misnomer, and some diurnal factor other than altered sensory input may explain the time of onset of confusion.

8. Why is it always important to recognize and evaluate acute confusion or delirium?

Delirium often is the only apparent clinical manifestation of a serious medical illness. For example, myocardial infarction or pulmonary embolus in older adults may present initially with confusion in the absence of chest pain or dyspnea. Urosepsis and pneumonia often occur in older adults without somatic complaints, fever, or leukocytosis, and delirium may be the sole initial clue to these and other infectious diseases. Similarly, abdominal catastrophes (e.g., bowel infarction, perforation, peritonitis) may be heralded by confusion in the very old. Thus, delirium can be an important clinical sign that leads to early recognition, diagnosis, and treatment of serious illness.

Even when delirium is caused by less serious conditions (mild dehydration, constipation, use of low-dose antihistamines), it can lead to significant, potentially reversible comorbidity and excess disability, especially in frail, older adults. When the underlying conditions are identified and are properly managed, the confusion and other cognitive disturbances associated with delirium are usually reversible. Treatment interventions can also alleviate comorbidity, reduce distress and disability, increase function, and improve quality of life. Recognition and evaluation of acute confusion or delirium is therefore essential for the identification and treatment of reversible conditions.

9. How should acute confusion be evaluated?

The workup for acute confusion or delirium should include:
Complete history
Chart review (with close attention to medications administered, including PRNs)
Physical and mental status examinations
Laboratory evaluation including:
Urinalysis
Complete blood count
Chemistry profile (with electrolytes including calcium and magnesium)
Electrocardiogram
The use of further tests, such as chest x-ray, CSF examination, electroencephalogram, or brain imaging, should be directed by the specific findings from the history, record review, and patient examination.

10. How is acute confusion or delirium treated?

Appropriate treatment of delirium begins with ensuring the patient's safety, attending to medical emergencies, and managing any other underlying medical conditions, medication effects, or environmental factors that are thought to be contributing to the delirium. Thus, the treatment of delirium and amelioration of the acute confusional state will depend on the specific etiologic factors identified.

11. When should psychotropic medications be used in the management of elders with acute confusion or delirium?

Psychotropic medications are often used in acute and long-term care settings when acute confusional states are associated with agitated or combative behaviors, psychotic symptoms (e.g., hallucinations and delusions), or severe disruption of the normal sleep-wake cycle. The medications usually used for calming these agitated patients are the high-potency neuroleptic/antipsychotics and the short half-life benzodiazepines. Unfortunately, controlled clinical trials have not been conducted to determine the efficacy or safety of these drugs in patients with delirium. In particular, it is not known whether such drugs diminish or exacerbate agitation, combativeness, psychosis, insomnia, or confusion; whether they shorten or prolong the course of the delirium; or whether they reduce the excess disability and mortality associated with delirium.

Although clinical experience suggests that some patients' agitation and psychosis may be effectively quieted with these medications, these agents can also complicate the course of delirium. They can cause sedation and worsen lethargy. The benzodiazepines can also cause increased confusion, anterograde amnesia, disinhibition, and paradoxical excitation. The neuroleptic/antipsychotics can induce akathisia, a syndrome of motor restlessness that may worsen the agitation. When this occurs, it is usually difficult to distinguish the effects of the drugs from the symptoms and signs of delirium.

For this reason, it is usually preferable to manage agitation, sleep disruption, and psychosis by first addressing medical conditions, medication effects, and environmental factors that may be causing these symptoms, with an emphasis on proper nursing care. Pharmacologic strategies should generally be reserved for those patients who are refractory to these measures and who remain highly distressed or physically unsafe without medication to calm them down. Benzo-diazepines and neuroleptics should not be used as a treatment for acute confusion when it is un-complicated by agitation, insomnia, or psychosis. Some clinicians report benefit from the use of chloral hydrate on an empiric basis to calm agitated patients and to treat insomnia when it is thought to be associated with severe sleep deprivation that complicates treatment.

12. What safety precautions should be observed for acutely confused patients?

For many patients with delirium, acute confusion will be accompanied by lethargy or agita-tion. Patients whose level of responsiveness is diminished may require airway protection or aspi-ration precautions. For those who are agitated, there may be a need for safeguards against injury: prevention of falls; restriction of access to arterial lines, urinary catheters, tracheostomy cannu-lae, and ventilator hoses; enforcement of precautions for new joint prostheses; avoidance of trauma from motor restlessness; and surveillance to avert wandering into unsafe situations.

13. What other nursing interventions are indicated to manage delirium?

Beyond immediate safety measures, nursing staff can be instrumental in reducing confusion by setting a calendar and clock in the patient's field of vision, providing frequent verbal reorien-tation cues, surrounding the patient with familiar personal possessions, pictures, and objects from home, and enlisting the help of family and friends in providing comfort and reassurance. Adjustment of the level of sensory stimulation may also be helpful, increasing the amount of stimulation for patients who have sensory impairment or deprivation and reducing the level for those who are overwhelmed by external stimuli. Nursing staff can also employ sleep hygiene measures to manage the disruption of sleep-wake cycles that typically occurs in patients with delirium.

14. Describe the follow-up care that should be provided after delirium has resolved.

Delirium is a traumatic experience for most patients. Although some are amnestic for events that occur during the course of delirium, many have distressing memories of their confusional state. Even after their acute confusion has resolved, their recollections of illusions, hallucinations, and delusions may be confusing and upsetting, and they may harbor misunderstandings about events and treatment, sometimes attributing malicious intentions to caregivers and family mem-bers. For those patients who are not persistently confused due to underlying dementia, it is usually helpful to conduct a debriefing session. This gives the patient an opportunity to express residual concerns, fears, and anger; and it gives the health care provider a chance to provide a medical ex-planation for the confusional state and to counsel the patient and family. It is especially important to reassure patients about the resolution of their confusion and to discuss prognosis, emphasizing that they are not expected "to go crazy" or "lose their mind," though they may be at risk for recur-rence of confusion if exposed to similar circumstances in the future. Therefore, patients and fami-lies should be advised to inform future health care providers about their history of confusion and any known causal or precipitating factors. This history can be extremely valuable for prevention.

15. Which conditions are most commonly associated with complaints of amnesia or memory impairment in older adults?

Depressive disorders, dementing illnesses, and effects of drugs and alcohol account for most of older adults' complaints about memory problems. When neuropsychological testing provides objective evidence of memory deficits, dementia is often the cause. However, **depression** can also impair performance on formal tests of cognitive function, and it accounts for a substantial proportion of subjective memory complaints among elders, with and without dementia (see also Chapter 24).

Alcohol can affect memory in several ways. Acute alcohol intoxication can cause "black-outs," with amnesia for the period of intoxication. Chronic alcohol abuse can lead to alcohol amnestic syndrome, though these patients seldom have insight into their memory impairment and rarely complain about it. Although this condition is also known as "Korsakoff's psychosis," it is actually a disorder of memory function and not a psychotic illness. It is also distinct from dementia in that cognitive functions other than memory are relatively spared.

Drugs other than alcohol can interfere with memory function. Elderly patients commonly receive anesthetic agents, narcotic analgesics, and benzodiazepines, all of which can cause amnesia.

Of note, the syndrome of **delirium** usually includes memory impairment, but memory difficulty is usually not a specific presenting complaint of patients suffering from delirium.

16. When does a patient with memory impairment qualify for a diagnosis of dementia?

Memory impairment, by itself, is not sufficient to diagnose dementia. At least three other criteria must be met:

- Mental status examination must demonstrate that other aspects of cognitive function are impaired. Evidence for this may include agnosia, aphasia, apraxia, or deficits in executive functions.
- The cognitive deficits must be clinically significant in that they interfere with social or occupational functioning or ability to care for oneself.
- The cognitive deficits must not be attributable to depression or delirium or other nondementing neuropsychiatric syndromes.

17. When is memory impairment reversible?

Numerous conditions associated with memory impairment are treatable and reversible. The memory deficits in **nondemented patients** with delirium almost always resolve when the condition causing the delirium is successfully treated. Memory complaints in nondemented patients with depression improve with effective treatment for the depression. Various drugs may impede memory without causing the full syndrome of delirium, dementia, or depression, and in these cases, memory often improves after reduction or discontinuation of the drug.

Approximately 10% of older adults with dementia may have a reversible component to their cognitive dysfunction. In **demented patients** with comorbid depression or delirium or adverse drug effects involving memory, treatment of the comorbid condition usually leads to some improvement in memory function. When the dementing process is due to such conditions as hypo- or hyperthyroidism, vitamin B12 or folic acid deficiency, neurosyphilis, Lyme disease, subdural hematoma, normal pressure hydrocephalus, or autoimmune disease, prompt treatment may help reverse memory impairment. However, when these conditions remain untreated for > 6 months to 1 year, clinical experience suggests that the prognosis for recovery of memory function becomes poor.

18. What is pseudodementia?

Pseudodementia is a term used to describe the reversible cognitive impairment commonly associated with major depressive disorder in older adults. However, this term is misleading, as there are several ways that memory problems appear to be related to depression. Some depressed patients have memory *complaints* despite intact cognitive *performance*, and others have poor memory *performance* due to apathy or lack of motivation despite intact cognitive *capacity*. However, there is evidence that some patients with onset of major depression in late life have measurable changes in cerebral function associated with diminished cognitive capacity. When depression is treated, many patients experience improvement in cognitive function, but a significant proportion have persistence of cognitive impairment consistent with a diagnosis of dementia, or they go on to develop dementia within 2 years of their episode of depression. For these patients, the dementia associated with their depression is clearly not simply "pseudo" dementia.

19. How are memory complaints evaluated?

If memory problems are evident, the evaluation should focus on identifying potentially reversible causes. A comprehensive evaluation includes a careful history, physical and mental status examination, and screening laboratory tests. It is often helpful to use standardized instruments for assessment of both cognitive function (e.g., Mini-Mental State Exam or Blessed Information-

Memory-Concentration Test) and affective status (e.g., Geriatric Depression Scale). Laboratory evaluation usually includes a urinalysis, complete blood count, chemistry profile including indices of hepatic and renal function, thyroid function tests, serum B12 and folic acid levels, and serologic test for syphilis. The need for borellia titers, erythrocyte sedimentation rate, or other laboratory tests depends on the findings from the history, physical, and mental status examinations. Although brain imaging (e.g., CT or MRI scan) is often done routinely, the need for this depends on the duration of memory problems as well as other findings from the history, physical, and mental status examination.

20. How should memory problems be managed?

As with confusion, appropriate management of memory loss begins with ensuring the safety of the patient and treating causal factors and comorbid conditions. Patients with mild memory loss may benefit from mnemonic aids (e.g., making lists and using signs or reminders) and cognitive strategies (self-cueing). Those with moderate and severe memory impairment usually require assistance of a caregiver who can provide cues, prompts, and supervision. Home safety includes measures to ensure that kitchen, plumbing, and electrical appliances are properly turned off. When memory problems are severe, patients usually require supervision or assistance with most activities of daily living.

Effective pharmacologic treatment of memory problems has been very limited. Some drugs have been shown to produce modest improvement in memory performance for some patients, but gains generally are not sustained and do not translate into substantial improvement in functional level (i.e., ability to perform activities of daily living).

BIBLIOGRAPHY

1. Conn DK: Delirium and other organic mental disorders. In Sadavoy J, Lazarus LW, Jarvik LF (eds): Comprehensive Review of Geriatric Psychiatry. Washington, DC, American Psychiatric Press, 1991, pp 311–336.
2. Diagnostic and Statistical Manual of Mental Disorders, 4th ed. Washington, DC, Amercian Psychiatric Association, 1994, pp 123–163.
3. Eisdorfer C, Sevush S, Barry PP, et al: Evaluation of the demented patient. Med Clin North Am 78:773–793, 1994.
4. Jones BN, Reifler BV: Depression coexisting with dementia: Evaluation and treatment. Med Clin North Am 78:823–840, 1994.
5. Lipowski ZJ: Delirium in the elderly patient. N Engl J Med 320:578–582, 1989.
6. Rabins PV: Psychosocial and management aspects of delirium. Int J Psychogeriatr 3:319–324, 1991.

3. FATIGUE AND WEAKNESS

Stephen I. Chavin, M.D.

1. Patients often present to their primary care physicians with a complaint of tiredness or weakness. What symptoms do these terms describe?

Features Distinguishing Between Fatigue and Weakness

FATIGUE	WEAKNESS
Feeling of extreme exhaustion not preceded by extraordinary physical activity	Usually accompanied by decreased muscle strength in single tasks
Difficulty concentrating on physical and mental tasks	Reduced endurance in repetitive muscle activity
Generalized inability to accomplish necessary daily activities	Often associated with ≥ 1 objective physical abnormalities of the neuromuscular system

Patients use a bewildering variety of terms to describe what appears to be the same subjective symptom complex. The terms include fatigue, exhaustion, tiredness, and weakness, in addition to malaise or lassitude. These terms are usually synonymous with **fatigue**, defined as the presence of one or more features listed in the above table.

Other patients use the term fatigue to describe what appears to be a **weakness**, or diminution of muscle strength and muscle function. In some instances, patients can accurately describe the nature of their complaint. In other cases, the physician must carefully probe both the patient and family members in order to elicit the history and formulate a differential diagnosis.

2. In the general population, how prevalent is fatigue?

A national survey completed 20 years ago showed that fatigue was the 7th most common complaint reported by patients. In a more recent study of 1159 consecutive adults attending two primary care clinics, 24% of patients reported fatigue as a major problem, although fatigue was not invariably the reason for the clinic visit. Of the 1159 patients surveyed, 31% were aged 65 years or older. In this group of elderly people, 34% of the women and 18% of the men reported fatigue as a major complaint. These prevalences were not significantly different from those in younger members of the cohort.

Other surveys of primary-care patients complaining of fatigue have indicated prevalences ranging from as low as 2–9% up to 17–47%. Overall, a reasonable estimate is that 1–11 million patient visits to physician offices per year are related to the symptom of fatigue.

3. Why do some patients with fatigue fail to report this symptom to the physician?

Some patients, because of personality or culture, may simply deny the presence of a symptom. Other patients remain unaware of the developing fatigue and unconsciously may reduce their levels of physical activity. Among these patients, there is no intention to deceive; they simply have modified their lifestyle to accommodate the fatigue. To identify such cases, the physician must have a suspicious mind and ask the patient detailed questions, e.g., about changes in amount and kinds of daytime physical and mental activities and alterations in sleeping habits.

4. Can fatigue and life events be associated?

Some life events, such as death, spousal illness, or concerns about personal finance, may lead to feelings of fatigue. Furthermore, the mere self–awareness of growing older may cause symptoms of fatigue. Finally, poor nutrition or extreme reduction in the amount of physical exercise also may lead to this symptom. The biochemical or physiologic mechanisms by which life events cause fatigue can only be speculated at this time. Clearly, a careful history plus the development of a mutually trusting relationship between patient and physician will facilitate identification and perhaps alleviation of the relevant factors.

5. Is depression often associated with fatigue?

Yes. Fatigue is included in the operational definitions for a number of psychiatric disorders, including major depression and dysthymia according to the DSM–IV. The symptom is also assessed in various depression rating scales used for elderly patients, such as the Beck, Yesavage, and Hamilton instruments. The Center for Epidemiologic Studies Depression Scale (CES–D) and the Profile of Mood States (POMS) are two especially useful tools because they separate fatigue–related questions from the total scale.

The inclusion of fatigue on these scales attests to the high prevalence of fatigue and related somatic symptoms in patients with psychiatric disorders, but it does not explain the etiologic relationships. Although there is considerable observational and experimental evidence linking the hypothalamic–pituitary axis to both fatigue and depression, the physiologic mechanisms of the linkage remain obscure. The important point is that the physician must seek out evidence of psychiatric disease in a patient complaining of fatigue.

6. What kinds of medical diseases are associated with fatigue?

In a study of 300 cases of "weakness and fatigue" in an urban referral medical clinic, 20% (61 patients) were found to have physical causes for the fatigue. These causes included chronic infection, metabolic disease such as diabetes mellitus, neurologic disease, and heart disease. Among the 61 patients with identifiable physical causes, 46% had an obvious disease, 21% had equivocal diagnostic findings, and 33% had occult disease. The remaining 80% of the 300 patients, for whom no physical causes could be identified, were given diagnoses of "nervous exhaustion or fatigue, psychoneurosis, or depression" (no demographic information was provided about these patients).

Thus, a variety of diseases have been linked to fatigue. In some, such as cardiac failure or atrial fibrillation, inadequate perfusion of peripheral tissues is the likely cause. In sleep disorders, an impairment of the reticular activating system may reasonably be inferred. In the majority of medical conditions—such as hypo- and hyperthyroidism, diabetes mellitus, hepatitis, cancers, lymphoma, tuberculosis, electrolyte disturbance, chronic obstructive pulmonary disease, and acute infection—plausible mechanisms often are not obvious. In fact, there may be a multiplicity of mechanisms that operate through a small number of common pathways and effectors, such as interleukin-6 and tumor necrosis factor.

7. Can medications cause fatigue?

Pharmacologic therapies are a common and often unpredictable cause of fatigue. The number of medications that have been linked to fatigue is legion, and few classes of drugs have escaped this notoriety. Nonetheless, accurate studies of incidence or prevalence are difficult to find in the literature.

In some cases, e.g., antihistamines, sedative tricyclic antidepressants, hypnotics, and psychotropic drugs, the cause–effect relationship between the drug's use and the development of fatigue is well-established, and plausible pharmacologic explanations are obvious. In the majority of cases, however, the causal connection may only be suspected, and this problem is compounded if the adverse effect is an idiosyncratic one. Even placebos have been associated with fatigue, indicating that the pharmacodynamics may involve a synergism between the drug and patient. The nearest one can come to proving that a medication has caused fatigue is to demonstrate a chronologic relationship between the start of therapy and the appearance of symptoms, as well as cessation of symptoms following discontinuation of the medication.

Commonly Prescribed Medications That May Cause Fatigue

Alcohol	Chemotherapeutic agents, cytotoxic drugs
Anticholinergic agents	Dopamine and dopamine agonists, e.g.,
Anticonvulsants	bromocriptine
Antiviral agents, e.g., amantidine	H_2 receptor antagonists
Beta-blockers, esp. lipophilic ones	Hypnotics
Biologic response modifiers, e.g.,	Neuroleptic agents
interferons	Nonsteroidal anti-inflammatory agents
Caffeine	Retinoic acid derivatives
Calcium channel blockers	Tricyclic antidepressants
Chemotherapeutic agents, antimetabolites	Vasodilators

8. Is anemia a common cause of fatigue in the elderly?

This is a widely held misconception. In fact, a low hemoglobin concentration is an *uncommon* cause of fatigue. As a general rule, symptoms from anemia seldom appear until the hemoglobin has fallen to levels considerably < 50% of normal. Also, with chronic anemias, their development may be slow enough to allow time for physiologic adaptions to ensure delivery of adequate O_2 and other nutrients to the peripheral tissues, thereby preventing symptoms.

When significant symptoms are noted in a patient with only moderate anemia, the physician should suspect some underlying pathology that either is interacting synergistically with anemia (e.g., congestive heart failure with poor cardiac output) or is itself causing both the symptoms and anemia (e.g., metastatic cancer). Anemia, however, may be directly responsible for the symptoms when it has developed acutely (e.g., severe autoimmune hemolytic anemia) with inadequate time for compensatory mechanisms to appear. A somewhat different situation occurs when the anemia has developed quickly as a result of blood loss; in this case, the signs and symptoms are those of hypovolemia, poor cardiac output, and inadequate perfusion of essential organs, such as brain and liver.

The definitive test for anemia as the cause of fatigue is a therapeutic trial transfusion of packed red blood cells adequate to raise the hemoglobin to a level of 7–8 gm/dl. A positive result is a significant reduction in the patient's symptoms sustained for the duration of the hemoglobin elevation (usually many days). If the beneficial effects are only transient (1–2 days), it is unlikely that a low hemoglobin concentration per se is causing the fatigue. Before choosing a therapeutic transfusion trial, the physician and patient should consider the risks and benefits of this approach, taking into account the severity of the symptoms, possibility of volume overload, and infectious complications.

9. Is it possible to distinguish between fatigue from physical causes and fatigue from psychologic ones?

Fatigue, like pain, is subjective and possesses no objective or easily demonstrable attributes or correlates. Therefore, the two types of fatigue are indistinguishable unless a cause can be identified. In another sense, however, certain characteristics may point toward one or the other etiology.

Physical Fatigue	*Psychologic Fatigue*
1. Worsens as day progresses	1. Varies unpredictably and rapidly in intensity
2. Diminished or eliminated after rest or sleep	2. Most severe on awakening
3. May be objectively demonstrated by muscle weakness, esp. after muscle use	3. May improve as day progresses
	4. No measurable muscle weakness or relation to muscle use

Finally, patients who appear to be fatigued but who deny or minimize the complaint are more likely to be suffering from a physical cause, whereas patients with psychologic fatigue rarely deny the presence of fatigue and may even exaggerate it. An important caveat is that a patient may be suffering simultaneously from both psychologic and physical causes of fatigue. For example, patients with lymphoma may suffer physical fatigue as well as depression.

10. Why should the primary care doctor pay serious attention to a common subjective complaint such as fatigue?

1. Patients with fatigue as a major complaint may have a persistent and striking degree of global dysfunction, comparable to that seen in patients with untreated hyperthyroidism or patients who have survived myocardial infarction. Thus, fatigue is not a trivial complaint but one with serious health implications.

2. The symptom may be a harbinger of a serious medical condition, e.g., chronic infection, overdose, or drug reaction, which may be diagnosed and treated at an early stage.

3. The attention paid to the patient's complaints may foster an improved patient–doctor relationship.

11. How should fatigue be evaluated in an ambulatory primary care setting?

When the patient presents initially with a complaint of fatigue, a minimal workup should include a comprehensive history (physical and psychological) and physical exam. If these investigations are unrevealing, then it probably is reasonable to defer further extensive laboratory testing until the fatigue has persisted for 4–8 weeks.

12. How do laboratory tests help elicit the causes of chronic fatigue?

In a survey of 102 patients (mean age, 57) with fatigue, the following laboratory tests were done: hematocrit, erythrocyte sedimentation rate (ESR), serum creatinine concentration, serum potassium concentration, urinalysis, serum thyroxine and triiodothyronine concentration, serum thyroid stimulating hormone, chest x-ray, mono-spot test, and stool for occult blood. Only the ESR showed a significant difference in fatigued versus control subjects; 12% of the fatigued subjects compared with 4% controls had abnormally elevated ESRs, although unequivocal causes for the elevation could not be found. Thus, in the absence of any cause readily identifiable from the initial history and physical examination, random laboratory investigations usually are not helpful in evaluating the causes of fatigue. In such cases, the best approach is periodic follow-up and clinical reassessments.

13. What is muscle weakness? How does it differ from fatigue?

Muscle weakness is an abnormal physical finding characterized by decreased muscle strength and reduced endurance in repetitive muscle activity. It can be demonstrated objectively and quantified, in contrast to fatigue, which is subjective and not easily measurable. A careful medical history and physical examination focusing on the neuromuscular system will often confirm the presence of muscle abnormalities, including diminished strength, wasting, contractures, fasciculation, and abnormal deep tendon reflexes. The clinical history may show a clear relationship between muscle usage and symptoms. Biochemical and pathologic studies may reveal additional structural and compositional changes in the muscle fibers and cells. In cases of pure fatigue, none of these features are present.

14. Name some common diseases that present with muscle weakness.

Metabolic diseases, such as Cushing's syndrome, should be considered. Conditions that cause myopathies or neuropathies, such as diabetes mellitus, vitamin deficiencies, and degenerative diseases of muscle, also should be weighed. Old cerebrovascular accidents with residual paresis may be difficult to identify from the history. Inadequate or excessive muscular exercise has been identified in some cases. Finally, a variety of rheumatologic or collagen-vascular diseases may be responsible.

15. Is there a relationship between fatigue and weakness?

Although they are the consequences of two separate processes, there may be inter–relationships between these two clinical findings. Patients who have true muscle weakness may have to work harder to accomplish activities of daily living and to maintain independent function; this extra work may lead to a perception of fatigue. On the other hand, a person initially suffering from psychologic fatigue may become less active or even immobile, which in turn may result in muscle atrophy and reduced functional capacity. Thus, the two conditions may mutually reinforce one another. The physician must look for both conditions and treat each one separately and appropriately.

BIBLIOGRAPHY

1. Allan FN: The differential diagnosis of weakness and fatigue. N Eng J Med 231:414–418, 1944.
2. Denollet J: Emotional distress and fatigue in coronary artery heart disease: The global scale (GMS). Psychol Med 23:111–121, 1993.
3. Downey JA, Myers SJ, Gonzales EG, Lieberman JS: The Physiological Basis of Rehabilitative Medicine, 2nd ed. Boston, Butterworth–Heinemann, 1994, pp 393–411.
4. Engel GL: Nervousness and fatigue. In MacBryde CM, Blacklow RS (eds): Signs and Symptoms: Applied Pathologic Physiology and Clinical Interpretation, 5th ed. Philadelphia, J.B. Lippincott, 1970, pp 632–649.
5. Fuhrer R, Wessely S: The epidemiology of fatigue and depression: A French primary care study. Psychol Med 25:895–905, 1995.
6. Kroenke K, Wood DR, Mangelsdorff AD, et al: Chronic fatigue in primary care: Prevalence, patient characteristics, and outcome. JAMA 260:929–934, 1988.
7. Matthews DA, Manu P, Lane TJ: Evaluation and management of patients with chronic fatigue. Am J Med Sci 302:269–277, 1991.
8. National Center for Health Statistics: The National Ambulatory Medical Care Survey: 1975 Summary, United States, January–December 1975. In Vital and Health Statistics series 13, no. 36 [DHHS publ no. (PHS)84-1717.] Hyattsville, MD, Public Health Service, 1978.
9. Seller RH: Fatigue. In Differential Diagnosis of Common Complaints. Philadelphia, W.B. Saunders, 1986, pp 139–148.
10. Waltman RE: Weakness. In Yoshikawa TT, Cobbs EL, Brummel–Smith K (eds): Ambulatory Geriatric Care. St. Louis, Mosby, 1993, pp 316–323.

4. INVOLUNTARY WEIGHT LOSS IN THE ELDERLY

Mary Ann Forciea, M.D.

1. What is significant weight loss in older patients?

A documented fall in weight of 4–5% in 1 year is the best standard to use in outpatients over age 65. Wallace et al. have demonstrated, in a prospective study of a population of community-dwelling men over age 65 who were eligible for care through the Veterans Administration (VA), that a 1-year documented weight loss of > 4% was the best single predictor of death within 2 years. Other standards used in the literature have ranged from 7.5–10% over 6 months, but these higher limits have not been as carefully correlated with future mortality as has the 4–5% limit. In Wallace et al.'s 2-year follow-up, mortality rates were 28% in weight losers, as compared with 11% in controls.

2. Is weight loss in the elderly different from that in other medical patients?

Diseases identified as the cause of weight loss in older patients are the same as those identified in middle-aged adults: **unknown causes** (approx 25% in most studies), **depression**, and **cancer** being the three most common diagnoses. The widely held belief that weight loss in older patients is more often due to malignant causes has not been validated in studies to date. Morley and others suggest that social or functional disorders which limit access to food (poverty, immobility, and isolation) may be more prevalent in older patients who lose weight than in younger persons.

Thompson and Morris have suggested that involuntary weight loss may be less serious in elderly outpatients than in younger patients. They found a 2-year mortality of 9% in their study of 45 elderly primary care patients who had lost 7.5% of their baseline body weight in the 6 months prior to the study. Wallace et al., in a VA clinic-based study, found a 2-year mortality of 28%, closely approximating mortality levels reported in younger patients losing weight. Differences in disease burden in the two populations may well explain the difference in mortality seen.

3. What is the differential diagnosis of involuntary weight loss in the elderly?

Common causes of weight loss in elderly outpatients can be more easily remembered with the portentous mnemonic **DEAD** (which refers of course to the outcome of excessive weight loss): drugs, eating, access, and disease.

Drugs. Medications can produce anorexia, xerostomia (due to anticholinergics), and nausea, which curb appetite. Taste and smell can be altered by a variety of medicines. Drugs such as antibiotics often result in diarrhea and caloric loss. In addition, the physical fact of taking 4 or more tablets shortly before a meal (once-a-day meds being ingested with breakfast) may inhibit normal appetite. Refer to the table for examples of specific medications.

Eating. Elderly patients may lack the manual dexterity to cut food or use standard silverware due to stroke, arthritis, or confusion. The amount of time required to consume a meal may leave the food cold and unappealing. Patients may have adopted unusual diets either to promote health or by overly enthusiastic efforts to reduce salt or cholesterol. Sullivan et al., in a study of elderly patients admitted to a VA evaluation unit, found > 80% to be affected by oral health problems that could interfere with normal mastication.

Access to food. Older patients can lose weight because they are too poor to buy enough nourishing food, too immobile to shop for food, or too confused to prepare appealing meals. They may be unaware of community assistance programs, such as "meals on wheels," or too proud to use such services. Liquid food supplements are not covered by federal (Medicare) or most state (Medicaid) assistance programs.

Disease. In the 75% of cases of weight loss where a cause is identified, a wide variety of illnesses may present (see Question 5).

Medications that May Affect Appetite and Digestion

Decreased appetite
  Anorexia—amphetamines (Ritalin), selegiline
  Xerostomia—anticholinergics, e.g., oxybutynin (Ditropan), flavoxate (Urispas), trihexyphenidyl
    (Artane), benztropine (Cogentin), pilocarpine
  Nausea—digoxin, quinidine

Altered taste and smell—antibiotics, steroid nasal sprays

Diarrhea—antibiotics, nonsteroidal anti-inflammatory drugs

---

4. List some oral problems seen in the elderly that may affect appetite and digestion.
Absent teeth
Missing teeth
Poorly fitting dentures
Dental caries with or without pain
Gingival infection or inflammation
Mucous membrane infection (candidiasis)
Temporomandibular joint pain

5. Which diseases are usually associated with weight loss in the elderly?
Depression was the most frequent single cause found by Thompson and Morris in their elderly family practice patients. Elderly patients must still be screened for alcohol use and can certainly be active alcoholics.

Malignancies, especially lung and GI tumors, are frequent causes of weight loss. Chronic leukemias and lymphoma can also be seen. Physiologic products of malignant cells, such as tumor necrosis factor, a cytokine, can interfere with the body's metabolism and caloric requirements.

Cardiopulmonary disorders, such as congestive heart failure or chronic obstructive pulmonary disease, can be associated with weight loss in late stages ("cardiac cachexia").

Renal failure and uremia may present with anorexia as one of the earliest symptoms.

Infection, especially with tuberculosis, is still seen in older patients, particularly those with compromised immune function. HIV should certainly be considered in those patients with risk factors.

Endocrine disorders may manifest with weight loss as a presenting symptom. Hyperthyroidism is the most notorious endocrine cause of weight loss, and in the variant of hyperthyroidism known as "apathetic hyperthyroidism," weight loss may be the presenting symptom. Patients with diabetes mellitus may lose weight from osmotic diuresis with severe hyperglycemia. In the late stages of either type I or type II diabetes mellitus, patients may lose weight due to a combination of renal disease, abnormal protein metabolism, and depression, but weight loss would rarely be the presenting symptom at this stage of the illness.

6. What information from the history is pertinent in evaluating weight loss?
Documentation of the weight loss is ideal, since Marton et al. described an inaccuracy rate of nearly 50% in patients complaining of weight loss. Evidence of weight change from the medical records is preferred but often unavailable. Many states require weight reporting on the drivers' license; although this is a self-report, the number can give some indication of "usual" weight. Evidence from clothing, such as wear on belt holes or safety pins on waist bands, can also support recent weight loss. Photographs are often useful, as is history provided by family.

Dietary review is important but often difficult. Older patients may be unwilling to complete dietary logs, and their recall of meal composition is unreliable. Caregivers may be more helpful in supplying dietary information.

Social information addressing the issues in access to food will be helpful. Information on **alcohol** use and **smoking** history are always relevant. Past **surgical history** can be important, especially if on the GI tract.

7. Which components of the physical exam are relevant?

Documentation of the **weight** is necessary, either to quantitate loss or to establish a new baseline. **Blood pressure** recordings should include orthostatic alterations, which might indicate dehydration as well as weight loss. **Temperature** should be recorded.

The **skin** should be examined for confirmation of weight loss and for jaundice, rash, or petechiae. Palpation of **lymph nodes** in the submandibular, supraclavicular, axillary, and inguinal regions is important, as is estimation of size of the **liver** and **spleen**.

Examination of the **eyes** may signal thyroid disease. Careful examination of the **oral cavity** is especially important, as Sullivan and colleagues found that the number of general oral problems was the best predictor of involuntary weight loss in the year preceding inpatient geriatric assessment in a group of elderly veterans.

The **thyroid** gland should be examined for size and consistency; a bruit overlying an enlarged gland usually indicates increased blood flow as is seen in Graves' Disease. **Chest** exam may disclose evidence of consolidation or obstruction. **Abdominal** examination should include assessment of organ size and consistency. **Pelvic** and **rectal** examinations are especially important in pursuing occult malignancy.

Neurologic assessment must include an evaluation of mental status, as well as muscle tone and strength as it pertains to mobility.

8. What constitutes a cost-effective workup?

In Thompson and Morris' study of elderly outpatients, the initial history and physical examination revealed a source for the weight loss when an organic cause was evident. Although no case-control studies have been conducted in the elderly, most authors recommend laboratory testing to include complete blood count, erythrocyte sedimentation rate, urinalysis, multiphasic chemistry panel (blood sugar, creatinine, liver function tests, calcium, phosphorus, and electrolytes), thyroid stimulating hormone, chest x-ray, and HIV testing (if risk factors are present). The role of the prostate-specific antigen screening test in elderly men has not yet been defined but is being offered in many practices as part of periodic screening in older men.

Specialized laboratory studies are sometimes ordered to evaluate whether weight loss has led to actual malnutrition. Measurement of serum albumin is often an initial screen; levels of transferrin, retinol-binding protein, or prealbumin have been proposed as indicators of visceral protein stores. Cutaneous delayed hypersensitivity is reduced in malnutrition, as are the numbers of total lymphocytes.

9. How can I treat weight loss?

If no specific cause of weight loss is identified (as happens in approximately 25% of patients), watchful waiting is best. In Thompson and Morris' study, 27% of patients stabilized their weight during the 2-year study period.

In patients in whom an organic cause is identified, clearly treatment should be offered. Medication regimens should be altered, when possible, if side effects are responsible. Dental referral is indicated for patients with contributing oral problems.

Collaboration with a skilled social worker can help to address not only societal services, such as meal service or homemaker services, but also help to educate patients and families about caregiving skills. Formal consultation with a dietician is of great value in educating families and patients about a nutritious diet but also in addressing special problems such as modified diets (low-salt or diabetic diets), texture-specific diets (soft, pureed), and in the use of liquid dietary supplements. (See also Chapter 16.)

BIBLIOGRAPHY

1. Marton KI, Sox HC, Krupp JR: Involuntary weight loss: Diagnostic and prognostic significance. Ann Intern Med 95:568–574, 1981.
2. Morley JE, Mooradian AD, Silver AJ, et al: Nutrition in the elderly. Ann Intern Med 109:890–904, 1988.
3. Pamuk ER, Williamson DF, Madans J, et al: Weight loss and mortality in a national cohort of adults, 1971–1987. Am J Epidemiol. 136:686–697, 1992.
4. Reife CM: Involuntary weight loss. Med Clin North Am 79:299–313, 1995.
5. Sullivan DH, Martin W, Flaxman N, Hagen JE: Oral health problems and involuntary weight loss in a population of frail elderly. J Am Geriatr Soc 41:725–731, 1995.
6. Thompson MP, Morris LK: Unexplained weight loss in the ambulatory elderly. J Am Geriatr Soc 39:497–500, 1991.
7. Wallace JI, Schwartz RS, LaCroix AZ, et al: Involuntary weight loss in older outpatients: Incidence and clinical significance. J Am Geriatr Soc 43:329–337, 1995.
8. Wise GR, Craig D: Evaluation of involuntary weight loss. Postgrad Med 95(4):145–151, 1994.

5. DIZZINESS AND VERTIGO

Dana L. Suskind, M.D., and Glenn W. Knox, M.D.

1. What is the clinical difference between dizziness and vertigo?
Dizziness and vertigo must be clinically differentiated; each has a distinct differential diagnosis. Dizziness describes a sense of light-headedness and unsteadiness; it may be multifactorial in origin. Dizziness is a common and often complicated complaint in geriatric patients. It is the most common reason for physician visits in patients over 75 years of age and the third most common reason in patients over 65 years. Vertigo, a specific type of dizziness described as a sense of rotational movement and spinning, suggests vestibular pathology. Approximately 50% of elderly patients with dizziness have a peripheral vestibular disorder, and 35% have a central or mixed diagnosis; in only 10% is the dizziness idiopathic. Oscillopsia—the inability to maintain a horizon while walking—is due to bilateral absence of vestibular function and usually results from ototoxic medication.

2. Can dizziness be a normal part of aging?
Presbystasis is the term used to describe the dysequilibrium of aging. It is thought to result from an overall decline in vestibular, visual, proprioceptive, and neuromuscular function. Although functional decrease in vestibular activity in elderly people is slight, the overall decline in compensatory mechanisms (i.e., proprioception, vision, and neuromuscular) leaves them vulnerable to unstable conditions to which a younger person could easily adapt. Presbystasis is a diagnosis of exclusion. The elderly patient with symptoms of vertigo or dizziness often has a definable etiology. Patients diagnosed with presbystasis are prime candidates for vestibular rehabilitation, during which they learn methods of compensation.

3. What major etiologies should be considered in vertigo or dizziness in the elderly?

Vertigo—acute
  Vertebrobasilar event
  Toxic (drugs/illness)
  Infectious
  Trauma
  Tumor
  Seizure
  Transient ischemic attack
  Cerebrovascular accident
  Cardiac arrhythmia
Vertigo—recurrent
  Meniere's disease
  Migraine
  Hypothyroidism
  Multiple sclerosis
  Presbylabyrinth
  Syphilis
  Diabetes mellitus
    Small vessel
    Peripheral neuropathy

Vertigo—positional
  Benign paroxysmal positional vertigo
  Infection
  Trauma
  Cervical vertigo
  Central causes
Imbalance
  Medication toxicity
  Sensory impairment
  Cervical spine dizziness
  Presbystasis
Presyncope
  Orthostasis
  Hyperventilation
  Muscle weakness

Adapted from Mader SL: Dizziness and syncope. In Yoshikawa T (ed): Ambulatory geriatric care. St. Louis, Mosby, 1993, pp 305–315.

4. What is vestibular rehabilitation? Who is a candidate?

Vestibular rehabilitation is a form of physical therapy designed specifically to help dizzy patients to cope in their environment through vestibular compensation. It is a multidisciplinary treatment program that uses vestibular provocation as well as conditioning and control exercises. It teaches the patient to use existing visual or proprioceptive cues. Although vestibular suppressants may be used as adjunctive therapy, preferably patients should avoid such medication during vestibular rehabilitation. Vestibular rehabilitation is most often used in patients with benign paroxysmal positional vertigo (BPPV) and dizziness secondary to presbystasis, vestibular surgery, or traumatic head injury. Although elderly patients make slower progress in vestibular rehabilitation than younger patients, they often derive significant benefit. Vestibular rehabilitation is inappropriate for patients in whom the cause of dizziness has not been defined. In addition, long-term benefits have not been found in patients with Meniere's disease.

5. What is Meniere's syndrome?

Meniere's syndrome is characterized by episodic vertigo, aural fullness, tinnitus, and fluctuating hearing loss. The pathophysiology is thought to be secondary endolymphatic hydrops. Diagnosis is made on the basis of the typical clinical history and documentation of fluctuating hearing loss as well as episodic vertigo. Medical management includes acute management with antivertiginous medication, prophylactic salt restriction, and diuretics in an effort to reduce the hydrops. Surgical treatments, such as labyrinthectomies, vestibular nerve sections, and endolymphatic shunts are not recommended in elderly patients, who tend to have more difficulty adapting after such procedures. Vestibular rehabilitation results in minimal improvement.

6. In taking a patient's history, what questions are important to differentiate etiologies?

A patient's history is often the most important factor in establishing the cause of dizziness or vertigo; therefore, probing for historical clues is critical. First, the differentiation between dizziness and vertigo should be made. This differentiation helps to distinguish vestibular from nonvestibular causes. Precipitating factors, such as head movement or sudden positional changes, are important etiologic clues—especially rolling over in bed. The time course and pattern of symptoms are also important. Vertigo with BPPV lasts only seconds, whereas vertigo in Meniere's syndrome lasts for 30 minutes to hours. Symptoms occurring in conjunction with vertiginous episodes, such as fluctuating hearing loss, tinnitus, and aural fullness, may indicate a vestibular origin. Visual loss, an inability to speak or swallow, and near syncope may indicate a central vascular origin. Pertinent medical history must include a history of trauma and prior use of medication, tobacco, and alcohol.

7. Which aspects of the physical exam need to be evaluated during the work-up for dizziness and vertigo in the elderly?

Initial evaluation should include traditional orthostatics, full cardiovascular exam, and a complete neurotologic work-up. Blood pressure and pulse should be measured in the lying, sitting, and standing positions, because orthostatic hypotension is a common cause of dizziness in the elderly. Orthostatic hypotension is defined as a drop in systolic blood pressure of ≥ 20 mmHg from lying to standing position. Cardiovascular exams are performed to investigate possible cardiac arrhythmias and carotid bruits.

A complete neurotologic exam should be performed, beginning with an otologic exam and including a cranial nerve exam, evaluation of the external and middle ear, and a fistula test. The fistula test is performed by applying pressure to the ear and evaluating for vertigo and nystagmus. A positive result indicates the presence of a fistula of the labyrinth due to cholesteatoma or infection. Evaluation for nystagmus, an objective finding that accompanies vertigo, is also important. Spontaneously induced nystagmus may indicate central or peripheral vestibular dysfunction. Nystagmus is named according to the direction of the rapid component. A Weber-Rinne test is performed to assess for sensorineural or conductive hearing loss. The Romberg test, which is performed with the patient's eyes closed, evaluates cerebellar function and gait.

The Hallpike maneuver is used to evaluate for BPPV. Nystagmus as well as vertigo is assessed after the head is turned to the left and the patient is quickly lowered from a sitting to a supine position. The head is held in the supine position for 1 minute. The procedure is repeated with the head turned to the right. The test should be repeated several times on the side which is most symptomatic to check for fatigability. A positive Hallpike test classically provokes the patient's symptoms and elicits nystagmus on the affected side.

8. Which adjunctive tests should be ordered to evaluate the dizzy or vertiginous patient?

Adjunctive tests may greatly facilitate a diagnostic work-up. They should be obtained, however, with a systematic rather than a "shotgun" approach. A complete audiogram should be obtained in all patients complaining of hearing loss and vertigo and in all patients with abnormal neurotologic exams. Electronystagmography (ENG), which evaluates the vestibular system by recording nystagmus, aids in differentiating central from peripheral vestibular dysfunction. It should be obtained in patients complaining of vertigo or patients with neurotologic findings such as nystagmus. Patients should avoid all vestibular suppressants for at least 48 hours before testing. Auditory brainstem-evoked responses should be obtained in patients with asymmetric sensorineural hearing loss to rule out acoustic neuroma. Posturography and magnetic resonance imaging (MRI) may be considered in selected patients. MRI examination of the temporal bone is often ordered in patients suspected of having acoustic neuromas or other cerebellopontine angle masses. Computed tomography (CT) of the temporal bones may be obtained when cholesteatomas or other middle ear lesions are suspected.

An EKG and possibly a Holter monitor should be obtained in patients with cardiac findings. In clinically suspicious histories, laboratory blood tests should include a fluorescent treponemal antibody absorbed test to rule out syphilis, thyroid function tests to rule out hypothyroidism, and glucose levels to rule out diabetes mellitus.

9. What is the role for vestibular suppressants such as valium and meclizine in elderly vertiginous patients?

The use of vestibular suppressants is not contraindicated in the elderly. An antiemetic may also aid patients with severe nausea and vomiting. Elderly patients, however, may be extremely sensitive to vestibular suppressants. In addition, they may be taking other medications that interact with or affect the metabolism of such medications.

10. Which medications are possible causes of dysequilibrium?

Geriatric patients are often on polypharmacy that may either cause or exacerbate baseline dizziness or vertigo. It is extremely important to obtain a thorough medication list, including as-needed prescriptions.

Class of Drug	Type of Dizziness	Mechanism
Alcohol	Positional	Cerebellar dysfunction
Sedatives	Disorientation	Depression of central processing
Antihypertensives	Lightheadedness	Orthostatic hypotension
Anticonvulsants	Dysequilibrium	Cerebellar dysfunction
Aminoglycosides	Dysequilibrium, oscillopsia/vertigo	Damage to labyrinthine hair cells
Diuretics	Positional	Orthostatic hypotension

From Baloh RW, Glorig A: Dysequilibrium of aging (presbystasis). J Laryngol Otol 100:1037–1041, 1986; with permission.

11. How does the time frame of the symptoms relate to the diagnostic etiology?

The time frame of the patient's symptoms may give an indication of the etiology. BPPV usually resolves within 30 seconds to a minute after the provoking positional change. In patients with vascular etiologies, such as transient ischemic attack, cerebrovascular accidents, orthostatic hypotension, or vasovagal hypotension, symptoms last for several minutes. Episodes of vertigo in Meniere's disease usually last from minutes to hours. The episodes of vertigo with neuronitis and labyrinthitis continue for days.

12. Define BPPV. How is it diagnosed?

BPPV is one of the most common causes of vertigo in elderly patients. It occurs usually after trauma or an episode of viral labyrinthitis. The pathophysiology is thought to be due to the release of otoconia (small calcium carbonate crystals in the saccule) into the posterior semicircular canal. With head movement the crystals are displaced, resulting in vertigo and nystagmus. Patients develop vertigo that occurs with positional changes and lasts less than 1 minute. BPPV is diagnosed by a suggestive history and a positive Hallpike maneuver on physical examination. Extensive diagnostic testing is not required. Although 90% of cases resolve spontaneously within a few months, exacerbations may last for years.

Treatment is directed toward active provocation of the vestibular system with the goal of vestibular habituation and resolution of symptoms. The Epley maneuver repositions free-floating endolymphatic particles in the posterior semicircular canal. The patient is placed in the provocative head-hanging position and remains there for several minutes. The patient is then rotated to the opposite side, with the head turned 45° downward. The patient should be aware that dizziness is exacerbated initially during the exercises but will subside with time. Theoretically this maneuver allows the floating particles to continue their course through the common crus into the utricle by rotating the posterior semicircular canal 180° in the plane of gravity. Meclizine may be useful in the short term for control of symptoms.

BIBLIOGRAPHY

1. Belal A, Glorig A: Dysequilibrium of aging (presbystasis). J Laryngol Otol 100:1037– 1041, 1986.
2. Bolah RW: Dizziness in older people. J Am Geriatr Soc 40:713–721, 1992.
3. Cohen H, Rubin AM, Gombash L: The team approach to treatment of the dizzy patient. Arch Phys Med Rehabil 73:703–708, 1992.
4. Cohen H: Vestibular rehabilitation reduces functional disability. Otolaryngol Head Neck Surg 107:638–643, 1992.
5. Katsarkas A: Dizziness in aging: A retrospective study of 1194 Cases. Otolaryngol Head Neck Surg 110:296–301, 1994.
6. Mader SL: Dizziness and syncope. In Yoshikawa T (ed): Ambulatory Geriatric Care. St. Louis, Mosby, 1993, pp 305–315.
7. Sloan PD, Baloh RW: Persistent dizziness in geriatric patients. J Am Geriatr Soc 37:1031, 1989.

6. SEXUAL FUNCTIONING

Fran E. Kaiser, M.D.

1. How does the sexual response cycle change with aging?

Changes in Human Sexual Response with Aging

PHASE	MALE	FEMALE
Excitement	Reduced scrotal vasocongestion Decreased testicular elevation Delayed penile erection	Reduced breast and genital vasocongestion Diminished vaginal secretions Delayed arousal
Plateau	Prolonged Diminished pre-ejaculatory secretions	Reduced elevation of uterus and labia majora
Orgasm	Short duration Reduction in prostatic and urethral contraction	Short duration Fewer and weaker uterine and vaginal contractions
Resolution	Rapid detumescence and testicular descent Prolonged refractory period	Rapid reversal to prearousal stage

As defined by Masters and Johnson, the stages of sexual response change with aging, although these changes do not preclude sexual activity. In 1992, the NIH defined erectile dysfunction as "the inability of the male to attain and maintain erection of the penis sufficient to permit satisfactory intercourse." Erectile dysfunction has replaced the emotionally charged term *impotence*.

2. Are loss of sexual function and erectile dysfunction normal consequences of the aging process?

No. While some older adults experience a decrease in sexual activity with age, many individuals remain sexually active. Erectile dysfunction, though common with age (occurring in 52% of all men aged 40–70 and > 95% of diabetic men > 70), indicates underlying organic disease. An estimated 30 million men in the United States have erectile dysfunction.

3. Is the most common cause of erectile dysfunction psychogenic?

No. Prior to the 1980s, it was thought that 90% of erectile dysfunction was due to psychogenic causes. Although underlying organic etiologies are more common than psychogenic problems, one cannot discount a psychological overlay to a chronic problem. Depression, performance anxiety (fear of failure), and "widower's syndrome" (a widower's entering a new relationship may evoke guilt about the deceased partner, as bereavement may not be completed) may occur.

We now know that the most common cause of erectile dysfunction is vascular. Over 50% of men have vascular dysfunction, which can relate to poor arterial inflow, excessive venous outflow, or a combination of these factors. Neurologic, hormonal, and medication effects can also play a role. Neurologic problems such as stroke, multiple sclerosis, spinal cord lesions/traumas, and peripheral and autonomic neuropathy may cause erectile dysfunction. Diabetes, hypo- and hyperthyroidism, hyperprolactinemia, and Cushing's syndrome are associated with erectile dysfunction. No one knows the frequency of these conditions— it depends on the setting. An endocrinologist will see more hormonal problems than an internist, and a psychiatrist may see more depression than another specialist.

Etiology of Impotence

Vascular	Psychologic	Medications *(cont.)*
Arteriosclerotic	Depression	Antidepressants
Venous leakage	"Madonna" syndrome	H$_2$ blockers
Arteriovenous malformations	Performance anxiety	**Systemic disorders**
Local trauma	Widower's syndrome	Renal failure
Nervous system	Stress	Chronic obstructive pulmonary
Central	**Endocrine**	disease
Stroke	Diabetes mellitus	Cirrhosis
Multiple sclerosis	Hypogonadism	Leprosy
Temporal lobe epilepsy	Hyperprolactinemia	Myotonia dystrophica
Spinal cord	Hypothyroidism	**Nutritional disorders**
Trauma	Hyperthyroidism	Obesity
Tumor	Cushing's syndrome	Protein-calorie malnutrition
Peripheral	**Medications**	Zinc deficiency
Autonomic neuropathy	Antihypertensive drugs	**Peyronie's disease**
Sensory neuropathy	Anticholinergics	**Prostatectomy**

4. What is the role of medication in causing erectile dysfunction?

Ten percent of commonly prescribed medications result in erectile dysfunction. In nearly 25% of men with erectile dysfunction, medications play a role. *All* antihypertensives, regardless of class, have been associated with impotence. The most common medications to cause potency problems are thiazide diuretics. These drugs drop penile pressures and lower testosterone and bioavailable testosterone levels.

5. How does hypogonadism cause erectile dysfunction?

Hypogonadism can be defined as a low testosterone (generally < 300 ng/dl) and a low bioavailable testosterone level. Bioavailable testosterone is the fraction of testosterone not bound to sex hormone-binding globulin (SHBG) and is the "testosterone equivalent" of the relationship of the free thyroxine index to total thyroxine. That is, since testosterone is bound to SHBG, a measure of the total testosterone alone is not especially helpful in defining gonadal status. Low testosterone and low bioavailable testosterone levels are linked to low libido (sex drive) but not, per se, to erectile dysfunction. Young men who have been castrated may get erections. However, improvement in libido with testosterone treatment may be enough to overcome sexual disinterest and erectile problems in some individuals.

6. What tests are helpful in diagnosing and determining the cause of erectile dysfunction?

All patients should be screened for sexual problems. A nonjudgmental question such as "Do you have any difficulty with your ability to have sex?" may be a good opener.

A careful sexual, medical, and medication history and a depression assessment using the Beck Depression Inventory or the Yesavage Geriatric Depression Scale are all beneficial. Penile tissue should be examined for fibrous plaques of bands that would occur with Peyronie's disease (plaques or bands causing penile bending). Small or soft testicles, gynecomastia, and increased hip girth suggest hypogonadism. Decreased penile sensitivity or abnormal cremasteric or bulbo-cavernosus reflexes suggest neuropathy. Penile Doppler testing can be helpful to diagnose abnormal vascular status, especially when an exercise component is added. This test measures pressure in the penis and compares it to pressure in the arm. A ratio < 0.65 (penis to brachial pressure) is diagnostic of vascular problems.

Testosterone, bioavailable testosterone, and luteinizing hormone should be measured. Thyroid function tests should be obtained. Nocturnal penile tumescence testing (sleep study of erectile function) is not especially helpful in those over age 50, as it is often impaired in older subjects despite an ability to get and maintain erections adequate for intercourse.

7. How can you treat erectile dysfunction?

When an etiology such as hypogonadism with decreased libido or depression is found, management is clear. However, in most cases, the etiology is often multifactional, and a variety of alternatives is available. **Vacuum tumescent devices** (the creation of negative pressure using a pump attached to a plastic tube placed over the penis) creates an erection; a band or ring is then placed at the base of the penis, the vacuum is released, the tube removed, and the individual has an erection lasting 15–30 minutes. The recently approved **Caverject** (prostaglandin E_1, alprostadil) is used as a penile injection when the individual wishes to get an erection. **Surgery** or the implantation of bendable or inflatable rods into the penis is another method of treatment. Each has benefits as well as problems, and often the lifestyle of the individual dictates the choice.

8. What is the effect of estrogen loss in women?

Estrogen deficiency is associated with a reduction in vaginal blood flow, decreased vaginal lubrication, and increased vaginal fragility with thinning of vaginal mucosa. These changes can result in dyspareunia (painful intercourse). To treat estrogen deficiency locally, Estrace cream (or its equivalent) is inserted into the vagina 2–4 gm once daily for 2 weeks and then as maintenance 1 gm 1–3 times a week. Estrogen and progesterone have minimal effects on libido, and levels do not predict desire, sexual function, or sexual response. Estrogen has a positive and beneficial effect on vaginal lubrication and tissue strength (stronger and less friable) and from that aspect can improve sexual function. Testosterone does seem to play a major role in libido in women.

9. Is hysterectomy associated with an alteration in sexual function?

Hysterectomy is the most commonly performed surgery in women, with one-third of women over age 60 having had this procedure. However, it tends not to be associated with a decline in sexual function. For women who feel that sex is primarily a procreative function, the loss of the uterus may impact on the psychological importance and influence sexual response.

10. Does medication use affect sexual function in women?

Essentially unknown, as few studies of medication effect explore sexual function in women.

11. What reasons do older people give for changes in their sexual activity?
- Lack of a partner
- Partner erectile dysfunction
- Personal health problems
- Vaginal dryness

Masturbation is a common form of sexual expression, especially when one does not have a partner or the partner's health or abilities are impaired. Many older individuals find this an acceptable and enjoyable experience.

12. What about sexuality in a long-term care setting?

There is no age at which sexual activity and expression ends. It is important to recognize that a nursing home is still home. Staff need to provide opportunities for privacy for mutually desired sexual activities or for masturbation. The only true problem is coercive or aggressive behavior.

BIBLIOGRAPHY

1. Bretschneider JG, McCoy NL: Sexual interest and behavior in healthy 80-50-102 year olds. Arch Sex Behav 17:109–129, 1988.
2. Diokno AC, Brown MB, Herzog AR: Sexual function in the elderly. Arch Intern Med 150:197–200, 1990.
3. Feldman HA, Goldstein I, Hatzchristou G, et al: Impotence and its medical and psychosocial correlates: Results of the Massachusetts Male Aging Study. J Urol 151:54–61, 1994.
4. Kaiser FE, Viosca SP, Morley JE, et al: Impotence and aging: Clinical and hormonal factors. J Am Geriatr Soc 36:511–519, 1988.
5. Kaplan HS, Owett T: The female androgen deficiency syndrome. J Sex Marital Ther 19:13–24, 1993.
6. Krane RJ, Goldstein I, de Tejada IS: Impotence. N Engl J Med 321:1648–1659, 1989.
7. Morley JE, Kaiser FE: Impotence: The internist's approach to diagnosis and treatment. Adv Intern Med 38:151–168, 1993.
8. Roughan PA, Kaiser FE, Morley JE: Sexuality and the older woman. Clin Geriatr Med 1:87–106, 1993.

7. CONSTIPATION

William F. Edwards, M.S.N., R.N., C.S., C.R.N.P

1. What is constipation?

From a medical perspective, constipation is often defined as a frequency of < 3 bowel movements a week. From the individual's perspective, constipation can mean that stools are difficult to expel, too hard, or too small, or there may be a sensation of incomplete evacuation. Although it is important to teach the patient about normal bowel function, successful management requires that the clinician also respect the patient's concerns.

2. Is constipation a normal part of aging?

The frequency of bowel movements in healthy older populations is essentially the same as it is in the younger population. Despite this fact, the use of laxatives is more common in the elderly, even if they are not having infrequent stools.

3. List the causes of constipation.

For most elderly individuals, there are likely to be multiple contributing factors:

Dietary
Inadequate caloric intake
Poor fluid intake
Low-fiber diet
High-fat diet
Refined foods
Poor dentition
Swallowing problems
Tube feedings
Psychological
Depression
Confusion
Emotional stress
Functional
Inadequate toileting
Poor bowel habits
Weakness
Immobility/lack of exercise
Colonic/anorectal disorders
Ischemia
Postsurgical obstruction
Rectocele or rectal prolapse

Colonic/anorectal disorders *(cont.)*
Tumors
Volvulus or megacolon
Barium or bezoars
Fissures or hemorrhoids
Fistula or abscess
Radiation fibrosis
Stricture
Prostatic enlargement
Diverticulosis
Neurogenic disorders
Spinal cord lesions
Parkinson's disease
Cerebrovascular accidents
Dementia
Endocrine/metabolic disorders
Diabetes
Hypothyroidism
Hyperparathyroidism
Hypokalemia
Hypercalcemia

4. What medications can cause constipation?

Aluminum: antacids (Amphojel, ALternaGEL), sucralfate
Anticonvulsants: phenytoin, carbamazepine, phenobarbital
Antidepressants: amitriptyline, nortriptyline, venlafaxine
Antihistamines: diphenhydramine, chlorpheniramine
Antihypertensives: acebutolol, prazosin
Antilipemics: cholestyramine, colestipol
Antiparkinsonian drugs: bromocriptine, Sinemet, amantadine
Antipsychotics: haloperidol, risperidone

Antispasmodics: oxybutynin, opiate or barbiturate compounds
Bismuth: Pepto-Bismol, Rectacort
Calcium: antacids (Tums), supplements (calcium carbonate)
Calcium channel blockers: verapamil, nifedipine
Diuretics: hydrochlorothiazide, furosemide, indapamide
Ganglionic blockers: trimethaphan
Iron supplements
Laxative misuse
Nonsteroidal anti-inflammatories: naproxen, sulindac, ketoprofen
Opiates: codeine, morphine, oxycodone
Phenothiazines: thioridazine, chlorpromazine, perphenazine
Sedatives: diazepam, flurazepam, thiothixene

5. Do all individuals complaining of constipation require a complete evaluation?
Individuals with a precipitous change in bowel habits (including the caliber or characteristics of the stool) require a thorough evaluation. For those with a history of constipation > 2 years, the focus should be on management. In obtaining the history, you must find out how the patient defines constipation and whether the patient has had a change in bowel function or is dealing with a long-term problem. Many elderly were reared with the idea that daily movements were essential to good health and that failure to move the bowels led to the buildup of dangerous toxins.

6. What other aspects of the history are most important?
- In patients with recent onset of constipation, the history should focus on excluding underlying causes such as malignancy, intestinal obstruction, or others.
- Exacerbation or complications of a known illness must be considered.
- A thorough evaluation of recent changes in diet, medications, emotional state, and level of activity is warranted.
- In evaluation of the diet, total caloric intake, fiber content, and fluid intake should receive special attention.
- The clinician needs to inquire about problems related to chewing and swallowing.
- It is essential to evaluate the patient's complaint of constipation as thoroughly as possible.
- The color, amount, consistency, frequency, size, and symptoms experienced during defecation are key components of the history.
- Brief screening tests for cognitive function and mood assist the clinician in detecting nonphysiologic causes of constipation.

7. Is a complete physical examination necessary in evaluating the patient with constipation?
If the patient is not known to the clinician, a complete physical exam is needed to rule out systemic causes. For most patients, the focus is on examination of the mouth, abdomen, and anorectal area and assessment for dehydration. The **oral** examination focuses on adequacy of dentition and detection of any lesions or tumors. The **abdomen** is examined for normal bowel sounds and detection of pain or localized masses. The **anorectal area** is evaluated for sphincter muscle tone; presence of stool in the vault; lesions such as hemorrhoids, strictures, fistulas, or masses; and prostatic enlargement.

8. How do you decide when to do additional diagnostic testing?
If the symptom of constipation began < 2 years ago or if the patient has pain or any evidence of rectal bleeding, colonoscopy or sigmoidoscopy and barium enema are mandatory. In addition to detecting cancer, endoscopy can also reveal the presence of diffuse dark pigmentation, melanosis coli, which is caused by chronic use of laxatives such as cascara, senna, and aloe.

If the patient has liquid stool leakage or symptoms of impaction with an empty rectal vault, abdominal x-rays can detect a high impaction or other signs of obstruction. Additional diagnostic testing, such as colonic transit time and motility studies, is needed only if the patient does not respond to treatment for constipation.

9. Are any serious complications associated with constipation?

Fecal impaction is the major complication, and it can be life-threatening. Fecal impaction can cause cognitive problems, malaise, fatigue, urinary retention, bowel and urine incontinence, anal fissure, hemorrhoids, stercoral ulcer, and intestinal obstruction. Watery diarrhea can occur around impacted stool. A mass of stool in the rectum can impair sensation and lead to the need for larger volumes of stool to stimulate the urge to defecate. Constipated patients, especially those who have chronically abused laxatives, can develop **megacolon** and **volvulus**. Straining during defecation affects cerebral and coronary circulation and can cause transient **ischemic attacks** and **syncope**, especially in the frail elderly. Finally, chronic constipation is a risk factor for **colon** and **rectal carcinoma**.

10. Discuss approaches to treating constipation.

The treatment of constipation is individualized for each patient according to the identified causes. The clinician must balance the need to make changes slowly with the patient's desire to get results quickly (as evidenced by the $400-million/year laxative industry). Patient outcome goals might include the passage of a soft formed stool at least 3 times a week without straining and the avoidance of complications associated with constipation.

1. The first step in managing constipation is to stop or switch any medications that may be contributing, including laxatives.

2. It is best to start a bowel program with an empty colon, which may require the use of enemas or even manual disimpaction. Aside from avoiding soap suds, there is no consensus on the best type of fluid to use for enemas. In patients who may require a series of enemas, normal saline is probably best. The temperature should be about 105° F, and the amount should not exceed 500 ml. For occasional use, the popular sodium phosphate enema is usually safe, but the amount should not exceed 120 ml.

3. Healthy bowel function requires an adequate **fluid intake**. If there are no fluid restrictions because of renal or cardiac problems, 2 to 3 liters/day is an appropriate goal. This needs to be done gradually to improve compliance. Water is the ideal fluid—caffeinated beverages and some fruit juices can cause diuresis, which can exacerbate constipation.

4. **Dietary fiber** should also be increased. This is done gradually to avoid the unpleasant bloating and gas pains and to give the patient's colon a chance to adapt. The amount of additional fiber required to improve bowel function varies greatly, from 6–30 gm.

5. Regular **exercise** is an important component of healthy bowel function. Ambulatory patients should be encouraged to walk for 20 minutes daily. Even those elderly individuals who are bed- or chair-bound can benefit from an exercise program that involves turning from side to side, twisting the trunk, or exercising the arms.

6. The clinician should instruct the patient in the importance of establishing a **routine** that promotes normal bowel function. This includes taking advantage of the gastrocolic reflex, which for most individuals, is most pronounced after breakfast or supper. Many individuals find it helpful to have a warm drink with breakfast. It is important that the patient have a private opportunity for about 10 minutes each day to attempt to have a bowel movement. It is also important to emphasize the need to respond as soon as possible to any urge to defecate. Proper position also facilitates bowel function. Squatting is the best position, but this is often not possible for the elderly who require high toilet seats. The squatting position can be emulated in these cases by using a foot stool. The patient should be instructed to lean forward and use the hand to apply firm pressure on the lower abdomen.

7. Institutionalized patients require close monitoring. It is not adequate simply to mark whether or not the person's bowels moved. It is important to note the amount, color, and consistency of the stool. Each care plan should include information about the individual's usual bowel habits, including the time of day that is most conducive to normal evacuation.

11. What are the most effective ways of adding fiber to the diet?

The best way to add fiber is by making subtle changes in the diet. The changes should be made gradually to avoid gas pains and bloating, which can occur with fiber. Switching to **whole-grain breads** and to **cereals** high in fiber might be the only change some individuals need to make. Lessons in label reading are often necessary because prominently advertised "wheat" breads are often not made of whole wheat.

Many brans have become popular, but wheat bran is the most effective type for promoting bowel function. For individuals who prefer hot cereals, wheat bran may be mixed in with the cereal. Institutional food is often low in fiber, and residents of such facilities may benefit from a **fiber supplement**. Supplements made from 2 parts wheat bran (sometimes given in the form of 100% bran cereal, which is more palatable but less effective than crude bran), 2 parts applesauce, and 1 part prune juice have been effective. The starting dose is 30 ml daily, and it costs significantly less than laxatives.

The common advice "eat more fruits and vegetables" may not be sufficient to add enough insoluble fiber to the diet. A dietary consultation may be appropriate to help an individual make changes that take into consideration traditional eating habits, cost, dentition, and taste.

12. Are there any precautions associated with adding fiber to the diet?

1. Fiber should not be added to the diets of individuals with **megacolon**. In fact, such patients should be on a fiber-restricted diet and may need to be managed with enemas.

2. Some elderly individuals are at risk for development of **bezoars**. Bezoars are hard, dense masses of fibrous materials that can cause irritation in the stomach or obstruction in the intestines. Individuals with poor dentition, history of surgery for peptic ulcer disease, or stomach cancer are at greater risk for bezoars.

3. Fiber should be avoided in patients with **intestinal stricture**.

4. Increased fiber can pose a hazard for **bed-bound patients** by increasing bulk in a colon that is already distended.

These exceptions aside, most elderly individuals who make dietary changes gradually to increase fiber will have no problem. Fiber supplements may carry a risk of decreased mineral absorption as well as the risk of overdosing. The risk for mineral depletion is virtually nonexistent for those who add fiber through their diet, because high-fiber foods tend to have greater amounts of the minerals in question. Individuals who use fiber supplements should be told not to expect overnight results. They also should not double-up on supplements because this can cause diarrhea or even obstruction. The latter is most likely to occur if the patient does not drink enough water.

13. What is the role of laxatives in the management of constipation?

For most patients, laxatives and enemas should not be a part of routine bowel management but should be used only occasionally to prevent the complications associated with constipation. Individuals who have used laxatives for years will require education about the harmful effects of laxatives and their role in causing constipation. However, patients with megacolon or with a medical condition which requires that they avoid straining may need to use laxatives or enemas.

14. What considerations influence choice of laxatives?

The choice of laxative is determined by:
• The cause of the problem
• Nature of the constipation (is the stool hard or soft, high in the colon or in the rectum?)
• Other medical conditions
• Other medications the patient may be taking
• Cost of treatment
• Patient preference

15. Describe the different types of laxatives and considerations in their usage.

Bulk laxative may benefit ambulatory individuals who do not respond to increases in dietary fiber and fluid. In choice of a specific agent, sugar and sodium content needs to be considered, as does taste and convenience. Bulk-forming laxatives can inhibit the absorption of drugs such as digoxin and salicylates. As with dietary fiber, these agents should be avoided in patients who are bed-bound, have swallowing difficulties, or have intestinal stricture, because bulk-forming laxatives may contribute to obstruction or get stuck in the throat. The patient must drink adequate amounts of fluid to avoid problems with these laxatives.

Osmotic or **saline laxatives** are good choices if bulk-forming agents cannot be used or are ineffective. These agents attract water into the bowel and stimulate peristalsis. They are popular because they empty the bowel within a few hours. Individuals with poor renal function should avoid magnesium-,phosphate-, or sulfate-based salts. Lactulose and sorbitol are hyperosmolar agents that increase fluid in the colon and promote formation of a soft stool. They are rather slow-acting in recommended doses. Lactulose is unpalatably sweet and is much more expensive than most other laxatives.

Emollient laxatives include mineral oil and docusate salts. Mineral oil should be avoided in the elderly because of the risk of aspiration, interference with absorption of fat-soluble vitamins, and risk of leakage through the anal sphincter. Stool softeners are popular, but studies of patients receiving them have shown no change in stool weight or water content, no increase in frequency of bowel movements, and no change in colonic transit time. They are especially ineffective in patients who have a large amount of soft stool in the colon. Stool softeners are often recommended in bed-bound patients with hard dry stool, in patients who must avoid straining, and as an adjunct to bulk agents. For most individuals, adding 8 oz of water to their daily intake would probably be more effective.

Stimulant or **irritant laxatives** should be rarely used because of the risk of damage to the colon and electrolyte imbalance. They are popular because of their efficacy, but they have a more toxic long-term effect than other laxatives. Castor oil and aloe should be avoided entirely because safer choices are available. Cascara is less irritating than senna, and bisacodyl is safer than phenolphthalein (Ex-Lax, Feen-a-Mint). The latter is commonly used by the elderly but should be avoided because its effects can last several days. It can impair vitamin D and calcium absorption and has been associated with dermatitis, photosensitivity reactions, and Stevens-Johnson syndrome.

Bisacodyl and **glycerin suppositories** are appropriate for occasional use when stool is present in the rectum and are usually effective within an hour. They may cause cramping and local irritation. **Enemas** should be reserved for constipation that does not respond to other approaches.

BIBLIOGRAPHY

1. Allison OC, Porter ME, Briggs GC: Chronic constipation: Assessment and management in the elderly. J Am Acad Nurse Pract 6:311–317, 1994.
2. Cheskin LJ, Schuster MM: Constipation. In Hazzard WR, Bierman EL, Blass JP, et al (eds): Principles of Geriatric Medicine and Gerontology, 3rd ed. New York, McGraw-Hill, 1994.
3. Ellickson EB: Bowel management plan for the homebound elderly. Gerontol Nurs 14:16–19, 1988.
4. Goldstein MK, Oliveira J: Constipation, diarrhea and fecal impaction. In Yoshikawa TT, Cobbs EL, Brummel-Smith K (eds): Ambulatory Geriatric Care. St. Louis, Mosby-Year Book, 1993.
5. Hogstel MO, Nelson M: Anticipation and early detection can reduce bowel elimination complications. Geriat Nurs 13:28–33, 1992.
6. Stone JK: Managing bowel function. In Chenitz WC, Stone JK, Salisbury SA (eds): Clinical Gerontological Nursing: A Guide to Advanced Practice. Philadelphia, W.B. Saunders, 1991.
7. Wald A: Constipation and fecal incontinence in the elderly. Gastroenterol Clin North Am 19:405–419, 1990.
8. Yakabowich M: Prescribe with care: The role of laxatives in the treatment of constipation. J Gerontol Nurs 16:4–11, 1990.

8. RHEUMATOLOGIC CONDITIONS IN THE ELDERLY

Edna P. Schwab, M.D.

1. What are the characteristic features of polymyalgia rheumatica?

Polymyalgia rheumatica is a common cause of musculoskeletal pain in older individuals. The etiology is unknown. In a survey of Olmsted County, Minnesota, conducted by the Mayo Clinic, its prevalence was found to be 500/100,000 persons over age 50. Most patients are at least 50 years old. Female sex predominates by a ratio of 2.5:1.

Bilateral aching and stiffness of the shoulder girdle, neck, and hip girdle muscles in association with constitutional symptoms and an elevated Westergren ESR characterize polymyalgia rheumatica. These symptoms are most common in the morning and frequently are associated with malaise, weight loss, and low-grade fever. Physical examination is remarkable for tenderness and limitation of motion of the shoulders and hips. Weakness, however, is not evident. Synovitis has been demonstrated by arthroscopy and biopsy of shoulder joints.

The onset of polymyalgia rheumatica may be gradual but more often is sudden. This condition rarely responds to nonsteroidal anti-inflammatory drugs and often requires the initiation of corticosteroids. Low doses of prednisone (10 mg/day) usually result in an excellent therapeutic response. Polymyalgia rheumatica is a self-limited disease but may also have a more prolonged course. In patients whose ESR is normal, the diagnosis is made if characteristic symptoms are present and the response to prednisone is rapid and complete. Sometimes, it may be difficult to distinguish between the diagnosis of polymyalgia rheumatica and rheumatoid arthritis because of the similarities in presentation and lack of positive serologies in older patients. A high index of suspicion should be maintained for the closely associated disease, temporal arteritis, which occurs in 6–45% of patients with polymyalgia rheumatica.

2. Which laboratory findings are characteristic of polymyalgia rheumatica?

The ESR is often elevated to > 40 mm/hr and commonly to > 100 mm/hr. Evidence of an anemia due to chronic disease along with mildly elevated liver function abnormalities is usually present. Radiographs of the joints may demonstrate soft tissue inflammation without evidence of erosions.

3. Define giant cell arteritis and describe its features.

Giant cell arteritis is a large-vessel vasculitis that often affects the vessels of the aortic arch. It has a reported prevalence of 133/100,000 people over age 50, as surveyed by the Mayo Clinic in Olmsted County, Minnesota. Superficial vessels, such as the occipital, external carotid and its branches, including the temporal, lingual, and facial arteries, may be involved. Deeper vessels may also be affected, including the vertebral artery and internal carotid along with its branches. Vessels lacking elastic tissue, such as the intracranial arteries, are spared. Most often, however, the branches of the aorta, occipital, or temporal artery become inflamed, with patients developing symptoms associated with the involved vessels.

Common symptoms consist of occipital or temporal headaches in 90% of patients, along with jaw claudication and tenderness over the temporal artery. Diplopia may occur as a result of ischemia to the extraocular muscles. The most dreaded complication is irreversible visual loss, which occurs in 15% of patients, most commonly due to ischemic optic neuritis with involvement of the ciliary branches of the internal carotid. Stroke is a rare complication of giant cell arteritis. As in polymyalgia rheumatica, these symptoms are often accompanied by constitutional symptoms of fever, malaise, anorexia and weight loss. These nonspecific symptons often prompt an evaluation for an occult malignancy. Polymyalgia rheumatica may be present in up to 50% of cases of giant cell arteritis.

4. What laboratory and histologic features are diagnostic for giant cell arteritis?

In a patient who has characteristic findings of giant cell arteritis, laboratory evaluation usually demonstrates an elevated ESR usually > 100 mm/hr. Anemia and mildly elevated liver function tests may also be present.

The diagnosis is made by a temporal artery biopsy demonstrating destruction of the internal elastic lamina associated with granulomatous inflammation. Histologic examination reveals areas of inflammation of the media and fragmentation of the elastic lamina of the artery. This pattern of involvement follows those vessels that contain internal elastic lamina. Granulomas contain lymphocytes, histiocytes, and giant cells. Inflammatory edema or thrombus may occlude the vessel, leading to ischemic symptoms typically seen in this disorder. It is important to remember that the entire vessel is generally not involved. Skip lesions, areas of inflammation interspersed with normal-appearing vessel, may be found on a temporal artery biopsy. Biopsies should include at least 1 inch of vessel.

5. How is giant cell arteritis treated?

When the diagnosis of giant cell arteritis is considered, treatment should be started with high-dose corticosteroids, at least 50 mg/day of prednisone, and continued after the diagnosis is confirmed. Symptoms, rather than ESR, should determine the tapering schedule. Clinicians should also start appropriate therapies, such as calcium and vitamin D, to lessen the toxicity of corticosteroids.

6. What are the characteristic features of elderly-onset rheumatoid arthritis?

Rheumatoid arthritis (RA) is a chronic inflammatory disease involving the synovium which may be accompanied by systemic manifestations of fever, malaise, fatigue, and weight loss. The etiology of the disease is unknown. Typically, it affects patients during the third to fifth decades of life with a prevalence rate of 0.3–3%. Females are affected more often than men with a ratio of 2:1 to 3:1. The prevalence of RA increases with age, occurring in 30–40% of people over age 60. The proportion of affected men also rises with age. Patients with long-standing RA often have more severe disease with extra-articular manifestations, joint deformities, and comorbidities.

Patients who develop RA after age 60 generally have milder arthritis, lack rheumatoid nodules, and are rheumatoid factor-positive in only 32–58%, unlike disease seen in younger patients. Most patients with RA gradually develop symmetric pain, swelling, and stiffness in peripheral joints, sparing the distal interphalangeal joints. Occasionally, RA presents acutely. In hemiplegic patients, the paralyzed side is not affected by the disease. In the elderly patient, large joints, such as shoulders, are commonly involved. Studies evaluating the prognosis of elderly-onset RA have been contradictory. Most early studies describe a rapid decline, while more recent reports describe a more benign course. Other diagnostic considerations in the elderly patient who develops an acute symmetric polyarticular synovitis include pseudogout, polyarticular gout (especially in women on diuretics), systemic lupus erythematosus, and paraneoplastic disease.

7. How often does systemic lupus erythematosus occur in older adults?

Systemic lupus erythematosus (SLE) may present in 15–20% of elderly patients with females being more frequently affected. Rather than a female-to-male ratio of 5–8:1 as found in the younger population, the ratio is 2:1 in the elderly. The disease in the elderly also is milder, with manifestations of serositis, joint pain, interstitial lung disease, and sicca symptoms being more common. CNS involvement and renal disease are less frequent. Laboratory tests may include a positive antinuclear antibody (ANA), low complement levels, and positive antibodies to ds-DNA, SS-A, SS-B or Sm. Healthy older adults may have a low-titer positive ANA present in their serum without evidence of any systemic disease.

Drug-induced SLE occurs more commonly in the elderly and should alert the physician to detect the causative agent. Inciting drugs include procainamide, hydralazine, and isoniazid. Anti-histone antibodies, in addition to a positive ANA, are found in 70–95% of patients. Symptoms resemble those seen in older-onset SLE.

8. What are the features of primary Sjögren's syndrome?

Primary Sjögren's syndrome is a frequent diagnosis in elderly patients who present with sicca symptoms. Patients often complain of grittiness in their eyes and dryness of their mouth associated with odynophagia. Polyarthritis, arthralgias, myalgias, fever, and fatigue may be accompanying symptoms. Systemic manifestations of vasculitis, interstitial nephritis, Raynaud's phenomenon, interstitial lung disease, hypothyroidism, and central and peripheral nervous system involvement occur infrequently.

9. Which conditions are associated with nonarticular or soft-tissue rheumatism?

Soft-tissue rheumatism is another entity frequently reported in the elderly. It refers to conditions such as fibromyalgia, bursitis, tendinitis, low back pain and cervical spine pain syndromes. It is important to realize that low back pain may be due simply to back strain but may also be due to more serious causes, including compression fractures secondary to osteoporosis or primary or secondary malignancies such as multiple myeloma and metastatic cancer. Other common soft-tissue conditions in the elderly include rotator cuff tendinitis, which can result in severe shoulder pain that radiates to the elbow and impairs range of motion of the shoulder. Elderly men and women may develop adhesive capsulitis which results following a period of inactivity of the shoulder. The presentation is that of progressive stiffness and discomfort of the shoulder with limitation of motion. Pain often occurs with movement.

10. How does reflex sympathetic dystrophy syndrome present?

Reflex sympathetic dystrophy occurs commonly in the elderly with diabetes or following trauma, cerebrovascular events, or peripheral nerve pathology. It presents with severe burning pain and swelling of an extremity, hand, or foot. Signs of vasomotor instability are often present, manifested by temperature changes, edema, sweating and trophic changes of hair, skin, and nails. As the disorder progresses, skin and muscle atrophy occur with the development of contractures and restricted motion. During the later stages of the disorder, radiographs of the extremity often reveal diffuse osteoporosis.

11. What are the common rheumatic manifestations of endocrinopathies and malignancies?

Endocrinopathies such as hypothyroidism may be associated with joint and muscle pain and stiffness. Weakness is not a prominent feature. Hyperthyroidism can present as a painless proximal myopathy or, infrequently, with soft-tissue swelling, clubbing, and periostitis called thyroid acropachy. Acromegaly frequently produces degenerative changes of cartilage. Carpal tunnel syndrome may be a manifestation of diabetes, hypothyroidism, and acromegaly. Diabetes has also been associated with diffuse idiopathic skeletal hyperostosis, Charcot joints, and limited joint mobility. Pseudogout has been associated with hypothyroidism and hyperparathyroidism.

Primary **malignancies** and metastatic tumors may present with polyarticular joint pain, and these diagnoses should be considered in patients with an abrupt onset of a rheumatologic condition. Lymphomas and leukemias may present with synovitis in the elderly that resembles rheumatoid arthritis or polymyalgia rheumatica. Hypertrophic osteoarthropathy can be seen with pulmonary malignancies and other cancers. Neoplasms have been associated with the development of polymyositis and dermatomyositis. In one series, 25% of cases of these disorders were associated with neoplasia of the breast, lung, ovary, colon, stomach, and uterus.

12. What are the features of remitting seronegative symmetric synovitis with pitting edema?

This disorder occasionally occurs in older men, with a male-to-female ratio of 2:1. It presents as an acute symmetric polyarthritis involving the wrists, metacarpophalangeal joints, tarsal and metatarsophalangeal joints and interphalangeal joints. There is associated pitting edema of the hands, soft tissue swelling of the distal upper and lower limbs, and morning stiffness. Constitutional symptoms are often absent. This disease may be closely related to seronegative rheumatoid arthritis. Synovial fluid is mildly inflammatory, and the ESR is often elevated. The disease occurs more often in the fall but can occur throughout the year. The overall prognosis is good following treatment with low-dose prednisone.

BIBLIOGRAPHY

1. Allen NB, Studenski SA: Polymyalgia rheumatica and temporal arteritis. Med Clin North Am 70:369–384, 1986.
2. Daly MP, Berman BM: Rehabilitation of the elderly patient with arthritis. Clin Geriatr Med 9:783–801, 1993.
3. Healy LA: The spectrum of polymyalgia rheumatica. Clin Geriatr Med 4:323–331, 1988.
4. Irby WR, Owen DS: Rheumatic Diseases in the Aged: Diagnosis and Management of Rheumatic Diseases. Philadelphia, J.B. Lippincott, 1988.
5. McCarty DJ, O'Duffy JD, Pearson L, Hunter JB. Remitting seronegative symmetrical synovitis with pitting edema: RS3PE syndrome. JAMA 254:2763–2767, 1985.
6. McGuire JL: The endocrine system and connective tissue disorders. Bull Rheum Dis 39(4):1–8, 1990.
7. Nesher G, Moore TL, Zuckner J: Rheumatoid arthritis in the elderly. Am J Geriatr Soc 39:284–294, 1991.
8. Stevens MB: Connective tissue disease in the elderly. Clin Rheum Dis 12:11–32, 1986.
9. Van Schaardenburg D, Breedveld F: Elderly-onset rheumatoid arthritis. Semin Arthritis Rheum 23:367–368, 1994.

9. ARTHRITIS AND MUSCULOSKELETAL PAIN IN THE ELDERLY

Edna P. Schwab, M.D.

1. What changes occur in the aging joint with osteoarthritis?

Aging is a risk factor for the development of osteoarthritis. There are biochemical differences between the aging joint and a joint affected by osteoarthritis. In normal joints, cartilage, which is 70% water, is maintained by the interaction of chondrocytes, proteoglycans, and type II and IX collagen. The composition of these proteoglycans is altered and the water content of cartilage diminishes in the aging joint. In the joint affected by osteoarthritis, the dominant feature is cartilage loss. The water content of cartilage is increased, and inflammatory mediators, either derived from chondrocytes or synovial fluid, decrease proteoglycan composition and synthesis while degrading proteoglycans and collagens.

2. How prevalent are arthritic conditions in the elderly?

Arthritis and musculoskeletal disorders are two of the most prevalent chronic conditions among the elderly and are important public health problems among adults of working age. As the population ages, the prevalence of arthritis, with its negative impact on function, is expected to rise. In a study by Hughes, the most frequent musculoskeletal conditions diagnosed among a sample of elderly persons over age 60 were osteoarthritis (in 83%), old fractures (in 32%), and soft-tissue rheumatism (in 13%). Joint impairment was most frequently observed in the upper and lower spine (92%), hands (58%), feet (55%), knees (35%), and hips (20%). Joint impairment, pain, and psychological status all had an effect on predicting future disability.

3. What is the impact of pain?

Pain and limitation in motion from arthritis can restrict the independence of older persons by impairing their performance of activities of daily living (ADLs). Upper extremity impairment is more pronounced in men and significantly related to inability in performing ADLs, while lower extremity impairment is more common in women and is significantly related to impairment in instrumental ADLs. Both upper and lower extremity impairments occur in increased frequency in both sexes over the age of 80.

The National Health Interview Survey revealed that elderly persons in the community with arthritis represent 70% of the population with 1 or more limitations in physical activity and represent two-thirds of those persons with 5 or more ADL impairments. Data from the Longitudinal Study on Aging indicate that the extent of arthritis-related disabilities increases with time. These impairments were found to be strong risk factors for predicting adverse outcome. Elderly people with 1 or more ADL impairments were 2.5 times more likely to die and 5 times more likely to end up in a nursing home when compared to those without any limitations. In the nursing home, pain as a result of musculoskeletal disorders is extremely common, often limiting the patient's ability to function.

The early diagnosis of musculoskeletal disorders and implementation of appropriate treatment often improve the older person's ability to perform daily tasks and enhances their quality of life. Symptoms in the elderly, however, may not be as apparent as in younger persons due to multiple coexisting conditions and cognitive impairment. A decline in function may not be perceived by a patient, family member, or staff members until impairment or disability is significant.

4. What are the causes of musculoskeletal symptoms in the elderly?

Symptoms of joint pain, limitation of motion, swelling, and morning stiffness are features of various arthritides. A thorough history with a review of systems and physical examination will help to differentiate the various rheumatic conditions in the elderly, such as those with articular or soft-tissue involvement (i.e., osteoarthritis, crystal arthropathies, periarthritis, tendinitis, bursitis, and entrapment neuropathies) from conditions which also have systemic manifestations. These conditions include infectious arthritides, polymyalgia rheumatica, giant cell arteritis, elderly-onset rheumatoid arthritis, and connective tissue disorders. Appropriate radiographs and laboratory tests including synovial fluid analysis help to establish an early and accurate diagnosis.

5. Which is the most common form of chronic arthritis?

By far, the most common and disabling rheumatic condition in patients over 55 years of age is **osteoarthritis**. Radiographic changes often precede symptoms and frequently may not correlate well with symptoms until marked progression and cartilage loss occur. Approximately 30–50% of elderly patients have symptoms of joint pain, stiffness, and limitation in range of motion. Studies have demonstrated that 12% of elderly patients cannot perform ADLs as a result of pain and limitation from osteoarthritis. About half of these individuals end up confined to the bed or wheelchair. Predictors of disability include the severity of other coexisting diseases, cardiopulmonary status, visual or hearing impairment, renal disease, functional capacity, social support, education level, income, and availability of social and home-care services.

6. Describe the common symptoms and findings characteristic of osteoarthritis.

Joints that are commonly involved in osteoarthritis include areas of weight-bearing, such as the lumbar spine, hips, and knees. Hands (especially the first carpometacarpal joint), cervical spine, and feet (primarily the first metatarsophalangeal joints) are also commonly involved. Early morning stiffness, when present, characteristically lasts 10–30 minutes. Stiffness may occur following periods of inactivity, while pain often increases with activity and improves with rest. Musculoskeletal examination may reveal swelling, deformities, bony overgrowth (referred to as Heberden's and Bouchard's nodes when involving the distal and proximal interphalangeal joints of the hands, respectively), crepitus, limitation of motion, and synovial effusions. Muscle spasm, tendon contractures, and capsular contractures may also be observed depending on the site of involvement.

Cervical and lumbar pain may result from arthritis of the apophyseal joints, osteophyte formation, pressure on surrounding tissue, and muscle spasm. Radicular symptoms are caused by nerve root impingement. Cervical and lumbar stenosis develops when facet joints and the ligamentum flavum hypertrophy as a result of disc degeneration, which narrows the spinal canal causing compression of the cord. Anterior vertebral osteophytes may also contribute to cord compression. Patients may develop localized pain, extremity weakness, gait ataxia, or abnormal neurologic findings. Pseudoclaudication is a characteristic feature of lumbar stenosis and is described as pain in the buttocks or thighs occurring with ambulation and relieved by rest or lumbar flexion. Hip pain is usually felt in the groin or the lateral or medial aspects of the thigh; however, it can be referred to the knee or buttocks and may be misdiagnosed as lumbar stenosis.

Pain from osteoarthritis may develop from any part of the involved joint or tissue. Ischemia and vascular pressure from subchondral bone, inflammation of the synovium, distention of the joint capsule, inflamed ligaments and bursae, cartilage destruction, and nerve terminal release of enzymes and inflammatory mediators, as well as increased volume of synovial fluid and muscle spasm, all contribute to pain. Sleep disruption as a result of pain may exacerbate the pain cycle, contributing to further disability and depression.

7. What are the laboratory and radiographic findings in osteoarthritis?

Laboratory findings in osteoarthritis are usually normal. Radiographs classically reveal the presence of joint-space narrowing with subchondral sclerosis as an early finding. As arthritis progresses, the development of marginal osteophytes, subchondral bone cysts with sclerosis, and subluxation occurs. In advanced disease, loose bodies and subchondral bone collapse may be evident. Synovial fluid analysis reveals noninflammatory fluid (< 500 cells/ml).

8. Have risk factors been associated with the development of osteoarthritis?

- Although age is a risk factor, osteoarthritis does not develop in all elderly people.
- Congenital abnormalities, such as Perthes' disease and congenital dislocation of the hip, have been associated with the development of osteoarthritis of the hip.
- Prior trauma to the joint, inflammatory conditions such as crystal arthropathies, septic arthritis, metabolic disorders (acromegaly and hemochromatosis), and hereditary factors have all been associated with the development of osteoarthritis.
- Obesity is a major factor associated with the development and progression of osteoarthritis.

9. How is osteoarthritis best managed?

Realistic goals need to be established with the patient. Pain often leads to deconditioning, loss of range, and disability. The physician should educate the patient about exercising, using joint protection, incorporating rest periods into the daily routine, and reducing or eliminating risk factors that may result in pain and disease progression. The patient should also be made aware of the various treatment options available for the management of osteoarthritis. The suggested course of management might include a combination of the following:

Exercise and rehabilitation: Resting the joint for prolonged periods, especially in the elderly, may result in deconditioning, muscle atrophy, contractures, and osteoporosis. A supervised exercise program with a physical therapist and occupational therapist will help to strengthen affected muscles and improve range of motion. An evaluation for appropriate assistive devices and appliances should be performed. Application of heat or cold packs following exercise is often beneficial.

Pharmacologic therapy: Initiation of drug therapy should take into account the side effect profile of the drug, comorbidities of the patient, and potential drug interactions. Acetaminophen is often an effective analgesic agent used to treat osteoarthritis. It has fewer side effects than nonsteroidal anti-inflammatory agents (NSAIDs) when used in therapeutic doses (4.0 gm/day) and is as effective as NSAIDs in many patients. NSAIDs are the most commonly prescribed agents used to treat arthritis, but the elderly are at increased risk of adverse effects from these drugs, including acute renal failure, gastric ulceration, cardiovascular effects, and cognitive impairment. When patients are using these agents, they should be monitored closely for evidence of adverse reactions. In addition to the drug's side effect profile, the choice of an NSAID should also consider dosing frequency.

Topical capsaicin cream, an inhibitor of the release of substance P from nerve terminals, has also been effective in alleviating joint pain. Narcotics such as codeine, propoxyphene, and oxycodone can be used if other modalities are ineffective. This usually occurs in situations where arthritis is associated with bony collapse, as in avascular necrosis, or when there is evidence of nerve impingement. The physician needs to monitor these drugs for constipating effects and for cognitive and respiratory alterations. Relaxation and biofeedback techniques may be effective in diminishing the degree of pain in some affected patients.

Intra-articular corticosteroid injections may also be used to alleviate the pain from arthritis. However, these agents should not be administered more than 3 to 4 times a year to a single joint. Antidepressants in low doses have been used to control chronic pain with some success. The blockage of serotonin reuptake augments the inhibitory pathways of the spinal tract, thereby inhibiting pain perception.

Psychological counseling: The older patient with osteoarthritis may require psychological counseling, especially if depression is evident. Persistent pain, disability, deformity, and a decline in function can often lead to depression. This depression can be exacerbated if the patient has sexual difficulties and/or is unable to work as a result of arthritis. The patient should receive psychiatric, sexual, or financial counseling if any of these situations arise.

Surgery: Patients who have not benefited from conservative measures may benefit from arthroscopy with joint debridement or lavage. Arthroplasty should be reserved for patients who continue to have persistent pain, loss of motion, and loss of function despite maximal medical management. Rehabilitation should follow surgery within 48 hours.

10. Which rheumatologic conditions can present with an acute monoarthritis in the elderly?

When a joint becomes acutely inflamed and painful, it requires an immediate evaluation. Several arthritides can present with a single acutely swollen and painful joint:

Infectious arthritis
  Bacteria
  Mycobacteria
  Fungi
  Spirochetes
  Viruses
Crystal-Induced Arthritis
  Gout
  Pseudogout
  Hydroxyapatite disease
    (Milwaukee shoulder)
Osteoarthritis
Foreign-body reaction

Neurogenic arthropathy (Charcot's joint)
Avascular necrosis
Tumor
Systematic disease with monoarticular flare
  (much less common)
  Rheumatoid arthritis
  Systematic lupus erythematosus
  Psoriatic arthritis
  AIDS
  Inflammatory bowel disease
  Behçet's disease
  Reiter's syndrome
  Reactive arthritis

11. What are the complications and mortality rate associated with septic arthritis?

Septic arthritis is the most life-threatening and destructive form of arthritis in all age groups. Joint destruction can occur in 1–2 days if the infection is unrecognized or inadequately treated. Approximately 25–40% of patients diagnosed with a septic arthritis are over age 60. Among the elderly, the mortality rate has been reported to be between 19–33%, as compared to 10% in the general adult population. Complications such as osteomyelitis, loss of joint motion and function, and osteoarthritis arise in the elderly.

12. Describe the clinical and diagnostic features of septic arthritis.

Physical findings include fever, joint swelling secondary to fluid distending the joint capsule, warmth, loss of motion, and severe pain. Constitutional symptoms may or may not be present. An investigation for an extra-articular site of infection should always be pursued.

Diagnosis is made by arthrocentesis of the involved joint. The presence of organisms on synovial fluid Gram stain or culture and evidence of an inflammatory synovial fluid help to confirm the diagnosis. Synovial fluid cell counts are often > 50,000 cells/mm3 with > 80–90% neurophils on the differential. Low white cell counts have also been reported, in the range of 6,000 cells/mm^3, but this is less frequent. Stains will be positive for organisms in approximately 75% of gram-positive infections and 50% of gram-negative infections. Other diagnostic tests include blood cultures, which may be positive in 25–78% of patients with nongonococcal bacterial arthritis but frequently negative in gonococcal arthritis. Appropriate imaging techniques, such as radiographs or MRI, should be obtained to evaluate for joint destruction and osteomyelitis. Antibiotic treatment should be started to cover organisms usually involved in septic arthritis. Treatment can be altered once culture results are available.

13. Which organisms are most commonly found in a septic arthritis?

Gram-positive aerobes cause infection in approximately 85% of cases; *Staphylococcus aureus* accounts for 67%, *Streptococcus pneumoniae* for 3%, and non-group A, β-hemolytic streptococci for 15%. *Staphylococcus epidermidis* is frequently found in prosthetic joint infections. Gram-negative bacteria account for 18% of infections but have also been reported to occur in up to 30% of geriatric patients. Gram-negative and anaerobic infections are also more commonly seen in parenteral drug users, immunocompromised hosts, and those with extremity wounds and GI cancers.

Although not considered common in the elderly, *Neisseria gonorrhoeae* can cause migratory arthritis, tendinitis, and an acute monoarthritis. This form of infectious arthritis is less destructive than that caused by nongonococcal organisms. *N. gonorrhoeae* needs to be considered in the elderly when appropriate clinical features are present. Tenosynovitis is the most frequent clinical presentation, although skin lesions in the form of pustules and macules may also be seen in two-thirds of the patients with disseminated gonococcal infection. In only 25% of patients with disseminated gonococcal infection will synovial fluid culture be positive.

Other agents, including fungi, viruses, spirochetes (Lyme disease), mycobacteria, and parasites, have also been reported to cause septic arthritis but usually have a more insidious course.

Microbiology of Septic Arthritis

ORGANISM	FREQUENCY
Gram-positive organisms	85%
Staphylococcus aureus	67%
Streptococcus pneumoniae	3%
Non-group A, β-hemolytic streptococci	15%
Gram-negative organisms	18%
Other agents	
Fungi	
Viruses	
Spirochetes	
Mycobacteria	
Parasites	

14. Discuss the pathogenesis of septic arthritis.

Septic arthritis most commonly occurs by hematogenous spread. Less frequent causes of infection include joint surgery, intra-articular injections, or penetrating trauma. The most common sites of infection involve the large joints, such as the knee and hip, but smaller joints may also be involved.

Risk factors predisposing the elderly patient to septic arthritis include:
Preexisting joint disease (rheumatoid arthritis and osteoarthritis)
Trauma
Intra-articular joint injection with glucocorticoids (infrequent, < 1/10,000 injections)
Concurrent extra-articular infection (skin, soft tissue, urinary tract, subacute bacterial
    endocarditis)
Illnesses or medications that impair host defenses:
    Diabetes mellitus
    Chronic renal failure
    Cirrhosis
    AIDS
    Corticosteroid therapy
    Cytotoxic agents

15. What are the common crystal-induced diseases in the elderly?

Crystal-induced arthritis often presents as a monoarticular arthritis. **Gout** is caused by the deposition of monosodium urate crystals. The prevalence of gout increases with aging and approaches 4% among patients in the 50–74 year-old range. It frequently occurs in the first metatarsophalangeal (MTP) joint, ankle, metatarsals, or knee, although any joint may be involved. The involved joint is often extremely tender, hot, swollen, and red, resembling an acute infection. Initial attacks are monoarticular, but subsequent flares may be polyarticular and accompanied by fever. Tophaceous gout often occurs in elderly men, while diuretic-induced gout has been observed in elderly women. Diagnosis is made by demonstrating urate crystals in synovial fluid with a polarizing light microscope. Radiographs in early disease are usually normal, but in chronic disease they may demonstrate classic erosions with overhanging edges.

The prevalence of **calcium pyrophosphate deposition** (CPPD) disease, also called **pseudogout**, increases with age. Between the ages of 65–75 years, 10–15% of individuals have evidence of CPPD. This rate increases to 30–60% after age 85. Joints most commonly affected include the wrists and knees, but other joints may also be involved. The typical presentation is that of an acute self-limiting monoarticular arthritis; however, asymptomatic disease with evidence of chondrocalcinosis on radiographs and a subacute chronic destructive arthropathy may develop. Radiographic changes often reveal the presence of chondrocalcinosis in the meniscus of the knee, the triangular ligament of the wrist, and occasionally the cartilage of the shoulder. Other findings resembling osteoarthritis include joint-space narrowing, bony sclerosis, subchondral cysts, and osteophyte formation. One should keep in mind that both gout and pseudogout can also present with a bursitis and tendinitis. Pseudogout has been associated with other conditions, including hypothyroidism, hyperparathyroidism, hemochromatosis, hypomagnesemia, and hypophosphatasia.

Apatite-induced arthritis, either secondary to hydroxyapatite (a component of bone) or other apatites, can cause an acute arthritis or periarthritis. A rapidly destructive arthritis due to hydroxyapatite has been found in the elderly and is called **Milwaukee shoulder syndrome**. It is typically seen in women over age 70. Other joints including the knee may also be involved. The synovial fluid is often bloody with evidence of apatite crystals.

Common Crystal-Induced Arthritis

TYPE	CRYSTAL	PREVALENCE	PRESENTATIONS
Gout	Monosodium urate crystals	4% of 50–70 year olds	Most commonly affects first MTP joint, metatarsals, ankle, knee. Other joints may be affected. May be monoarticular or polyarticular
CPPD	CPPD crystals	10–15% of 65–75 year olds 30–60% after age 85	Commonly affects wrists, knees, but other joints may be affected. Usually monoarticular but can be polyarticular.
Apatite-induced arthritis	Hydroxyapatite or other apatite	Most common in 65–75 year olds	Acute arthritis or periarthritis Rapidly destructive arthritis called Milwaukee shoulder

16. How do you treat a crystal-induced arthritis?

Treatment of gout, pseudogout, and apatite disease is very similar. The first line of therapy is often an NSAID, which should be used cautiously in the elderly person, especially if other coexisting diseases are present. Prostaglandin analogs should be considered for gastric protection. Colchicine is less often used for the acute flare of crystal-induced arthritis but may be used for prophylaxis for gout and pseudogout. Systemic glucocorticoids may also be used in the acute attack, especially if polyarticular joint involvement is present or contraindications to NSAID use are present. Intra-articular corticosteroid injection is an alternative treatment if a single joint is involved. In chronic arthritis, treatment modalities are similar to those used for osteoarthritis. Allopurinol and probenicid are reserved for use in chronic gouty arthritis.

17. Define osteonecrosis and discuss its features.

Osteonecrosis is another possible cause of pain in elderly patients. Pain develops as a result of impaired circulation to the affected bone, resulting in bony necrosis. Commonly involved sites include the knee, hip, or shoulder, but small joints may also be affected. Osteonecrosis is associated with a wide range of disorders, including systemic lupus erythematosus, systemic corticosteroids, trauma, alcoholism, cigarette smoking, and osteoarthritis, but it may also be idiopathic.

18. What risk factors are associated with the development of Charcot's joint?

Charcot's joint or neurogenic arthropathy may occur in patients who have peripheral sensory neuropathies, such as in diabetes mellitus, tabes dorsalis, pernicious anemia, and leprosy. Joint destruction occurs as a result of loss of pain perception. Other sensations may also be compromised, such as proprioception, touch, and temperature perception. Foot, ankle, and metatarsal joints are most commonly affected in diabetics, while larger joints are involved in those with tabes dorsalis.

BIBLIOGRAPHY

1. Bagge E, Bjelle A, Eden S, Svanborg A: A longitudinal study of the occurrence of joint complaints in elderly people. Age Aging 21:160–167, 1992.
2. Baker DG, Schumacher HR: Acute monoarthritis. N Engl J Med 329:1013–1020, 1993.
3. Bomalaski JS: Acute rheumatologic disorders in the elderly. Emerg Med Clin North Am 8:341–359, 1990.
4. Bradley JD, Brandt KD, Katz BP, et al: Comparison of an anti-inflammatory dose of ibuprofen, an analgesic dose of ibuprofen, and acetaminophen in the treatment of patients with osteoarthritis of the knee. N Engl J Med 325:87–91, 1991.
5. Bridwell KH: Lumbar spinal stenosis: Diagnosis, management, and treatment. Clin Geriatr Med 10: 677–701, 1994.
6. Chang CC, Greenspan A, Gershwin ME: Osteonecrosis: Current perspectives on pathogenesis and treatment. Semin Arthritis Rheum 23:47–69, 1993.
7. Hamerman D: Aging and osteoarthritis: Basic mechanisms. J Am Geriatr Soc 41:760–770, 1993.
8. Norman DC, Yoshikawa TT: Infections of the bone, joint, and bursa. Clin Geriatr Med 10:703–718, 1994.
9. Pierron RL, Perry HM III, Grossberg G, et al: The aging hip. J Am Geriatr Soc 38:1339–1352, 1990.

10. BEREAVEMENT

Margaret Yetter-Pritchard, M.S.W., L.S.W.

1. What is bereavement?

Bereavement is a process of mourning and grief that occurs after the death of a loved one. People who are bereaved experience grief reactions and periods of mourning and have feelings of intense sorrow and loss. Many of these experiences or reactions vary from person to person and in accordance with religious custom or cultural ritual.

Although the basis of this chapter is loss through death, death is not the only event that can create feelings of loss or grief in older persons or their families. The elderly often experience compounding losses through illness, disability, and role changes as well as death of family members and friends. The family can also experience its own sense of loss and grief in watching parents or loved ones decline. Caregivers have described dementing illnesses as similar to a "slow death" because of the insidious nature of the decline and the loss of personhood and memory.

Although this discussion is designed to help the practitioner help the patient, it also includes references to helping the families. In working with older people, it is vitally important to remember that they often are part of a larger family system. Treating older people requires a keen awareness of the level of involvement and importance of family.

Practitioners also need to understand their own feelings about dying, death, and loss. Often the death of a patient evokes strong feelings in the clinician. This discussion also addresses how practitioners can help themselves.

2. How do age, gender, relationship, and type of death affect bereavement?

The degree of emotional trauma in the event of anticipated or age-appropriate death may be altered by emotional and psychological preparation for the event. Some elderly people, as well as family members and caregivers, do not suffer protracted grieving periods with age-appropriate death. Conversely, the death of an adult child and unanticipated deaths from suicide, traffic accidents, or plane crashes are rated as involving the greatest degree of emotional and psychological trauma. The degrees of bereavement thus may vary with the circumstances of the death. Nonetheless, the theories of anticipated loss and age-appropriate death must be approached cautiously. Every situation needs to be assessed on an individual basis.

Men or widowers are at a slightly higher risk for increased health problems and social isolation after the death of a wife or companion, presumably because men have not cultivated the necessary social supports or networks to help them. It is also believed that men are more reluctant to reach out for help or to attend support groups. Widows generally tend to have larger support networks and to seek informal as well as formal supports more readily. Women have also been shown to have greater attachment to siblings; the death of a brother or sister can have great significance.

The many close and significant relationships formed among the elderly often go beyond the affection for first-degree relatives. Such relationships include "adopted" children, friends, neighbors, caregivers, and pets. Also, in an age of changing definitions of "family" and gender, it is important to assess the family structure and gender roles beyond the more conventional definitions in order to understand the significance of relationships and the impact of loss.

3. What medical complications are associated with bereavement?

- Increased incidence of physical and mental illness
- Increased somatization
- Increased risk for abuse of alcohol, tobacco, and medication (including prescription medication)
- Increased risk of suicide

A patient who has experienced the loss of a loved one may be at risk for exacerbation of existing medical or psychiatric problems as well as increased complaints of physical problems. A person in the grieving process should be assessed carefully for signs of abnormal or pathologic grieving as well as any medical issues that may need attention.

4. What are the differences between normal and abnormal grief reactions?

One of the better-known models that explain the normal grieving process is proposed by Elizabeth Kubler-Ross in her seminal work entitled *On Death and Dying*. She outlines five stages of "normal" bereavement. It must be stressed that the stages are fluid and variable. Not everyone proceeds categorically through each stage. The stages are interchangeable and vary in duration and sequence. In rare instances, some stages are not experienced at all.

Stage one: denial—"not me"
- This coping mechanism is used to buffer the unexpected shock of bad or unwelcome news. It is usually a temporary defense, replaced by some degree of acceptance.
- Denial may persist in degrees throughout an illness and up to the time of death. It is not necessary to challenge a patient's use of denial.
- A protracted or fixated use of complete denial is not a normal part of the grieving process and should be addressed by a mental health professional.

Stage two: anger—"why me?"
- Indication that mortality is beginning to become real to the patient.
- Rational and irrational components: rational in that patients may be in pain and discomfort, going through procedures and tests, and realizing that time is running out; irrational in that patients may take out their anger on family or staff who are trying to be helpful (e.g, by accusing staff of incompetence).
- One of the more difficult stages in which to maintain a relationship with the patient.
- May persist in varying degrees throughout the illness until death.
- Generally yields to other stages, such as bargaining and depression.
- Family and staff may need help from mental health professionals in maintaining a caring relationship with the patient during this stage.

Stage three: bargaining
- Attempt to postpone death through bargaining with a higher power.
- Generally not a prolonged stage.
- A more mystical or spiritual component to the dying process—belief that past good deeds, promises of exemplary behavior, or self-imposed time frames ("one more year") will delay death.
- Generally a more private process and not discussed with clinicians.

Stage four: depression
- Final stage before acceptance.
- May continue until time of death.
- The impact of loss is being absorbed and a grieving for past, present, and future begins.
- Considered a necessary preparation for death.
- Patients at this stage sometimes need quiet support. Chaplains, social workers, hospice workers, and other mental health professional may be helpful.
- This form of depression is relative to a normal course of bereavement and dying as opposed to a clinical syndrome requiring treatment.
- Possible consultation with a geriatric psychiatrist if this stage persists over a protracted period or if treatment may improve quality of life.

Stage five: acceptance
- Described as the final "rest" before death occurs.
- Patients are generally able to express their feelings about their death.
- Occurs closer to the end-stage of an illness. Often quiet reassurance is the basic need, including counseling, emotional support, and making sure the patient does not feel left alone.

Although these stages describe the terminally ill patient, they also relate to families or loved ones who may experience similar feelings. But remember: there is no "right" grieving process. Bereavement is highly individualized and has many religious and cultural variations. The five stages are also variable and may occur within each other, side by side, or out of the outlined sequence.

Normal grief reactions need to be understood. Although they are sometimes disturbing and sad, grief reactions are necessary and need to be experienced. Understanding them as normal may indicate that intense treatment, such as psychotherapy, antidepressant medication, or hospitalization, may not be needed. More appropriate are supportive services that may enhance and supplement the patient's natural healing course.

According to the DSM IV, normal grieving may present some of the same characteristics as a major depressive episode, such as feelings of sadness, crying, disruption of sleep patterns, poor appetite, weight loss, and social withdrawal. Abnormal grieving is generally of a longer duration with a greater intensity of symptoms and can lead to pathologic grief and depression. Generally the diagnosis of a major depressive episode is not assigned until the depressive symptoms have a duration longer than 2–4 months. According to the DSM IV, the following characteristics are not part of the normal grief reaction:

- **Guilt about things other than actions taken or not taken by the survivor at the time of death.** Statements such as "If I had called the doctor sooner," or "If I hadn't gone to the store I might have heard him," are normal, reflective statements.
- **Thoughts of death other than the survivor's feeling that he or she would be better off dead or should have died with the deceased person.** It is not unusual for bereaved or grieving people to wish they were with their loved ones or to feel some guilt the "it should have been me" (especially in the death of an adult child). Any actively developed plan for suicide, however, must receive immediate attention from a mental health care provider.
- **Morbid preoccupation with worthlessness.** It is not unusual for bereaved people to feel a personal loss or a loss of part of themselves. However, if there is a persistent message of "I'm not worth anything anymore," "I have no purpose in my life and am no good to anyone," or a continuous message of hopelessness about the future, a mental health professional should be consulted.
- **Marked psychomotor retardation.** Bereaved persons may not appear spry and energetic. However, if their motor activity seems markedly changed or severely lethargic or if there appears to be a discontinuity between desired and actual movement, a mental health professional should be consulted.
- **Prolonged or marked functional impairment.** Some social isolation and apathy toward physical appearance and housekeeping are normal for bereaved people. However, if this pattern persists and worsens as time goes on, it may be a sign of abnormal grieving and a mental health professional should be consulted.

There are certain signs that a clinician can look for to assess a person's positive processing of grief. Within the first several months of loss a person should resume some normal functioning. If the person begins to resume social contact, voicing hope about the future, a normal grieving process is most likely. For many older people, especially those who have lost a spouse, their roles and functions need to be redefined. This process can take a great deal of emotional energy, and patients may need support and counseling to help them through this period of redefinition.

5. When is treatment for abnormal grief reaction required?

The clinician must be aware of any exacerbation of existing medical or psychiatric symptoms of a bereaved person. Also, every person reacts differently and needs treatment accordingly. According to the definition of abnormal grieving in the DSM IV, if symptoms go beyond 2–4 months and remain at the same or increased intensity, a geriatric psychiatrist should be consulted for assessment.

In the initial stages of bereavement supportive counseling and support group information should be offered. If the patient or family is in the hospital at the time, the clinician can consult the hospital social work department or hospice department to find out about in-patient counseling and other community services.

Attention should be paid to the bereaved people as early as possible after the loss. If an ongoing relationship has been established, interventions and information about supports should be given after burial and other related arrangements have been made. If little or no contact with the bereaved person is expected, information should be given for future reference.

Just as there is no complete definition of "normal" grieving, commencement of treatment must also be individualized. When a patient sends messages that he or she is having a difficult time in adjusting to the loss or if there is a stark absence of any grief reaction, help should be offered. Many people may desire medications for symptoms such as sleeplessness, anxiety, or depression. Such requests should be addressed and assessed on case-by-case basis. If a patient complains of excessive physical symptoms, with few or no physiologic findings, a mental health professional should be consulted and the patient referred for assessment.

6. What is the most important thing to do or say to a patient who is grieving?

More important than knowing what to say to a bereaved person is knowing what not to say. The natural instinct is to try to make people who suffer feel better. In the case of death, nothing that anyone can say will make the feelings of sadness or loss go away. The best approach is recognition of the loss, validation of the feelings, and an open door to talk about it if a patient so desires. Statements such as "Well, it was a blessing," or "He had a long life," or "It was God's will," are not universally accepted and should be avoided. They are reflective of particular orientations and may tend to minimize the loss for some people. Simple statements such as "I'm very sorry about your loss," "I know this must be a very difficult time for you," or "I am going to miss them too," validate the loss without trying to minimize it.

Some clinicians struggle with how much to do when a patient dies. Frequently asked questions include "Should I send a card?," "Should I send flowers to the family?," and "Should I go to the funeral?" Again there is no right or wrong answer. All practitioners must keep a sense of professional boundaries, but they are human nonetheless. In some cases, especially if a clinician has developed a good relationship or has had a long ongoing relationship with the family, some gesture, whether it be a card, flowers, or attending the funeral, is appropriate. However, practitioners should not feel a sense of guilt if they decide not to do any of the above. In general, there should be some point at which clinicians have closure, not only for themselves but also for the family.

7. Is the family my patient?

Clinicians cannot overlook the family members or caregivers of their elderly patients. Often caregivers who have been caring for a parent or loved one experience a tremendous amount of loss, not only for their loved one, but also for their role and investment in the caregiving. Such families may need special attention and should be referred to the appropriate clinician for counseling, support, and information about resources to help them.

It is not unusual for some families to express anger at the clinicians involved with the care of the deceased. The phenomenon of "shooting the messenger" is a common reaction to an unexpected or unwelcome patient outcome. Allowing families to express their feelings without taking it personally or reacting defensively can help diffuse some of these reactions.

8. How do I handle my own feelings about death?

We all have our own fears and reactions to our own mortality as well as the mortality of our patients. It is normal for clinicians to feel a certain sense of sadness, loss, and helplessness when a patient dies. It is equally as normal to have appropriate distancing and coping mechanisms to allow emotional and psychological safety in a field where death and illness can be regular occurrences. If clinicians are to remain healthy and to provide sound and appropriate help to patients facing death or coping with the loss of a loved one, it is just as important to explore their own feelings about death and bereavement as it is to assess the patient's feelings and beliefs.

BIBLIOGRAPHY

1. Birren J, Shaie KW: Handbook of the Psychology of Aging. New York, Van Nostrand Reinhold Co., 1985.
2. Cleiren M: Bereavement and Adaptation. Philadelphia, Hemisphere Publishing Corp., 1992.
3. Holmes TH, Rahe RH: The Social Readjustment Rating Scale. J Psychosom Res 11:213–218, 1967.
4. Kubler-Ross E: On Death and Dying. New York, MacMillan, 1969.
5. Lamm M: The Jewish Way in Death and Mourning. New York, Jonathan David Publishers, 1969.
6. Rando TA: Grief, Dying and Death: Clinical Interventions for Caregivers. Champaign, IL, Research Press, 1984.

III: *Prevention and Health Promotions*

11. PRINCIPLES OF SCREENING

Susan Day, M.D., M.P.H.

1. Why screen?

The fundamental principle behind screening is that the quality and duration of an individual's life can be improved by identifying early or asymptomatic disease, by modifying behavior to achieve a more healthy lifestyle, and by maximizing function when disease exists. Interventions for these purposes fall into three categories:

1. **Primary prevention** is targeted toward identifying and reversing risk factors that may predispose individuals to developing a disease in the future. Examples include nutrition, exercise, and accident prevention. Interventions at this stage often involve counseling, immunizations, or chemoprophylaxis.

2. **Secondary prevention** efforts, including most screening programs, are aimed at preventing disease in the preclinical or asymptomatic phase. Hypertension and breast cancer screening are examples.

3. **Tertiary prevention** includes measures that identify symptomatic but untreated disease. Rehabilitation programs fall into this category.

2. Why make separate recommendations for screening the elderly?

1. **The benefit from screening/preventive interventions is greater in the elderly.** With the higher prevalence of disease in this population, more true-positive results will be obtained with a screening test. Of course, these tests may be less specific as well—an individual may have multiple possible causes of a positive occult blood stool sample, ranging from benign to malignant.

2. **There is evidence of under-utilization of screening/preventive programs in the elderly.** Despite the benefit of screening in the elderly, evidence indicates that older individuals do not receive the recommended screening tests as often as they should. There are both provider and patient reasons for this underuse. There is also disturbing evidence that sociodemographic factors, such as race and education, further affect access to screening services, making the indigent elderly an important target group for screening efforts.

3. **The measure of a successful program differs in the elderly.** In reviewing the evidence that screening benefits the elderly, a number of different outcome measures are used, since identifying conditions that affect the quality of life and functional status may be more important than those that shorten life. In addition to morbidity and mortality, consideration should be given to the ability to live independently and avoid nursing home placement, the number of acute care visits and hospitalizations required, and the psychological sense of well-being. All these factors have been shown to improve with an effective screening program.

4. **The level of intervention is different.** Primary prevention, with lifestyle modification, has the greatest impact on reducing disease for the population as a whole. In teenagers, prevention of motor vehicle accidents and sexually transmitted diseases are areas of prime concern, but in older patients, other causes of morbidity and mortality must be considered. Primary prevention is still crucial; the value of exercise in maintaining functional status, preventing osteoporosis, and reducing the risks of falls is a good example. However, secondary and tertiary prevention interventions become increasingly important. Efforts to maximize functional status

in older patients with existing disease may have the greatest effect on the quality and duration of life.

3. What is the physician's role in screening?

The traditional role of a physician has been as healer, but as medical knowledge has grown, so has appreciation of the importance of preventing illness and maintaining health. As a member of the primary care team, the physician helps in teaching patients about healthy behaviors and ensuring that appropriate screening procedures are carried out in a timely fashion. Research indicates the importance of physician counseling in areas such as smoking cessation and exercise, as well as in performing diagnostic screening procedures such as rectal and breast exams and Pap smears. Other healthcare personnel also play important roles: e.g., nurse-initiated community-based screening for hypertension and breast cancer, counseling by nutritionists, and psychological screening by mental health providers.

4. What criteria are used to identify conditions suitable for screening?

Expert panels have reviewed the literature to formulate recommendations for timing and frequency of screening interventions. These panels have increasingly included the elderly as a group for whom distinct recommendations need to be derived. The following list includes elements generally agreed upon as being essential in the decision to screen.

1. **The condition must have a significant effect on the quality or quantity of a patient's life.** Screening should be targeted toward identifying conditions associated with significant morbidity, i.e. the "burden of suffering." Screening for hypertension and breast cancer help reduce mortality and morbidity, and screening for glaucoma and hearing impairment in the older individual can improve the quality of life.

2. **The condition must be treatable.** Clinical interventions studied across a range of patient ages often demonstrate an age-related response to therapy. Evidence of effectiveness in older patients should be sought.

3. **The disease must have an asymptomatic period during which detection and treatment significantly reduce morbidity and/or mortality.** For any screening program to be effective, early detection of risk factors or disease must lead to an intervention which has a positive impact on outcome. Advancing detection of disease by 5 years will only be useful if the resulting treatment prevents or delays disease development by > 5 years.

4. **Tests for detection of disease must be affordable, safe, and have known test characteristics.** Both the cost of initial screening and the subsequent evaluation must be taken into account. The costs of evaluating a positive stool test for blood, an elevated serum prostate specific antigen, or an elevated serum CA-125 have been assessed and led to a general caution about using inexpensive but nonspecific tests which may lead to further expensive and risky diagnostic interventions.

5. **The incidence of the condition must be sufficient to justify the cost of screening.** No matter how dramatic the effect of early treatment in a specific condition, mass screening is not warranted if the disease is so rare that only a few individuals will benefit.

5. What are good test characteristics for a screening instrument?

1. **High sensitivity:** The ideal screening test should identify a high proportion of patients having the condition being sought. Since screening takes place at an early stage in the disease and because test sensitivity may vary according to the stage of disease, documentation on the sensitivity of the test in a given screening setting should be sought.

2. **High specificity:** The test should be normal in patients not having the condition being sought. In a low-prevalence situation, as often encountered in a screening setting, specificity is the key to reducing false-positive and false-negative results.

3. **High positive predictive value in the population being screened:** Some screening tests are designed to be used in low-prevalence situations, meaning that there will be many more people without the disease than with the disease. However, all patients who are told that their test is positive will need to receive further testing and/or treatment. The cost of follow-up of false-positive

test results must be considered, both in terms of actual dollars and the psychological cost to the patient. The possibility of a false-positive result is reduced when the prevalence of disease increases.

4. **High negative predictive value:** A patient having a negative screening test should feel reassured that he or she does not have the condition of concern and not worry that the test could be in error. Thus, a normal result should be a reliable indicator that no disease exists. The cost of a false-negative test includes the loss of the benefit of screening (including, perhaps, a tendency to delay the reporting of symptoms) and the psychological costs of false reassurance.

6. How should general screening recommendations be applied to individual patients?

For people of all ages, screening programs must be adapted for the individual, taking into account the presence of risk factors and comorbid conditions. Public policy analyses, however, understate the risks and benefits to the individual patient, particularly the older patient. Functional status, presence of existing diseases, and attitudes toward screening can all appropriately influence the screening and preventive care interventions recommended for a given patient. It would not be reasonable to screen a 90-year-old woman with severe congestive heart failure for preclinical cervical cancer because her survival is already limited by her cardiac disease. However, screening for decreased visual acuity might result in an intervention that would improve that patient's eyesight and allow her to enjoy more sedentary activities such as reading.

Patient preferences for treatment must also be considered. Recommendations for mass screening are based on aggregate data and assume that an individual would pursue treatment, if indicated. Individuals may have very strong preferences about what treatments they would consider acceptable, and these preferences should be respected. A patient's ability to undergo treatment must also be taken into consideration. If the optimum cancer treatment would be too toxic for a given individual, screening would not be appropriate unless a less toxic alternative was available.

7. Why don't physicians comply with screening recommendations?

Physicians give several reasons when asked why they do not carry out the preventive services recommended in their patients:

1. **They are unaware of the recommendations.** The need for physician education has been a long-standing problem. In addition, since recommendations change frequently, physicians must be motivated to keep up to date on the frequency and indications for screening.

2. **They do not have the time.** Particularly in the elderly, patients often may have multiple active problems that must be addressed during each interval visit. Procedures such as pelvic or rectal exams, which involve disrobing and sometimes special examination rooms, require additional time. Counseling is also time-consuming, especially if patients and their families wish to discuss and review the recommendations.

3. **They forget.** Despite the best intentions, providers may not remember to include preventive measures into a routine health check, or if they do remember, they forget which measures are due for a given patient.

4. **They disagree with the recommendations.** Physicians sometimes disagree with formal recommendations if these differ from what they were taught or their current practice protocol. For example, a physician may be following the recommendations of the American Cancer Society, which are significantly more interventionist than those of the U.S. Preventive Services Task Force. Discrepancies among programs endorsed by expert panels and individual providers need to be resolved by careful review of the basis for the recommendations.

8. Why don't patients participate in screening programs?

In general, elderly patients are more likely than their younger colleagues to pursue healthy behaviors, such as regular blood pressure checks, dietary modifications, and accident prevention. They also appear to have a greater belief in the importance of lifestyle modification (diet, exercise, smoking) in reducing the risk of future morbidity, as well as heightened awareness of available interventions. Reasons leading to lower compliance include:

1. **Misunderstanding about normal aging:** The elderly may accept new symptoms as part of normal aging and consider the development of disease as inevitable.

2. **Cost of screening:** There has been progress in insurance coverage for some preventive health measures, such as flu shots, pneumococcal vaccines, and mammograms which are now covered through Medicare. In addition, the increased participation of the elderly in managed-care systems which emphasize preventive measures has helped to reduce the cost of prevention to the individual. However, there are still the costs (and availability) of transportation and subsequent testing which must be considered.

3. **Fear:** Patients may be reluctant to enter a program that might detect an illness. They might be apprehensive about the actual tests involved. Many patients dread mammograms and sigmoidoscopy because of lack of dignity and discomfort involved or because of negative experiences reported by others.

4. **Lack of a primary care provider:** Many elderly have been cared for by physicians older than themselves. When these physicians retire from practice, healthy community-dwelling patients may not have contact with a primary care provider who can ensure that they receive routine preventive care.

9. What do you do when a patient refuses a screening procedure?

If a patient refuses a recommended screening test, the physician's first responsibility is to be sure that the patient understands the reason screening is being suggested and next to explore the patient's reasons. If the refusal is based on misinformation or logistic concerns, these should be addressed. Population-based estimates of disease should be translated into terms relevant to the individual; e.g., what is their risk of developing the condition, with and without screening? What are the chances of a false-positive or false-negative test? Do they understand the consequences of not participating? If an informed, competent patient refuses a screening test, the physician should respect that decision. The physician's recommendation and reasons for the patient's refusal should be documented on the patient's chart.

10. How can you improve the preventive care your elderly patients receive?

1. Work as a team to screen for preventable disease. Take advantage of community-based programs whenever possible.

2. Educate yourself and your patients about which conditions are worth screening for and what statistical rationales and emotional forces are involved.

3. Integrate screening into routine visits when possible, but do not hesitate to schedule a separate visit if more time is needed.

4. Develop a reminder system and flow sheet that is part of each individual's record.

5. Find out what barriers exist for the individual (language, transportation, cost, need for a companion) and work to fix them.

11. So what are the preventive interventions recommended for the general population aged 65 and older?

According to the 1995 recommendations of the U.S. Preventive Services Task Force, asymptomatic individuals ages 65 and over should receive the following screening and counseling interventions as part of routine care. The frequency of the individual services is left to clinical discretion, except where indicated.

Screening
> Blood pressure
> Height and weight
> Fecal occult blood test (annually) and or sigmoidoscopy
> Mammography + clinical breast exam (every 1–2 years)(women < 69)
> Papanicolaou test (all women who are or have been sexually active and who have a
> > cervix. Consider discontinuation of testing after age 65 if previous regular screening
> > provided consistently normal results.)

Vision screening
Assess for hearing impairment
Assess for problem drinking
Counseling
Substance abuse
 Tobacco cessation
 Avoid alcohol/drug use while driving, swimming, boating, etc.
Diet and exercise
 Limit fat and cholesterol
 Maintain caloric balance
 Emphasize grains, fruits, and vegetables
 Adequate calcium intake (women)
 Regular physical activity
Injury prevention
 Lap/shoulder belts
 Motorcycle and bicycle helmets
 Fall prevention
 Safe storage/removal of firearms
 Smoke detector
 Set hot water heater to < 120–130°F
 CPR training for household members
Dental health
 Regular visits to dental care provider
 Floss, brush with fluoride toothpaste daily
Sexual behavior (STD prevention)
 Avoid high-risk sexual behavior
 Use condoms
Immunizations
 Pneumococcal vaccine
 Influenza (annually)
 Tetanus-diphtheria (Td) boosters (every 10 years)
Chemoprophylaxis
 Discuss hormone prophylaxis (peri- and postmenopausal women)

BIBLIOGRAPHY

1. Asch DA, Hershey JC: Why some health policies don't make sense at the bedside. Ann Intern Med 122:846–850, 1995.
2. Hendriksen C, Lung E, Stromgard E: Consequences of assessment and intervention among elderly people: A three year randomized controlled trial. BMJ 289:1522–1524, 1984.
3. Lianov L, Kohatsu N, Bohnstedt M: Referral outcomes from a community-based preventive health care program for elderly people. Gerontologist 31:543–547, 1991.
4. Leventhal EA, Prohaska TR: Age, symptom interpretation and health behavior. J Am Geriatr Soc 34:185–191, 1986.
5. Prohaska TR, Leventhal EA, Leventhal H, Keller ML: Health practice and illness cognition in young, middle aged, and elderly adults. J Gerontol 40:569–578, 1985.
6. Rubenstein LZ, Josephson KR, et al: Comprehensive health screening of well elderly adults: An analysis of a community program. J Gerontol 41(3):342–352, 1986.
7. Sackett, DL, Haynes RB, Tugwell P: A Basic Science for Clinical Medicine. Boston, Little, Brown and Company, 1985.
8. Sox HC: Preventive health services in adults. N Engl J Med 330:1589–1595, 1994.
9. U.S. Preventive Services Task Force: Guide to Clinical Preventive Services: An Assessment of the Effectiveness of 169 Interventions. Baltimore, Williams & Wilkins, 1995.

12. CANCER SCREENING

Richard H. Greenberg, M.D., and David J. Vaughn, M.D.

1. Why screen for cancer in the elderly?

Cancer in persons > 65 years of age accounts for the majority of cancer incidence (58%) and a disproportionate amount of cancer deaths (67%) in the United States. By the year 2030, the elderly's share of all cancer incidence will increase from the current 58% to 70%. The incidence of cancer per 100,000 population is 10 times greater for the elderly versus those < 65 years of age (2085.3 vs. 193.9). Thus, screening the elderly for cancer makes sense: screening tests are widely available, early detection improves the length and quality of survival in this population, and effective treatments are available for those malignancies detectable by screening. (See also Chapter 11 on principles of screening.)

2. Why do the elderly get more cancer?

Many theories exist.

1. Aging generally leads to a **decline in immune function.** Involution of the thymus leads to T-cell deficiency, and interleukin-2 levels also decline with age. The overall decline in cell-mediated immunity is believed to impair immunologic surveillance against the appearance of spontaneous malignancies and to increase the susceptibility to environmental and infectious (e.g., viral) insults and carcinogenesis over time.

2. The appearance of cancer in response to **environmental exposures** may require long periods of time that favor an increased incidence in the elderly. Many known carcinogens require prolonged or cumulative exposures or lengthy time delays between the initial exposure and the appearance of the neoplasm. Strong evidence now exists to support the "multiple hit" hypothesis of carcinogenesis, in which a series of cumulative genetic mutations and alterations are necessary to transform normal tissues into malignancies.

3. The elderly also experience a wide range of **physiologic changes** that include alterations in hormone and enzyme levels which may influence normal cell growth and maturation; abnormalities of DNA transcription, proofreading, and repair; and alterations in the metabolic clearance of toxins.

3. How does ageism affect cancer care?

Ageism is prejudice or discrimination against a particular age group, especially the elderly. Such attitudes, whether overt or subtle, often lead to an **ultraconservative** or **nihilistic** approach to the management of cancer in the elderly. Education of the public and health care providers and the implementation of properly designed studies can help to overcome some of the misconceptions that undermine the detection and care of cancer in the elderly.

4. Does age increase the extent of cancer at diagnosis?

In general, the stage of cancer at presentation is not significantly different according to age, with the exception of ovarian cancer in which older women are more likely to have more advanced disease. However, when considering the yearly incidence of malignancy in the United States, the elderly account for a disproportionate number of cases:

- In men:
  - 84% of 200,000 annual cases of prostate cancer
  - 63% of 100,000 cases of male lung cancer
  - 70% of 75,000 cases of male colorectal cancer
  - 69% of the combined 66,000 cases of gastric, pancreatic, and urinary bladder cancers in men

• In women:

50% of 182,000 annual cases of breast cancer

76% of 74,000 cases of female colorectal cancer

61% of 72,000 cases of female lung cancer

65% of the combined 60,200 cases of gastric, pancreatic, ovarian, and urinary bladder cancers in women

Cancer in the elderly should be considered neither less aggressive, less metastatic, nor less of a public health problem than malignancies in younger patients.

5. With their frequent visits to doctors' offices, are the elderly adequately screened for cancer?

Despite having more physician visits and a progressively greater incidence of cancer than younger people, the elderly generally have a poorer participation in screening procedures. For example, more than half of women age > 65 did not have a mammogram in the preceding year, and nearly 40% have *never* had a mammogram. Similarly, such women are less likely to have had a Pap smear in the preceding year than their younger counterparts (41% vs. 67%).

6. What are the current recommendations for cancer screening?

True consensus has not yet been reached for all tumor types, but general guidelines are as follows:

Breast	Breast self exam monthly from age 20
	Physician breast exam annually from age 40
	Mammogram every 1–2 years starting at age 40 and annually starting at age 50 (see Question 7)
Colorectal	Annual physician digital rectal exam from age 40
	Annual fecal occult blood testing and flexible sigmoidoscopy every 3–5 years from age 50
	Because the efficacy of these screening measures outside high-risk populations has not been conclusively demonstrated, some policy-making groups offer no recommendation for this tumor type (see Question 8).
Uterine cervix	Annual Pap smear and pelvic examination starting at age 18–25 or at start of sexual activity in some populations
	Interval may be decreased to every 3 years after 3 negative yearly examinations
Prostate	Annual digital rectal exam and serum prostate-specific antigen level determination starting at age 50 are controversial
	Some higher-risk groups, such as men with family histories of prostate cancer or African-American men (2-fold higher incidence and mortality compared to whites) may warrant yearly screening starting at age 40.
	Transrectal ultrasound is generally an ineffective screening tool (see Questions 10 and 11).
Lung	Routine chest x-rays or sputum cytology in asymptomatic populations are not presently recommended.
	Smoking prevention/cessation should be encouraged.
Skin	Complete skin examination for populations at risk (family history, increased sun exposure, presence of precursor lesions)
	Interval of screening is at physician discretion
	Public education regarding minimizing sun exposure and skin self-examination
Ovary	No current recommendations for screening asymptomatic women other than examination of adnexa during a pelvic exam done for other reasons
	Pelvic ultrasound and serum CA-125 levels may eventually prove useful, especially in postmenopausal women.

Oral	Physician gloved examination of the oral cavity routinely (preferably yearly) for high-risk populations only (tobacco/alcohol use, presence of precursor lesions)
	Encourage regular dental examinations and cessation of risk exposures
Gastric	Upper GI barium fluoroscopy not generally applicable as a screening tool in the United States (This study has proven useful in endemic areas, such as Japan.)
Urinary bladder, pancreatic	No recommendation

7. Is there justification to continue breast cancer screening past age 69?

Prospective trials have not yet answered this question. However, the incidence of breast cancer continues to rise past age 70 and remains high past age 85. Sensitivity and specificity of mammography and physician examination of the breast improve as the breast ages and glandular tissue is replaced by fat. Cost-effectiveness analysis supports physician breast examination annually and mammography every 2 years after age 65 and continuing indefinitely. Such surveillance would terminate only in those who are very ill and deemed to have a minimal life-expectancy.

8. How should colorectal cancer screening be applied to the elderly population?

Colorectal cancer incidence continues to rise steadily with age, particularly past age 65, with continued increases past age 85. Although the limitations of current screening techniques apply to the elderly population, the increased cancer incidence in this subgroup may make these screening methods somewhat more cost-effective. Current screening recommendations do not specify a particular age cut-off but generally favor application to patient populations considered at risk (due to positive family history, presence of prior colorectal cancer, or presence of adenomatous polyp of > 1 cm size or villous/tubulovillous histology). Conversely, some researchers suggest efforts to identify low-risk populations who would not require further intensive screening. Some suggestions include consideration of discontinuing all colorectal cancer screening procedures for asymptomatic patients who have had two normal flexible sigmoidoscopies or a single normal colonoscopy. The management of patients with small (< 1 cm) adenomatous polyps remains controversial because little is known about their risk of future carcinoma. Future screening methods may utilize measures of colonic mucosal proliferation or the presence of genetic markers to stratify risk of future bowel neoplasia.

9. Is there justification to continue cervical cancer screening past age 64?

Almost 43% of deaths from cervical cancer occur in women aged > 65 years. Cervical cancer in the elderly appears to progress more rapidly to invasive disease. In addition, many elderly women have *never* had a Pap smear. Surveillance for cancer of the uterine cervix should continue to the point of minimal life-expectancy, rather than an arbitrary age cut-off.

10. Does age influence the interpretation of the serum PSA level?

Prostate-specific antigen (PSA) concentrations correlate directly with age. The normal serum PSA concentration of a 60-year-old man increases approximately 0.04 ng/ml/yr. This rise is attributed to a typical increase in prostate volume of 0.5 ml/yr. Based on these trends, age-specific normal reference ranges for the serum PSA (based on the 95th percentile) for most modern assays are:

Age 40–49	0–2.5 ng/ml
50–59	0–3.5 ng/ml
60–69	0–4.5 ng/ml
70–79	0–6.5 ng/ml

Use of age-specific reference ranges makes the serum PSA level a more sensitive tumor marker in men < 60 years of age and a more specific tumor marker for men > 60 years of age.

11. How are serum PSA determinations and digital rectal exam used in prostate cancer screening?

No clear consensus exists. Some cost-benefit analyses suggest the appropriateness of digital rectal exam (DRE) and serum PSA determination for prostate cancer screening limited by the end points of age > 75 or the presence of significant pre-existing medical conditions that would predict a life-expectancy of < 10 years. A screening algorithm for the early detection of significant prostate cancer is:

Serum PSA Level	DRE	Diagnostic Action
≤ age-specific range	Negative	Continue annual serum PSA and DRE
> age-specific range	Negative	TRUS* Biopsy visible lesions Sextant biopsies of remaining prostate, with two cores including transition zone tissue
Any value	Positive	TRUS Biopsy palpable and visible lesions Sextant biopsies of remaining prostate

* TRUS=transrectal ultrasound.

Additional cost savings per cancer discovered can be obtained by determining prostate gland volume at the time of TRUS and not biopsying patients whose only abnormality is an elevated absolute serum PSA that corrects to normal range when prostate volume is considered (i.e., presence of normal PSA density ≤ 0.12 ng/ml serum/ml prostate)

12. What socioeconomic barriers must be overcome to enhance cancer screening in the elderly?

This area has attracted increased research interest, particularly in light of the demographic shifts that are predicting for increased elderly populations at risk for cancer in future years. The decline in physical mobility and financial resources associated with aging may be a significant barrier for access to or participation in screening efforts. Four factors have been identified as being important to the success of screening efforts in such a population:

1. **Education and recruitment:** Subpopulations at risk are identified and educational programs are introduced into local communities in a succinct and culturally sensitive fashion. Television is a particularly effective medium for reaching the elderly, especially the economically disadvantaged. Importantly, the format of the presentation may need modifications to be understood and remembered by a population who often has increased sensory or cognitive deficits. Recruitment to participate should be active and communicated through trusted community figures such as medical professionals, primary caregivers, community leaders, and friend/family "word of mouth." A common reason given for the failure of elderly individuals to participate in screening efforts is the lack of recommendations by their physicians. Specialists frequently visited by the elderly (e.g., ophthalmologists, rheumatologists) should share responsibility with primary care physicians to help educate and direct the elderly in proper cancer screening procedures.

2. **Accessible screening:** To be successful, the method of screening selected must be affordable and geographically accessible. The cost of testing and follow-up evaluation must not create a financial burden that would interfere with compliance. Patients should be informed of the screening benefits available to them through their insurance or Medicare programs. Education regarding cancer prevention behaviors should be integrated into such an outreach program. Mobile vans are particularly useful to reach the elderly who often have difficulty traveling to remote screening sites due to physical and sensory handicaps. The screening sites must also be easily accessible to this population.

3. **Efficient diagnosis and treatment:** Geographic and chronologic integration of the interpretation of test results, provision of diagnostic studies, and initiation of definitive management

are important components of a successful screening program for the elderly. Patient compliance is enhanced by decreasing time delays and providing management in a convenient manner that enhances bonding with a consistent health care team.

4. **Multidisciplinary treatment team:** Coordination of diagnosis, treatment, education, psychosocial support, and follow-up are important to a successful screening and treatment program for cancer in the elderly.

13. What misconceptions do the elderly have about screening?

Studies have identified a range of misconceptions that could deter an elderly person from participating in screening efforts. For example, many elderly persons believe that it is always "too late" when cancer is found and that cancer onset and curability are random processes or determined entirely by individual physiology and habits. They often do not perceive a potential benefit to be gained by early detection nor recognize the distinction between treating cancer at early versus late or terminal stages. Some persons avoid cancer screening centers because they believe cancer is contagious, or they have concerns about privacy or embarrassment. Additionally, some persons believe that if they are pain-free, they cannot have cancer, and others dismiss symptoms such as pain, anorexia, weight loss, and fatigue as being caused by progressive age or comorbid conditions. Few older adults realize that they are actually at increased risk of developing a wide range of malignancies.

Clearly, the elderly must be convinced that they are appropriate candidates for screening and that they can safely benefit from participation. Educational programs to address these issues should be sensitive to the older patients' concerns about appearing or becoming vulnerable, losing empowerment to control their lives, and becoming a burden to their families.

BIBLIOGRAPHY

1. Byrne A, Carney DN: Cancer in the elderly. Curr Probl Cancer 17:147–218, 1993.
2. Costanza M: Issues in breast cancer screening in older women. Cancer 74:2009–2015, 1994.
3. Littrup PJ, Kane RA, Mettlin CJ, et al: Cost-effective prostate cancer detection—reduction of low-yield biopsies. Cancer 74:3146–3158, 1994.
4. Oddone EZ, Feussner JR, Cohen HJ: Can screening older patients for cancer save lives? Clin Geriatr Med 8:5167, 1992.
5. Rubenstein L: Strategies to overcome barriers to early detection of cancer among older adults. Cancer 74:2190–2193, 1994.
6. Stamey TA, Ekman PE, Blankenstein MA, et al: Tumor markers: Consensus conference on diagnosis and prognostic parameters in localized prostate cancer. Scand J Urol Nephrol, Suppl 162:73–87, 1994.
7. U.S. Preventive Services Task Force: Guide to Clinical Preventive Services: An Assessment of 169 Interventions: Report of the U.S. Preventive Services Task Force. Baltimore, William & Wilkins, 1989.

13. IMMUNIZATIONS

Risa Lavizzo-Mourey, M.D., M.B.A.

1. Which immunizations are recommended routinely for persons over 65 years of age?

Influenza vaccine should be given annually during the fall to all persons over age 65. Because even healthy elderly persons have a reduced antibody response to the vaccine as compared with younger adults, it is recommended that the vaccine be given late in the fall—between Halloween and Thanksgiving. This timing allows a maximal antibody titer during the winter months of January and February, when the probability of influenza infection is greatest.

Pneumococcal vaccination should be given once at age 65 (with the 23 valent preparation). As a rule, it need be given only once. Data suggest that antibody levels begin to wane after 6 years. Revaccination is recommended at 6 years for those with the highest risk for fatal pneumococcal infection (those receiving dialysis or asplenic patients). The data are inadequate, however, to recommend revaccination for all elderly persons. Because the adverse reactions associated with revaccination are minimal (soreness at the injection site), the decision to revaccinate after 6 years should be based on clinical judgment and patient preference. Similarly, if pneumococcal vaccination cannot be documented, it is better to give the immunization and risk injection site soreness.

Tetanus and diphtheria should be given every 10 years during adulthood. Although both of these diseases are extremely rare in the United States today, more than half of the reported cases occur in persons over 60 years old. Often this is because the patient never received a primary series and has low antibody titers. For these reasons, it is important to obtain a vaccination history and give the primary series if necessary.

2. Why is it important to immunize older people against influenza and pneumococcus?

1. Older persons are particularly **susceptible** to infections of the lower respiratory tract. As a result, pneumonia and influenza are the fifth leading cause of death among the elderly. Even when respiratory infections do not cause death, they are associated with significant morbidity, including deconditioning, prolonged recovery times, and cardiac abnormalities such as arrhythmia. Elderly persons with cardiac disease, dementia, or chronic pulmonary diseases are at even higher risk for infection. Overall, 80–90% of the deaths caused by influenza occur in older persons. The incidence of pneumococcal pneumonia in persons over 65 is 50 cases/100,000 population compared with an overall incidence of 15–19 cases/100,000 persons/year in younger age groups.

2. Situations associated with a **greater risk of exposure** are common among today's elderly. Examples include nursing home residents, individuals living in other congregant situations, such as retirement communities or assisted-living homes, as well as those attending adult daycare or senior centers. Elders living in households with young or school-aged children are likely to be exposed to a variety of respiratory pathogens.

3. The vaccines for pneumococcal infection and influenza are **efficacious**. Based on case-control and epidemiologic studies, the efficacy of the pneumococcal vaccine is reported to be between 55–75% effective in preventing life-threatening pneumococcal diseases in the elderly. Similarly, the efficacy of influenza vaccine in preventing death in the elderly is between 70–100%. A recent meta-analysis confirms the cost-effectiveness of influenza vaccination in older persons. Finally, both vaccines are safe with relatively low risk of adverse reactions.

3. List the contraindications to influenza and pneumococcal immunizations.

• Severe allergic reaction to the pneumococcal vaccine in the past. This occurs in < 1% of the population.

- Anaphylactic reactions to eggs (hives, wheezing, or angioedema). The influenza vaccine virus is raised in egg media.
- History of Guillain-Barré or other neurologic syndromes after previous influenza vaccination.

4. About which adverse reactions should one warn patients?

- Two types of **systemic reactions** occur commonly:
    Fever, myalgia, malaise 6–12 hours after vaccination, which resolves in 1–2 days
    Mild, immediate hypersensitivity reaction
- **Altered hepatic clearance** of certain medications (warfarin, theophylline and phenytoin) may occur. This is rarely clinically significant.
- Many older patients may remember the 1976 outbreak of Guillain-Barré syndrome following the swine flu vaccinations, so the risk of **Guillain-Barré** after flu vaccination should be addressed. The risk is remote. Between 1976 and 1990, there was no association between flu vaccination and Guillain-Barré. In 1991, there was a slight increase in the incidence of Guillain-Barré in vaccinated adults < 65 years of age, but the incidence was lower than expected in those > 65. These observations are not believed to indicate a causal relationship.

5. Are there any other vaccine-related issues about which one should counsel patients?

One cannot stress too strongly that these vaccines protect against *specific causes* of respiratory illness, not *all* viral infections or pneumonia. A common reason patients give for not seeking an annual flu shot is that "they got a flu shot one year and then got the flu anyway." The most likely explanation for such an occurrence is that the patient had already been exposed to the influenza virus at the time of immunization or that the patient was afflicted with a viral illness other than the flu. Similarly, the pneumococcal vaccine is antigen-specific: It does not protect against pneumonia caused by organisms other than pneumococcus.

6. What are the most common misconceptions about contraindications to immunization in the elderly?

Contrary to common wisdom, immunization can be given in the following situations:
- The patient has had a previous reaction to a vaccination consisting of mild to moderate local tenderness and swelling or fever < 40°C.
- The patient experienced a mild acute illness following immunization.
- The patient is currently receiving antimicrobial therapy or is recovering from an acute illness.
- The patient has been recently exposed to an infectious disease.
- The patient has an atopic history including allergies to some antibiotics.
- The patient has a family history of allergies.
- The patient is scheduled to receive both the influenza and the pneumococcal vaccines on the same day. (Different sites should be chosen.)

7. Why is it necessary to immunize for flu annually?

The surface of the virus is continually changing. Influenza A has multiple subtypes based on its hemagglutinin ($H_1H_2H_3$) and neuraminidase (N_1N_2) antigens. These antigens drift with time, resulting in lost immunity and ineffectiveness of "old" vaccines.

Influenza B drifts less frequently, but when it does, the change is substantial and generally results in a major outbreak. Typically, the influenza vaccine includes the two subtypes of influenza A that are not prevalent that season and the type B strain.

8. What underlying diseases put elderly patients at risk for death due to influenza or pneumonia?

- Chronic respiratory disease
- Renal failure—especially those on dialysis
- Hemoglobinopathies
- Congestive heart failure

9. What is the recommendation concerning influenza prophylaxis of long-term care residents and workers?

All residents and workers should be immunized annually. Eighty percent must be immunized to achieve "herd" immunity. Once herd immunity is achieved, unvaccinated individuals are at lower risk because the probability of infection within the whole group has been reduced. This includes residents of retirement communities, assisted-living facilities, and participants in senior daycare.

Health care providers are a significant source of infection. Therefore, they must be immunized as well to achieve herd immunity. Because many health care providers are young women of child-bearing age, it is important to know that pregnancy and breast-feeding are not contraindications to immunization.

When an exposure occurs before the 2 weeks required to achieve adequate antibodies titers (> 1:40), **antiviral prophylaxis** should be administered using amantadine or rimantadine. This prophylaxis can be discontinued:

After 2 weeks if the patient has been immunized.

When the flu season is over, if the patient has not been immunized. If the exposure occurs early in the season, simultaneous immunization is advised to limit the course of prophylaxis.

If exposure is known to be to influenza type B. Although amantadine or rimantadine are 70–90% effective in preventing influenza A, they are ineffective against type B.

The maximum dose of amantadine is 100 mg/day, less if the patient has renal insufficiency. Rimantadine is usually dosed at 100 mg/day. Significant **neurologic symptoms** occur with both drugs, even at the recommended doses. As many as 30% of nursing home residents receiving prophylaxis have been reported to have psychosis, ataxia (with falls), seizures, or hallucinations. These are not benign medications in the frail, long-term care resident. However, an outbreak of influenza A is life-threatening to many residents.

10. What are effective strategies for increasing immunization rates?

Data from 1994 suggest that, at best, 58% of elders got annual influenza vaccines, and only 40% received pneumococcal vaccines. Several strategies have been shown to improve immunization rates, and in most studies, reduce hospitalization and mortality rates as well:

1. A policy of immunizing against pneumococcal infection in all elders on discharge from the hospital, with clear documentation on the chart cover.

2. Mailing pneumococcal vaccine reminder cards to everyone at age 65.

3. Mailing flu shot reminder cards to all ambulatory elders annually in the fall.

4. Having walk-in hours for influenza immunizations.

5. Involving all staff (housestaff, office staff, nurses, and physicians) in a fall campaign to immunize elders against the flu.

11. Do elderly travelers require any special immunizations?

No, not special ones. But older travelers should receive the World Health Organization–recommended immunizations or chemoprophylaxis for the area they plan to visit.

BIBLIOGRAPHY

1. Centers for Disease Control and Prevention: Control of influenza A outbreaks in nursing homes: Amantadine as adjunct to vaccine—1989–1990. JAMA 267:344–346, 1992.
2. Foster DA, Talsma AN, Furomoto-Dawson A, et al: Influenza vaccine effectiveness in preventing hospitalization for pneumonia in the elderly. Am J Epidemiol 136:296–307, 1992.
3. Gross PA, Hermogenes AW, Sacks HS, et al: The efficacy of influenza vaccine in elderly persons. Ann Intern Med 123:518–527, 1995.
4. Immunizations for Special Groups of Patients. In Guide for Adult Immunizations, 3rd ed. Philadelphia, American College of Physicians, 1994.
5. Sims RV, Steinmann WC, McConville JH, et al: The clinical effectiveness of pneumococcal vaccine in the elderly. Ann Intern Med 108:653–657, 1988.

14. REDUCING CARDIOVASCULAR RISK

Bruce T. Liang, M.D.

1. Why has the mortality rate for coronary artery disease (CAD) declined?

CAD remains the major cause of mortality and morbidity in the United States and the western world. Nearly 5.4 million individuals are diagnosed as having CAD, and close to half a million deaths per year are attributable to coronary atherosclerosis. Estimates place the treatment of this disease at nearly $8 billion annually.

Fortunately, a variety of factors have contributed to the decline in the death rate from CAD over the past 25 years, as treatment programs designed to prevent modifiable risk factors have been developed. There has been a decrease in **serum cholesterol** levels in general and an improvement in the detection and treatment of **hypertension** over the past two decades. The proportion of patients, irrespective of gender or race, whose hypertension has been treated and controlled has increased, especially among African-Americans and women. **Cigarette smoking** in middle-aged men has declined, and there has been a remarkable increase in the general level of **physical activity**. There has been some change in **diet**, with a decrease in the consumption of saturated fats, certain red meats, eggs, butter, and cream as well as an increase in the use of vegetable fats and low fat milk.

Other factors contributing to the decline in CAD deaths include the early use of **thrombolytic therapy** in the treatment of acute myocardial infarction (MI), or the use of various adjunctive therapies such as **aspirin** and **heparin**. The availability of coronary care units as well as improved medical and surgical therapy for patients with acute coronary syndrome have also improved survival rates.

2. Define the various coronary risk factors.

Risk factors for CAD refer to conditions that predispose individuals to the morbidity and mortality of coronary atherosclerosis. The primary modifiable risk factors for CAD are:
- Hypercholesterolemia
- Hypertension
- Tobacco smoking
- Diabetes mellitus
- Low levels of high-density lipoprotein (HDL) cholesterol

Other potential risk factors whose importance is still being established include:
- Serum triglyceride levels
- Personality type
- Level of physical activity (see Chapter 15)
- Obesity and body habitus

3. What is the importance of hypercholesterolemia in the progression of coronary atherosclerosis?

Hypercholesterolemia is one of the most extensively studied risk factors for the development of CAD. The level of serum cholesterol correlates directly with the CAD mortality rate. Every major epidemiologic study performed has shown this correlation. The Framingham Heart Study and the more recent Multiple Risk Factor Intervention Trial (MRFIT) have confirmed this relationship.

4. Does prevention of atherosclerosis result in decreased risk for CAD?

Meta-analysis of available clinical trials demonstrates that reducing serum cholesterol will diminish the overall risk for coronary atherosclerosis. Reduction methods include lowering total fat consumption, substituting polyunsaturated for saturated fat in diets, and the use of pharmacologic agents. For every 1% reduction in cholesterol level, there was a 2% decrease in the incidence of CAD in clinical trials that treated subjects for > 4 years (determined by the lengthy time taken to build up atherosclerotic plaque). The reduction in the number of nonfatal and fatal myocardial infarctions (MIs) as a consequence of lowering cholesterol levels has been found in meta-analysis of both primary and secondary prevention trials.

5. What is an elevated triglyceride level?

A number of genetic, epidemiologic, and clinical studies have correlated elevated triglyceride levels to increased CAD risk. However, such links may be secondary to other disorders. Various disease entities associated with hypertriglyceridemia, such as diabetes mellitus and chronic renal failure, are complicated by additional atherosclerosis risk. Current treatment guidelines for hypertriglyceridemia, based on an NIH-sponsored consensus conference in 1984, classify triglyceride levels as:

< 250 mg/dl	Normal
250–500 mg/dl	Borderline
> 500 mg/dl	High risk

Patients who have borderline-elevated triglyceride levels should be examined for possible secondary causes (such as diabetes), excessive alcohol consumption, obesity, or the use of nonselective beta-adrenergic blockers. Such patients should be placed on a low-fat diet, or if dietary therapy is ineffective, treatment with a fibric acid derivative such as gemfibrozil may be warranted.

6. How do lipid-lowering interventions affect blood flow and myocardial ischemia?

Often, patients without CAD have abnormal endothelial vasodilator function associated with elevated serum cholesterol levels, which may predispose them to myocardial ischemia. Studies demonstrate that cholesterol-lowering can improve endothelium-mediated vasodilator function, and this in turn may have important implications for reduced tendency toward myocardial ischemia. In addition to regression of coronary atherosclerosis, such results may explain the beneficial effect of cholesterol-lowering therapy.

7. Does tobacco use predispose to CAD?

The use of tobacco products is a major risk factor in patients prone to the development of CAD (see Chapter 18). A number of mechanisms may be responsible for the deleterious effect of tobacco use, including:
- Decreased level of HDL
- Higher level of low-density lipoprotein (LDL) triglycerides
- Acute effect on blood pressure
- Higher fibrinogen level
- Increased platelet aggregability
- Prolongation in bleeding time
- Increased plasma norepinephrine levels

8. Explain the relationship between hypertension and the risk for CAD.

Hypertension is a major modifiable risk factor for the development of coronary atherosclerosis. It may impact synergistically with hyperlipidemia to increase this risk. The term *dyslipidemic hypertension* has been used to describe patients with hyperlipidemia in the presence of hypertension. This condition may be related to increased triglycerides, decreased HDL, increased insulin levels, and insulin resistance.

When considering drug therapy for hypertension, one must bear in mind that antihypertensive medications may have an adverse effect on glucose tolerance, lipid levels, and insulin resistance that counteract the beneficial effects of blood pressure lowering. Furthermore, overly aggressive pharmacologic lowering of blood pressure has been reported to increase risk for cardiac events,

especially in men with established coronary atherosclerosis, suggesting that the relationship between hypertension treatment and CAD mortality follows a J-shaped curve.

9. Is dietary therapy for hypertension effective?

While the precise correlation between high sodium intake and hypertension is not defini-
tively established, clinical evidence suggests that a 100-mmol/day decrease in sodium intake leads
to an average decline of 6 mm Hg in blood pressure. An average American consumes 10–15 gm
of salt per day, an amount that far exceeds the body's needs. In addition, decreased consumption of saturated fat and an increased intake of potassium both contribute to a lowering of
blood pressure.

10. How does treating hypertension affect the risk for stroke and coronary disease?

A meta-analysis of major blood pressure-lowering trials evaluated 14 trials involving
45,000 patients for an average of 5 years. In 9 of the 14, benefits were seen in stroke reduction,
though the impact on CAD was not clear. In the Hypertension Detection and Follow-up
Program, > 7800 patients with a diastolic pressure between 90–104 mm Hg were enrolled.
Patients who received a diuretic, followed by an adrenergic blocker and then hydralazine,
demonstrated a 20% lower overall mortality rate, including 40% fewer deaths due to cerebral
vascular disease, 40% fewer deaths due to acute MI, and 20% fewer deaths due to CAD. On the
basis of these findings, the Second U.S. Joint National Committee recommended that the initial
goal of antihypertensive therapy be to maintain diastolic pressure at approximately 90 mm Hg.
Similarly, a large study enrolling 3,234 men demonstrated a significant reduction in CAD,
stroke, and overall mortality in the group receiving metoprolol. Although the drug was administered in a nonblinded open trial, the data suggested benefit from the use of this cardioselective
beta-blocker.

Thus far, only diuretics and beta-blockers have been shown to be effective in reducing hypertension with a subsequent decrease in morbidity and mortality. While well-tolerated and effective
in lowering blood pressure, angiotensin converting enzyme (ACE) inhibitors and calcium channel antagonists have not been studied in a prospective, controlled, primary prevention trial.
Therefore, their impact on CAD in hypertensive patients is not known. Caution should be exercised to ensure that metabolic abnormalities, such as hyperglycemia, hyperlipidemia, or electrolyte disorders, are corrected and that overzealous reduction of blood pressure is avoided so
that coronary perfusion is not jeopardized.

11. What evaluations are needed before an elderly person begins an exercise program?

In general, long-term physical activity plays an important role in maintaining ideal body
weight and muscle mass and perhaps in maintaining normal blood pressure and lowering lipid
levels. However, people who have been sedentary and wish to start regular exercise must be cau-
tious, because their sudden switch from a sedentary lifestyle to regular physical exercise may
induce ventricular arrhythmias or acute MI. This concern is especially important in the elderly,
because an age-related decline in physical activity may mean that symptoms of myocardial ischemia are not evident. Such patients should undergo a thorough physical exam and exercise
stress test before undertaking a program of vigorous physical activity. However, many elderly patients may not be able to reach 85% of predicted maximal heart rate during an exercise stress test.
In this case, a thallium perfusion scan following dipyridamole administration may provide equivalent information on the presence or severity of coronary disease.

12. What is an appropriate level of exercise?

The optimal level of exercise required to protect against CAD has not been established.
Exercise expenditures of about 2000 kcal/wk, or the equivalent of running 20 miles/wk, correlate
with protection from the development of CAD. If, after undergoing a thorough history, physical
exam, and treadmill testing, the patient has no evidence or history of ischemic heart disease, then
the exercise program probably does not need close monitoring. Another way to look at a desired

level of exercise is that three sessions per week, each lasting 20–30 minutes, is necessary to bring about a significant improvement in aerobic capacity. Five sessions can produce the maximal result, which is usually achieved after 4–6 weeks of training. In both men and women, there may be considerable additional reductions in risk factors for CAD if the level of physical activity exceeds the recommended guidelines.[11] The same general strategy should be applicable to the elderly, except that the intensity of exercise at each level of progression should be less; it should be individualized also on the basis of the results of screening procedures for coronary disease and the patient's general physical condition.

13. What is the relationship between obesity and CAD?

An NIH consensus conference on obesity concluded that obesity is associated with poorer health and decreased longevity. Although the precise role of obesity as an independent risk factor for CAD is unclear, analysis of the Framingham data reveals its contribution to the overall risk for CAD. Blood cholesterol, blood pressure, glucose, and uric acid levels all increase with a greater body mass index. Obesity has a strong positive correlation with blood pressure, triglyceride, and insulin levels and is inversely related to the concentration of HDL cholesterol. All of these abnormalities are associated with an increased risk for coronary atherosclerosis.

14. Explain the relationship between family history and the risk for CAD.

There is a clear tendency for familial aggregation of CAD, likely due to aggregation of risk factors among family members. In an evaluation of siblings of patients with documented premature atherosclerosis, it was demonstrated that 48% of brothers and 41% of sisters were hypertensive and that 45% of brothers and 22% of sisters had a lipid abnormality. In addition to the risk of developing premature atherosclerosis from a positive family history, familial aggregation of risk factors implies a predisposition for development of CAD ultimately manifesting late in life. Fortunately, such risk factors in first-degree relatives of affected family members are mostly modifiable and lend themselves to preventive strategies aimed at reducing risk early on.

15. How should diabetic patients be treated to reduce their risk for CAD?

In diabetic patients, mortality associated with coronary atherosclerosis is increased. In the first National Health and Nutrition Examination Survey, age-adjusted death rates for diabetics were twice those seen in nondiabetics. Three-quarters of the increase in mortality among diabetic men was due to CAD.

Type 2 diabetic patients with hyperinsulinemia are predisposed to coronary atherosclerosis. Insulin is a growth factor that enhances synthesis and uptake of lipids by smooth muscle cells. Epidemiologic studies have demonstrated that elevated fasting insulin levels predict the development of coronary atherosclerosis, even in nondiabetic patients, independent of all other CAD risk factors. Other studies demonstrate that hyperinsulinemia and insulin resistance, such as occur in Type 2 diabetics, result in an increased frequency of CAD. Hypertension and obesity also tend to be associated with diabetes and glucose intolerance. In fact, the frequency of hypertension is about twice that in patients with altered glucose tolerance.

Control of hypertension is particularly important in diabetic patients, as it leads to a decrease in microvascular complications. Because formation of glycosylated LDL has been implicated in the development of macrovascular disease, control of blood glucose may also help to reduce macrovascular or atherosclerotic complications in diabetics. Weight reduction can improve glucose-associated lipid abnormalities in Type 2 diabetics. However, medications that decrease glucose tolerance, such as diuretics, should be avoided.

16. How does the incidence of CAD differ between men and women?

CAD is much less prevalent in premenopausal women than in age-matched men. After menopause, however, rates for men and women begin to converge. The fundamental process of atherosclerosis does not appear to differ between men and women, and the usual risk factors correlate with the development of coronary atherosclerosis in both sexes.

17. How do hormones and replacement therapy affect the development of CAD in women?

The underlying hypothesis is that the differing rates of coronary atherosclerosis between men and women are due to differences in levels of estrogen and androgen hormones. Until puberty, HDL levels are about equivalent in males and females. At puberty, the level of testosterone increases in males, while estrogen production increases in females. The increase in testosterone correlates with a decrease in HDL level. In women undergoing natural menopause, serum levels of HDL gradually decline, and the total serum cholesterol and LDL levels gradually increase. Because estrogen replacement therapy favorably reverses these changes, it has been suggested that this therapy may achieve its salutary effect by altering the cholesterol and LDL/HDL levels.

The benefit of CAD reduction versus the risk of developing endometrial and breast cancer in postmenopausal women receiving estrogen replacement therapy remains controversial. Therefore, estrogen and progesterone use should be determined on an individual basis, especially for women at risk for thromboembolic disease or with associated coronary risk factors such as hypertension or tobacco use.

18. Can alcohol consumption help to prevent CAD?

Alcohol has a number of cardiovascular effects. Studies have shown an inverse relationship between regular consumption of small to moderate amounts of alcohol and coronary events. The Framingham study demonstrates a relative risk of 0.7 in subjects consuming at least 30 oz of alcohol per month. However, *excessive* alcohol use on a *chronic* basis is associated with the development of high blood pressure, dilated cardiomyopathy, as well as arrhythmias (the holiday heart syndrome). Alcoholism is associated with overt CAD, and heavy alcohol intake is positively associated with the prevalence of acute MI. Given the adverse effects of chronic alcohol use on overall mortality, consumption of alcohol as a preventive measure against coronary atherosclerosis remains controversial.

19. What pharmacologic measures can be taken to prevent a second MI?

A number of specific pharmacologic interventions can reduce mortality *after* the onset of acute MI, including the angiotensin-converting enzyme (ACE) inhibitors and beta-adrenergic blocking agents.

The CONSENSUS II study, conducted over 1 year at 103 Scandinavian centers enrolling 6,090 patients, demonstrated that patients receiving the ACE inhibitor **enalapril** within 24 hours of a confirmed MI failed to show improved survival during the next 6 months. However, there was a small but significant beneficial effect of enalapril on the progression of congestive heart failure.

In the SAVE (Survival and Ventricular Enlargement) trial in the United States and Canada, 2231 patients with an ejection fraction ≤ 40% following an acute MI were randomized in a double-blind fashion to receive placebo or **captopril** and then were followed for an average of 42 months. Captopril-treated patients had a 19% reduction in risk of all-cause mortality and a 21% reduction in the risk of fatal and nonfatal major cardiovascular events. There was also a 25% reduction in risk for recurrent MI.

Beta-blockers also may confer a survival benefit. Large clinical trials have shown that **atenolol, propranolol** and **metoprolol** improve survival in a wide spectrum of post-MI patients and reduce the incidence of sudden death and reinfarction. Results with **oxprenolol**, a beta-blocker with intrinsic sympathomimetic activity, are far less encouraging; at least one trial shows a slight increase in mortality.

Patients without contraindications to the beta-blockers (e.g., asthma, moderate or severe congestive heart failure, arrhythmias) should receive prophylactic treatment with one after acute MI. Data are conflicting over the benefit of continuing this therapy beyond 2 years; but if beta-blockers are well tolerated and if there is no reason to discontinue therapy, then they should be continued in most patients. For patients with an extremely good prognosis—e.g., those who have a first acute MI with good left ventricular function, negative stress testing and no significant ventricular ectopy—beta-blockers need not be given.

20. What about aspirin?

Anticoagulants should be used in patients at risk for thromboembolic complications, including thrombophlebitis, history of pulmonary embolism or systemic embolism, evidence of mural left ventricular thrombus, and severe heart failure. Although the evidence for the use of aspirin in preventing a second or recurrent MI is not definitive, data in all eight trials suggest that aspirin prophylaxis can result in a 10–15% reduction in total deaths and a 20–30% decrease in recurrent MI. Therefore, the current recommendation is that, in the absence of contraindications, aspirin in the dose of 80–325 mg/day should be given.

21. Can risk factor reduction provide any benefits in the elderly?

The reduction of risk factors has been deemed less beneficial in older patients because of their shorter life expectancy. Recent evidence, though, indicates that successful treatment of hypertension and smoking cessation will decrease cardiovascular mortality in the elderly. Furthermore, atherosclerosis is a progressive disease that is in fact more prevalent in older patients. More than one-half of all deaths in people aged 65 years or older are due to CAD. Thus, slowing the progression of atherosclerosis by reducing its risk factors may well be beneficial in the elderly as well.

BIBLIOGRAPHY

1. Anderson TJ, Meredith IT, Yeung AC, et al: The effect of cholesterol-lowering and antioxidant therapy on endothelium-dependent coronary vasomotion. N Engl J Med 332:488, 1995.
2. Blair SN, Kohl HW, Paffenberger RS Jr, et al: Physical fitness and all-cause mortality: A prospective study of healthy men and women. JAMA 262:2395, 1989.
3. Caspersen CJ, Bloemberg BPM, Saris WHM, et al: The prevalence of selected physical activities and their relation with coronary heart disease risk factors in elderly men: The Zutphen study, 1985. Am J Epidemiol 133:1078, 1991.
4. Goldman L, Cook EF: The decline in ischemic heart disease mortality rates: An analysis of the comparative effects of medical interventions and changes in lifestyle. Ann Intern Med 101:825, 1984.
5. Levine GN, Keaney JF Jr, Vita JA: Cholesterol reduction in cardiovascular disease. N Engl J Med 332:512, 1995.
6. MacMahon SM, Cutler JA, Furburg CD, Payne GH: The effects of drug treatment for hypertension on morbidity and mortality from cardiovascular disease: A review of randomized controlled trials. Prog Cardiovasc Dis 29(3 suppl 1):99, 1986.
7. Meade TW, Imeson J, Stirling Y: Effects of changes in smoking and other characteristics on clotting factors and the risk of ischemic heart disease. Lancet 2:986, 1987.
8. Reaven GM, Lithell H, Landsberg L: Hypertension and associated metabolic abnormalities—The role of insulin resistance and the sympathoadrenal system. N Engl J Med 334:374, 1996.
9. 1988 Report of the Joint National Committee on Detection, Evaluation and Treatment of High Blood Pressure. Arch Intern Med 148:1023, 1988.
10. Treasure CB, Klein JL, Weintraub WS, et al: Beneficial effects of cholesterol-lowering therapy on the coronary endothelium in patients with coronary artery disease. N Engl J Med 332:481, 1995.
11. Williams PT: High-density lipoprotein cholesterol and other risk factors for coronary heart disease in female runners. N Engl J Med 334:1298–1303, 1996.

15. EXERCISE IN THE ELDERLY: CAN IT IMPROVE FUNCTION?

Grace A. Cordts, M.D., M.S., M.P.H.

All parts of the body which have function, if used in moderation and exercised in labors to which each is accustomed, become thereby well developed and age slowly, but if unused and left idle, they become liable to disease, defective in growth and age quickly.

—Hippocrates

1. Can exercise improve functional status in the elderly?

Data from the Canadian Health Survey showed that an inevitable functional decline creates functional dependency starting 8–10 years before death. Most elderly people are totally dependent the year before death. The social and economic consequences of this dependency are staggering if one thinks of the projected increase in numbers of persons 65 years or older.

There is evidence that much of what was once viewed as aging is actually secondary to disuse. There are striking similarities between structural and functional declines associated with aging and the effects of enforced inactivity.

At age 65, women have an average of 19 more years of life, and men have an average of 15 more years. There is interest in looking at exercise as a potential way to minimize future functional decline or at least to compress the period of dependency into the last year of life—the concept of **compression of morbidity**. The potential benefit of improving quality of life is combined with the potential societal and economic benefits of decreasing institutionalization of our aging society.

Physical fitness is a determinant of functional status; intuitively, exercise should improve functional status. A preponderance of data supports this hypothesis. Exercise has been shown to improve multiple physiologic functions and has been used in the treatment of various diseases. Exercise improves cardiorespiratory capacity, muscle strength, endurance, flexibility, body composition (increases lean body mass and decreases fat), range of motion (ROM), sleep, and cognitive function. It has been shown to decrease patients' sensitivity to dyspnea and to improve lipid profiles. Exercise has been used to treat patients with cardiovascular disease, chronic obstructive pulmonary disease, diabetes mellitus, depression, osteoporosis, arthritis, Parkinson's disease, and falls, all with some degree of success.

Epidemiologic and observational studies show that people who exercise regularly require less support and institutionalization at any given age than nonexercisers. Abundant evidence indicates improvement in physical fitness when healthy older individuals take part in controlled, vigorous exercise.

It is not known whether sedentary, infirm elderly people can maintain or improve functional status by commencing exercise. Certain experimental data support the role of exercise in improving function, but some of the studies lack randomization, have inadequate statistical power, and fail to target people who are physically unfit or infirm. More experimental studies are needed to understand how exercise might improve functional status.

2. What are the goals of an exercise program for the elderly patient?

Ward describes six objectives for an exercise program for the elderly:

1. Increased energy to cope with normal daily tasks
2. Improved capacity for unusual or unexpected demands
3. Quicker recovery from illness or stress
4. Improved balance
5. Greater opportunity to meet new people
6. More fun

3. When is it too late to start exercising?

It is not clear when it is too late to start exercising or if it is ever too late to start. Certainly the epidemiologic data suggest that people 70 years or older who report low levels of exercise have an increased risk of death. People who maintain activity in their lives do better. In a randomized trial, Posner took healthy older sedentary adults and showed that exercise reduced new cardiovascular events in the next 2 years. A study of nursing home residents found that people even in their 90s can improve functional capacity, grip strength, chair-to-stand time, and self-ratings of depression. There certainly are anecdotal reports of people starting to exercise in their 80s and doing well into their 90s and 100s. Even bedridden individuals can be given ROM exercises to prevent contractures or bed mobility exercises that facilitate the tasks of caregivers.

4. Who should be assessed for cardiovascular risk before initiating exercise?

How detailed an exam and how much testing are needed before starting an exercise program are controversial. Some believe that all people should have a complete physical exam and cardiopulmonary stress test before initiating exercise, whereas others believe that exercise is a normal part of life and that no screening is required for asymptomatic healthy individuals. The American Heart Association recommends an exercise stress test for sedentary men over 45 years of age, sedentary women over 50, and anyone with hypertension or heart disease. The Royal College of Physicians and British Cardiology Society recommend minimal use of special evaluations and believe that a medical exam is not necessary before starting an exercise program as long as the work-out begins at a low level and progresses slowly.

The degree of work-up depends on the patient and the intensity of the program to be undertaken. Asymptomatic patients who are beginning a low level of activity that gradually builds intensity probably do not need special evaluation. Patients with active cardiopulmonary symptoms or a history of angina, myocardial infarction, or palpitations should undergo a thorough history and physical exam, focusing on cardiac and pulmonary symptoms. These patients and asymptomatic older persons who are planning to take up a competitive sport or to become involved in a vigorous exercise program should have a stress test. If the stress test is positive, further evaluation is necessary before exercise is undertaken.

5. Are any medical conditions a contraindication to exercise?

Patients with aortic stenosis, severe congestive heart failure, hypertrophic cardiomyopathy, or uncontrolled hypertension should be cautioned against exercise because of the adverse consequences.

6. How do exercise programs for the elderly differ from general exercise programs?

Physical fitness is the goal of exercise programs for younger individuals. Although physical fitness is an important aspect of all exercise programs, focusing on performance of activities of daily living and quality of life are more important for the elderly.

7. What does an exercise prescription include?

The content of an exercise prescription depends on whether its purpose is to increase physical fitness or improve, maintain, or regain functional status. Historically, an exercise prescription for physical fitness included the type, intensity, and frequency of exercise. Exactly what should be included to alter functional status is unknown, largely because it is not known what level of physical fitness is necessary to maintain functional status.

Most agree that improvement in physical fitness requires at least 20 minutes of aerobic exercise 3 times per week. For optimal benefit, the heart rate should be maintained at 60–80% of its maximum for the person's age for 20 minutes. A quick calculation for maximal heart rate is 220 minus age.

8. What should be included in an exercise program for the elderly?

The ideal program should include a warm-up period, an aerobic period, and a cool-down period. Flexibility exercises and strengthening exercises round out the program. The warm-up and cool-down periods should be extended, because steady state levels of blood pressure, heart rate, and ventilation are reached more slowly. The warm-up and cool-down periods should be about 20 minutes in duration.

9. What kind of exercise is best?

Walking is probably the cheapest and easiest form of exercise. Incorporating recreational activities into exercise helps to maintain compliance and participation. Water activities such as swimming, water aerobics, or water walking can be beneficial for patients with musculoskeletal problems. Water activities, however, do not have the beneficial effects of gravity for increasing bone density.

The type of exercise must take into account the patient and his or her potential problems as well as maximize safety, compliance, and enjoyment. Frail elders may have poor vision, unsteady gait, or musculoskeletal problems that limit the type of activity in which they can participate. In general, activities should be enjoyable and affordable, involve low impact with less force on joints, and use skills the patient already has. One study of exercise and mobility showed that any physical activity, including gardening, was beneficial as long as it was done 3 or more times per week.

Muscle-strengthening exercises should involve low resistance to prevent orthopedic injuries. They should be done with caution to avoid straining against a closed glottis to prevent cardiovascular complications. The patient should be instructed to exhale while performing the active phase of exercise and to inhale while relaxing. This strategy prevents straining against a closed glottis.

Isometric exercises should be avoided because they increase blood pressure and cardiac workload, creating the potential for adverse cardiac events.

10. What are the recommended intensity, frequency, and duration of exercise for elderly people?

The recommendations for achieving physical fitness in healthy younger people are well known. For cardiovascular fitness, the American Heart Association recommends activity 3 days per week for 20 minutes at 50% of $\dot{V}O_2$ max. The American College of Sports Medicine recommends activity 3–5 days per week at 60–90% of maximal heart rate or 50–85% of $\dot{V}O_2$ max. For the elderly who want to improve physical fitness, the intensity of exercise should be reduced and the duration and frequency increased to prevent injury. The same level of physical fitness can be achieved; it will simply take longer. Some evidence indicates that the intensity can be 40–50% of $\dot{V}O_2$ max and still have an effect. Future studies must address the issue of how intense a work-out is necessary.

From a practical standpoint, a good rule of thumb to monitor intensity is to tell patients that if they cannot talk during exercise, they are doing too much. The exercise program should leave the person feeling pleasantly aware of their muscles the next day. The amount of exercise should be increased gradually each week.

11. Do the elderly sustain more injuries and adverse effects from exercise?

No direct evidence addresses this question. If an exercise program is undertaken prudently, risk of injury or adverse complication should be minimized. The risk of injury seems to be related to high-intensity training and high-impact activities. Reviews of cardiovascular complications in cardiac rehabilitation programs show relatively low rates of adverse events: 1 in 112,000 patient hours for cardiac arrest; 1 in 294,000 patient hours for myocardial infarction; and 1 in 784,000 patient hours for death. The following recommendations may help to prevent injury:

- Emphasize warm-up period.
- Strengthen weakened joints, especially rotator cuff and wrists, if golf or tennis is to be undertaken.
- Emphasize low-impact activities, such as walking, bicycling, rowing, and cross-country skiing.
- In hot weather, exercise in air conditioning; in cold weather, exercise indoors.
- Ensure adequate hydration.
- Avoid exercising on hard surfaces.

• Use adequate footwear.
• For exercising in pools, make sure that adequate hand rails and nonslip decks are available.
• If balance is poor, avoid exercises such as cycling or skiing, which require balance skills.
• If symptoms occur, stop the activity immediately and contact a physician; go to the emergency department if symptoms do not resolve when exercise is stopped.
• Take antianginal medication before exercise.

12. How do you motivate and help patients comply with an exercise regimen?

Motivating patients and encouraging participation in exercise are major challenges. Emphasizing the benefits in terms of maintaining and increasing functional status is probably most successful. Specific examples include being able to get down on the floor to play with grandchildren, possibly preventing institutionalization, and recovering from illness quickly. Despite the lack of controlled studies, the following characteristics probably make an exercise program more appealing:

• Formal structure
• Demonstration of objective improvement (e.g, by keeping logs)
• Slow increase in exercise so that patient does not overdo it or become frustrated
• Easy ways to monitor intensity of work
• Grouping people according to ability and disability
• Use of enjoyable activities
• Supervision by older rather than young instructors

13. What community resources are available?

Because of a greater interest and emphasis on physical activity, more exercise programs aimed at older persons are being offered by various organizations. Local colleges and universities, community centers, YM or YWCAs, and rehabilitation hospitals with community outreach programs are good resources. The National Association for Human Development, American Physical Therapy Association, American Association of Retired Persons, and American College of Sports Medicine are valuable sources of information.

14. Is there a role for exercise in elderly hospitalized patients?

Often immobilization and bedrest are prescribed for hospitalized elders; both can cause an acute deterioration in function, which at times may be impossible to reverse. Elderly patients should be mobilized as soon as possible. ROM exercises should be initiated immediately to promote activity and to prevent contractures. Physical therapy and occupational therapy should be initiated as soon as medically possible to help prevent functional decline. Bedrest should not be prescribed unless it is essential for recovery from illness.

15. What is the role of rehabilitation hospital or outpatient programs for the elderly?

Elderly patients who have had any acute or semiacute deterioration in function may benefit from a rehabilitation program as an inpatient or outpatient. These patients are usually patients who have had an acute medical problem which has lead to immobilization and deterioration of function.

16. Does Medicare reimburse for rehabilitation?

Medicare reimburses for rehabilitation if the benefit from the program is functionally significant. For example, programs that teach patients how to toilet themselves or to fix a meal—skills that allow them to remain at home—and programs that teach family members how to transfer a bedridden patient so that the patient can be maintained at home are covered. The patient has to show improvement. Medicare reimburses for inpatient and outpatient services. Programs include in-home services, rehabilitation hospitals, skilled nursing facilities, and outpatient services. The type of program depends on patients' needs and their abilities to participate in activities. For inpatient programs to be reimbursed, the patient must need medical supervision and 24-hour nursing care as well as be able to participate in 3 hours of physical therapy, occupational therapy, or speech therapy 5 days per week. This intensity of activity may be too taxing for some patients.

17. What is the role of the primary care physician or geriatrician in promoting exercise?
Geriatricians and primary care physicians should take an active role in encouraging people to maintain physical activity or to begin an exercise program at any age. They can point out the benefits of exercise, know what community resources are available, help motivate patients, and know who needs further testing before initiating an exercise program. The physician should ask about physical activity at every office visit, including any symptoms associated with exercise, and encourage continued participation.

BIBLIOGRAPHY

1. Buchner DM, Beresford SA, Larson EB, LaCroix AZ, Wagner EH: Effects of physical activity on health status in older adults. II: Intervention studies. Annu Rev Public Health 13:469–488, 1992.
2. Elward K, Larson EB: Benefits of exercise for older adults. Clin Geriatr Med 8:35–51, 1992.
3. McMurdo ME, Rennie L: A controlled trial of exercise by residents of old people's homes. Age Aging 22:11–15, 1993.
4. Pollock ML, Graves JE, Sewart DL, Lowenthal DT: Exercise training and prescription for the elderly. South Med J 87:588–595, 1994.
5. Shephard RJ: The scientific basis of exercise prescribing for the very old. J Am Geriatr Soc 38:62–70, 1990.
6. Wagner EH, La Croix AZ, Buckner DM, Larson EB: Effects of physical activity on health status in older adults. I: Observational studies. Ann Rev Public Health 13:451–468, 1992.
7. Ward J: Exercise and the older person. Aust Fam Physician 23:642–649, 1994.

16. NUTRITION

Marie Bernard, M.D.

1. Name the most common nutritional problem among elderly individuals.

In studies of elderly individuals in hospitals and nursing homes, **protein-calorie malnutrition** is found in 30–50% of the population. Borderline protein-calorie malnutrition is common in elderly outpatients. Multiple epidemiologic studies have demonstrated that elderly individuals commonly consume less than two-thirds of the recommended daily allowance (RDA) for multiple nutrients. This, combined with the effects of accumulated illnesses, medications, and social circumstances, depletes body caloric reserves for the stress of acute illness or surgery. Thus, with hospitalization, elderly individuals have often developed protein-calorie malnutrition and its associated morbidity and mortality. Elderly outpatients are much less likely to have overt malnutrition, unless they are recuperating from an acute illness.

2. Why do many elderly have reduced calorie intakes?

A number of factors contribute to elderly individuals' becoming protein-calorie malnourished:

1. As one ages, the senses of smell and taste diminish, thus rendering foods less palatable.

2. Accumulated illnesses and medications may suppress the appetite or impair the absorption of nutrients.

3. Many elderly individuals suffer from functional problems, making it difficult to get proper access to food or to prepare food properly.

4. Many elderly individuals suffer from social factors that impair their ability to obtain food or their desire to consume it:

    Decreased income

    Social isolation

    Depression

All of these factors combine to lead to suboptimal intake among elderly individuals, often leading to protein-calorie malnutrition upon their presentation to a hospital or long-term care institution.

3. How does malnutrition affect outcome of care in the elderly?

In protein-calorie malnourished patients, the length of stay in the hospital, cost of hospital care, and mortality are all 30–100% greater than in normally nourished individuals. Malnourished elderly outpatients also have poorer health and greater morbidity than normally nourished individuals. Morbidity associated with protein-calorie malnutrition includes increased infections, longer recovery time for wound healing, and less recovery of function.

4. When should you evaluate the nutritional status of elderly individuals? How?

Nutritional assessment can be difficult in elderly patients because aging and disease cause decreases in lean body mass that can mimic those seen with malnutrition. Although weight loss is seen with aging, recent unintentional weight loss—especially if it is > 5–10% of one's usual weight or > 10 lbs in 6 months—is significant.

A recent expert panel of nutritionists and gerontologists has developed a consensus regarding the nutritional assessment of elderly individuals. Their Nutrition Screening Initiative provides the first generally agreed-on standards for determining the nutritional status of elderly individuals. They also recommend proper interventions once risk factors for malnutrition are identified.

5. When should nutritional intervention be initiated for elderly individuals?

Most experts would not advise allowing a thin, frail, elderly person to go for 10 days with suboptimal intake. There are no firm guidelines, but the more underweight the patient and the greater the metabolic stress (particularly if the albumin level is < 3.5 gm/dl), the earlier nutritional intervention should be considered. Early identification of patients with intake significantly below 1000 kcal/day is therefore necessary.

A registered dietitian is often helpful in guiding the assessment of the nutritional needs of hospitalized or institutionalized elderly individuals and in assessing how closely spontaneous intake approximates those needs. This task is more difficult in ambulatory elderly. However, the guidelines of the Nutrition Screening Initiative for the Level 1 screen can help in identifying elderly individuals at risk for borderline intake.

Risk Factors for Poor Nutritional Status

Inappropriate food intake	Acute/chronic diseases or conditions
Poverty	Chronic medication use
Social Isolation	Advanced age
Dependency/disability	

Modified from The Nutrition Screening Initiative, a project of the American Academy of Family Physicians, The American Dietetic Association and the National Council on the Aging, Inc., and funded in part by a grant from Ross, Laboratories, a division of Abbott Laboratories.

Medicare does not pay for a home nutritional assessment. However, such assessments can be performed easily by a number of individuals.

- Checklists of risk factors can be administered by lay persons or home health aides. These should be considered for every elderly individual.
- Level I screens can be performed by nurses, social workers, and other health professionals in regular contact with elders. This screen should be performed if an elder is found to be at risk of nutritional deficiency, based on responses to the checklist.
- The Level II screen is intended for physicians to evaluate elderly individuals who appear nutritionally deficient based on the checklist and Level I screen.

(See figures on pages 76–79.)

6. What is unique about providing dietary supplements to elderly individuals?

Supplementation of the diet with enteral formulas is the first intervention to be provided (after problems with depression, social isolation, and/or difficulties with access to food have been addressed). Unfortunately, no medications have been identified that are clearly beneficial in stimulating appetite in the elderly. Food supplements have limited benefit in many elderly, due to the development of early satiety and/or taste fatigue. In addition, many elderly substitute enteral formulas intended for diet supplementation for their usual intake, thus deriving no net benefit from the intervention. In cases when spontaneous and supplemented intake cannot bring calorie and protein intake to goal levels, nutritional support via a nasoenteric or enteric tube is indicated.

7. How are the enteral nutrition formulas classified?

A plethora of formulas is available for nutritional support of the elderly. Each formula claims special properties that purportedly benefit diverse populations. However, based on review of the literature, there are few indications in the elderly for specialized formulas.

Formulas can be classified according to **protein form** as polymeric (blenderized), elemental, or free amino acids. Polymeric formulas are preferable to elemental formulas for simple diet supplementation, as they are more palatable. Polymeric formulas appear to be better tolerated in most elderly than elemental or amino acid formulas, which are more costly and unnecessary in most instances. The source of the protein does not appear to affect tolerance of feedings, with the exception of milk-based formulas. (The elderly have a higher prevalence of lactase deficiency than younger individuals, making milk-based formulas poorly tolerated by many.) Formulas that are high in osmolality and/or fiber do not appear to influence the occurrence of diarrhea. One recent study with a very small number of patients suggests that elemental formulas are beneficial for diarrhea in hypoalbuminemic patients because of their easier absorption.

Enteral Formula Comparison Chart

	BLENDERIZED		ELEMENTAL	FIBER CONTAINING		LACTOSE-FREE
Product	Compleat Regular	Vitaneed	Travasorb	Enrich	Ensure Plus	Isocal
Cal/ml	1.07	1.0	1.0	1.1	1.5	1.06
mOsm/kg water	450	300	560	480	690	270
Calories to meet 100% RDA for vitamins and minerals	1600	1500	2000	1530	2130	2000
Flavors	Natural food	Natural food	Unflavored	Varied	Varied	Unflavored
Cal/protein per 8-oz can	250/9	250/8	250/11	250/9	360/13	250/8

8. How is an appropriate formula selected?

In general, the elderly require 0.8–1.0 gm protein and 25 kcal/kg body weight. Patients recuperating from hip fracture or major surgery may have higher protein needs, up to 1.0 gm/kg body weight. Thus, you should select a formula that provides an appropriate quantity of calories and protein over the course of 24 hours in an isosmolar form, or more concentrated form if there are concerns regarding fluid retention. Formulas that have a mixture of carbohydrate, long-chain triglycerides, and intact protein (i.e., formulas that mimic real food) are usually well-tolerated. Although the elderly have a high prevalence of disorders of the GI tract that can affect fat absorption, recent data suggest that many elderly individuals can tolerate enteral formulas with as much as 67% of calories provided as fat.

In intensive care unit patients, a low non-protein calorie to nitrogen ratio (e.g., 97:1) may be beneficial in promoting nitrogen retention. In metabolically stable patients, there may also be a role for providing more nitrogen-dense formulas to compensate for the fact that patients often do not receive the full amount of enteral nutrition prescribed (due to technical difficulties, cessation of feedings for diagnostic testing, etc.).

9. Is nutritional intervention effective in elderly individuals?

Few studies actually have demonstrated the efficacy of nutritional intervention in this or any age group. One study evaluated a group of 122 "thin" and "very thin" elderly women with hip fractures. In their randomized, controlled trial, they provided 1000 cal and 28 gm of protein by overnight tube feeding, in addition to a regular diet throughout the day. This intervention led to more rapid ambulation than in control patients. Another study demonstrated similar benefit of simple oral supplementation in 59 elderly hip fracture patients. In a prospective, controlled trial, the daily addition of 250 cal and 20 gm of protein to the usual diet resulted in fewer hospital complications, increased mobility, and fewer nursing home placements at 6-month follow-up than in the controls.

Several studies of long-term feedings in chronically ill elderly in nursing homes have failed to show the benefits demonstrated in shorter studies of elderly who have undergone surgical procedures. However, many of the long-term evaluation studies are retrospective, without clear documentation of the degree to which nutritional needs were matched with the nutrition support provided.

In sum, nutritional deficits would appear to be reversible in many cases. Adverse outcomes associated with malnutrition in the elderly are well-documented. Thus, the potential benefits of nutritional intervention appear worthy of the effort.

10. What type of enteral feeding tube is preferable for short-term use in elderly patients?

Patients anticipated to require enteral nutrition support for a short time should have a **small-bore, pliable, nasoenteric tube placed**. These are often weighted to facilitate placement and

Level 1 Screen

Body Weight

Measure height to the nearest inch and weight to the nearest pound. Record the values below and mark them on the Body Mass Index (BMI) scale to the right. Then use a straight edge (ruler) to connect the two points and circle the spot where this straight line crosses the center line (body mass index). Record the number below.

Healthy older adults should have a BMI between 24 and 27.

Height (in):_____
Weight (lbs):_____
Body Mass Index:_____
(number from center column)

Check any boxes that are true for the individual:

☐ Has lost or gained 10 pounds (or more) in the past 6 months.

☐ Body mass index <24

☐ Body mass index >27

For the remaining sections, please ask the individual which of the statements (if any) is true for him or her and place a check by each that applies.

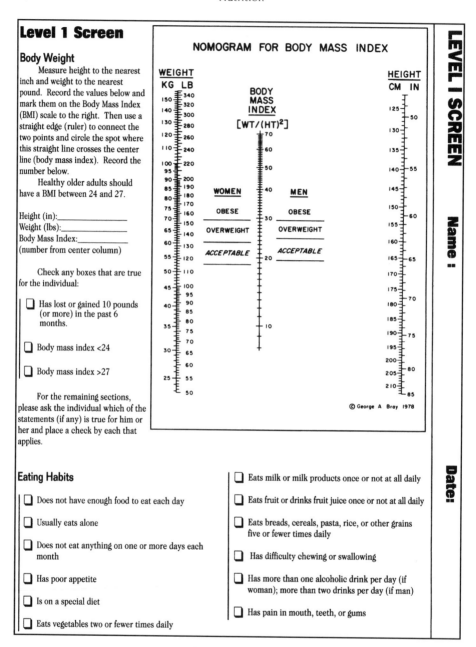

NOMOGRAM FOR BODY MASS INDEX

WEIGHT KG LB

BODY MASS INDEX [WT/(HT)²]

HEIGHT CM IN

WOMEN — OBESE / OVERWEIGHT / ACCEPTABLE

MEN — OBESE / OVERWEIGHT / ACCEPTABLE

© George A Bray 1978

LEVEL I SCREEN   Name: Date:

Eating Habits

☐ Does not have enough food to eat each day

☐ Usually eats alone

☐ Does not eat anything on one or more days each month

☐ Has poor appetite

☐ Is on a special diet

☐ Eats vegetables two or fewer times daily

☐ Eats milk or milk products once or not at all daily

☐ Eats fruit or drinks fruit juice once or not at all daily

☐ Eats breads, cereals, pasta, rice, or other grains five or fewer times daily

☐ Has difficulty chewing or swallowing

☐ Has more than one alcoholic drink per day (if woman); more than two drinks per day (if man)

☐ Has pain in mouth, teeth, or gums

The Level I and II screens. Reprinted with permission of the Nutrition Screening Initiative, a project of the American Academy of Family Physicians, The American Dietetic Association, and the National Council on the Aging, Inc., and funded in part by a grant from Ross Laboratories, a division of Abbott Laboratories.

(Figure continues on following pages.)

identification by x-ray. Before feedings are initiated, the tube tip must be confirmed to be in the stomach, either by aspiration of gastric contents or by x-ray. Inadvertent placement of the feeding tube into the tracheobronchial tree may not induce coughing in the elderly. Nasoenteric tube

A physician should be contacted if the individual has gained or lost 10 pounds unexpectedly or without intending to during the past 6 months. A physician should also be notified if the individual's body mass index is above 27 or below 24.

Living Environment

☐ Lives on an income of less than $6000 per year (per individual in the household)

☐ Lives alone

☐ Is housebound

☐ Is concerned about home security

☐ Lives in a home with inadequate heating or cooling

☐ Does not have a stove and/or refrigerator

☐ Is unable or prefers not to spend money on food (<$25-30 per person spent on food each week)

Functional Status
Usually or always needs assistance with (check each that apply):

☐ Bathing

☐ Dressing

☐ Grooming

☐ Toileting

☐ Eating

☐ Walking or moving about

☐ Traveling (outside the home)

☐ Preparing food

☐ Shopping for food or other necessities

If you have checked one or more statements on this screen, the individual you have interviewed may be at risk for poor nutritional status. Please refer this individual to the appropriate health care or social service professional in your area. For example, a dietitian should be contacted for problems with selecting, preparing, or eating a healthy diet, or a dentist if the individual experiences pain or difficulty when chewing or swallowing. Those individuals whose income, lifestyle, or functional status may endanger their nutritional and overall health should be referred to available community services: home-delivered meals, congregate meal programs, transportation services, counseling services (alcohol abuse, depression, bereavement, etc.), home health care agencies, day care programs, etc.

Please repeat this screen at least once each year--sooner if the individual has a major change in his or her health, income, immediate family (e.g., spouse dies), or functional status.

malposition may occur in up to 1.3% of the population receiving tube feedings, while as many as 35% of tube-fed patients may have clogged tubes. Such clogging may be resolved with water or pancreatic enzyme. At least one case report has described an elderly individual post-stroke who became an obligate nasal breather, leading to an inability to tolerate nasoenteric feedings.

11. Which type of enteral feeding tube is preferrable for long-term use?

In an individual who may require feedings for a prolonged period, **percutaneous endoscopic gastrostomy** (PEG) is the preferred method of feeding. **Surgical gastrostomies** are reserved for individuals at risk of complications with PEG placement (e.g., morbid obesity, esophageal obstruction, bleeding diathesis). Both procedures are associated with minimal complications. Morbidity and mortality associated with placement of these tubes may be due to the frail state of elders generally selected for this form of feeding. Occasionally, life-threatening complications of gastrostomies may arise, such as wound dehiscence, sepsis, or peritonitis.

Percutaneous non-endoscopic gastrostomies have been developed recently, and are probably comparable in morbidity and mortality to surgical gastrostomies in the hands of experienced physicians. An additional innovation is the **skin-level gastrostomy**. This form of gastrostomy has a short stoma, at the skin level, which is more aesthetically satisfying than the standard PEG

Nutrition

Level II Screen

Complete the following screen by interviewing the patient directly and/or by referring to the patient chart. If you do not routinely perform all of the described tests or ask all of the listed questions, please consider including them but do not be concerned if the entire screen is not completed. Please try to conduct a minimal screen on as many older patients as possible, and please try to collect serial measurements, which are extremely valuable in monitoring nutritional status. Please refer to the manual for additional information.

Anthropometrics

Measure height to the nearest inch and weight to the nearest pound. Record the values below and mark them on the Body Mass Index (BMI) scale to the right. Then use a straight edge (paper, ruler) to connect the two points and circle the spot where this straight line crosses the center line (body mass index). Record the number below; healthy older adults should have a BMI between 24 and 27; check the appropriate box to flag an abnormally high or low value.

NOMOGRAM FOR BODY MASS INDEX

WEIGHT KG LB

BODY MASS INDEX $[WT/(HT)^2]$

WOMEN — OBESE / OVERWEIGHT / ACCEPTABLE

MEN — OBESE / OVERWEIGHT / ACCEPTABLE

HEIGHT CM IN

© George A Bray 1978

LEVEL II SCREEN   Name: Date:

Height (in):_____
Weight (lbs):_____
Body Mass Index
(weight/height²):_____

Please place a check by any statement regarding BMI and recent weight loss that is true for the patient.

☐ Body mass index <24

☐ Body mass index >27

☐ Has lost or gained 10 pounds (or more) of body weight in the past 6 months

Record the measurement of mid-arm circumference to the nearest 0.1 centimeter and of triceps skinfold to the nearest 2 millimeters.

Mid-Arm Circumference (cm):_____
Triceps Skinfold (mm):_____
Mid-Arm Muscle Circumference (cm):_____

Refer to the table and check any abnormal values:

☐ Mid-arm muscle circumference <10th percentile

☐ Triceps skinfold <10th percentile

☐ Triceps skinfold >95th percentile

Note: mid-arm circumference (cm) - [0.314 x triceps skinfold (mm)]= mid-arm *muscle* circumference (cm)

For the remaining sections, please place a check by any statements that are true for the patient.

Laboratory Data

☐ Serum albumin below 3.5 g/dl

☐ Serum cholesterol below 160 mg/dl

☐ Serum cholesterol above 240 mg/dl

Drug Use

☐ Three or more prescription drugs, OTC medications, and/or vitamin/mineral supplements daily

or surgical gastrostomy. This may become the preferred gastrostomy for long-term feeding in ambulatory patients.

Percutaneous endoscopic gastrojejunostomies and surgical jejunostomies have been recommended in the past to limit problems with aspiration pneumonia, but these procedures do not necessarily limit aspiration. They are associated with a number of complications, such as bleeding, infections, and wound dehiscence.

Clinical Features

Presence of (check each that apply):

- ❏ Problems with mouth, teeth, or gums
- ❏ Difficulty chewing
- ❏ Difficulty swallowing
- ❏ Angular stomatitis
- ❏ Glossitis
- ❏ History of bone pain
- ❏ History of bone fractures
- ❏ Skin changes (dry, loose, nonspecific lesions, edema)

Percentile	Men 55-65 y	Men 65-75 y	Women 55-65 y	Women 65-75 y
Arm circumference (cm)				
10th	27.3	26.3	25.7	25.2
50th	31.7	30.7	30.3	29.9
95th	36.9	35.5	38.5	37.3
Arm muscle circumference (cm)				
10th	24.5	23.5	19.6	19.5
50th	27.8	26.8	22.5	22.5
95th	32.0	30.6	28.0	27.9
Triceps skinfold (mm)				
10th	6	6	16	14
50th	11	11	25	24
95th	22	22	38	36

From: Frisancho AR. New norms of upper limb fat and muscle areas for assessment of nutritional status. Am J Clin Nutr 1981; 34:2540-2545. © 1981 American Society for Clinical Nutrition.

Eating Habits

- ❏ Does not have enough food to eat each day
- ❏ Usually eats alone
- ❏ Does not eat anything on one or more days each month
- ❏ Has poor appetite
- ❏ Is on a special diet
- ❏ Eats vegetables two or fewer times daily
- ❏ Eats milk or milk products once or not at all daily
- ❏ Eats fruit or drinks fruit juice once or not at all daily
- ❏ Eats breads, cereals, pasta, rice, or other grains five or fewer times daily
- ❏ Has more than one alcoholic drink per day (if woman); more than two drinks per day (if man)

Living Environment

- ❏ Lives on an income of less than $6000 per year (per individual in the household)
- ❏ Lives alone
- ❏ Is housebound
- ❏ Is concerned about home security

- ❏ Lives in a home with inadequate heating or cooling
- ❏ Does not have a stove and/or refrigerator
- ❏ Is unable or prefers not to spend money on food (<$25-30 per person spent on food each week)

Functional Status

Usually or always needs assistance with (check each that apply):

- ❏ Bathing
- ❏ Dressing
- ❏ Grooming
- ❏ Toileting
- ❏ Eating
- ❏ Walking or moving about
- ❏ Traveling (outside the home)
- ❏ Preparing food
- ❏ Shopping for food or other necessities

Mental/Cognitive Status

- ❏ Clinical evidence of impairment, e.g. Folstein<26
- ❏ Clinical evidence of depressive illness, e.g. Beck Depression Inventory>15, Geriatric Depression Scale>5

Patients in whom you have identified one or more major indicator (see pg 2) of poor nutritional status require immediate medical attention; if minor indicators are found, ensure that they are known to a health professional or to the patient's own physician. Patients who display risk factors (see pg 2) of poor nutritional status should be referred to the appropriate health care or social service professional (dietitian, nurse, dentist, case manager, etc.).

12. How should enteral feedings be provided to the elderly?

Continuous enteral feedings are most commonly provided for individuals receiving naso-enteral feedings and often for individuals receiving gastrostomy or jejunostomy feedings. Continuous feedings are more easily administered through small-bore tubes than intermittent feedings. They may also decrease nausea, vomiting, and diarrhea. They have in the past been thought to be associated with a lower risk of aspiration pneumonia than intermittent feedings, but recent data challenge this assumption. Data suggest that intermittent feedings allow for better protein synthesis than do continuous feedings. However, at present, there is no conclusive evidence that one form of feeding should be preferred over another.

Continuous feedings are generally administered starting at 25–50 ml/hr and progressively increased to 100–125 ml/hr, depending on the predicted caloric needs of the individual and the caloric density of the formula. Intermittent feedings are generally started at 200 ml four times daily and progressively increased to as much as 400–500 ml every 4–6 hours, depending on caloric needs. Formulas with a high tonicity are often diluted initially and then progressively increased to full strength and eventually full volume.

13. What is the most dangerous complication of tube feeding in elderly individuals?

Aspiration pneumonia is the one complication that can lead to mortality. In the literature, its incidence ranges from 3–33%. In the past, experts believed that this complication could be limited by continuous feedings (which limit the volume of fluid in the stomach at any one time) and by feedings below the pyloric junction. However, recent studies suggest that continuous feedings may in fact increase the risk of aspiration pneumonia. Risk factors for pneumonia associated with tube feedings appear to be a history of pneumonia, esophagitis, and/or advanced age. The present literature suggests that gastrostomies and jejunostomies do not necessarily protect against the development of aspiration pneumonia.

All elderly patients, and especially those at high risk, should be monitored for clinical signs of aspiration, such as shortness of breath, rales, increased leukocyte count or shift, or simple confusion in a previously alert individual. If possible, avoid continuous tube feedings in individuals at risk for aspiration (with a prior history of aspiration or stroke).

14. What is the most common problem associated with tube feeding in elderly individuals?

Diarrhea. The development of diarrhea is particularly risky in the elderly, as it can predispose to skin irritation and the development of pressure ulcers. Risk factors for diarrhea in tube-fed patients include low serum albumin, antibiotic usage, hypertonicity of the formula, or low fiber content of the formula. However, several recent studies have disputed the role of low serum albumin level, tonicity of the formula, and fiber content of the formula. The major risk factor appears to be antibiotic usage.

15. Can frail elderly become infected as a result of contaminated tube feedings?

Recent studies have shown that manipulation of formulas (e.g., mixing of powdered formulas) leads to contamination. However, contamination does not appear to be related to the development of diarrhea or sepsis. One series found that pneumonia developed in 2 patients out of 24, with the organism found in respiratory secretions being the same organism found in the enteral formula. In this study, similar organisms were also found on the hands of nurses caring for these patients. Several other studies have had similar findings.

BIBLIOGRAPHY

1. Bastow MD, Rawlings J, Allison SP: Benefits of supplementary tube feeding after fractured neck of femur: A randomized controlled trial. BMJ 287:1589–1591, 1983.
2. Delmi M, Rapin C-H, Bengoa J-M, et al: Dietary supplementation in elderly patients with fractured neck of the femur. Lancet 335:1013–1016, 1990.
3. Dwyer J: Nutrition Screening Initiative. Washington, D.C., Nutritional Screening Initiative, 1991.
4. Morley JE, Glick Z, Rubenstein LZ: Geriatric Nutrition: A Comprehensive Review. New York, Raven Press, 1990.
5. Mowe M, Bohmer T. The prevalence of undiagnosed protein-calorie undernutrition in a population of hospitalized elderly patients. J Am Geriatr Soc 39:1089–1092, 1991.
6. Sullivan DH, Walls RC: Impact of nutritional status on morbidity in a population of geriatric rehabilitation patients. J Am Geriatr Soc 42:471–477, 1994.
7. Sullivan DH, Walls RC, Lipschitz DA: Protein-energy undernutrition and the risk of mortality within one year of hospital discharge in a select population of geriatric rehabilitation patients. Am J Clin Nutr 53:599–605, 1991.

17. ALCOHOL

David Oslin, M.D.

1. Is alcohol use safe in late life?

Generally, most people over age 65 do not have problems associated with alcohol consumption. No evidence suggests that the responsible use of alcohol in moderate amounts is deleterious to one's physical health. In fact, it may reduce cardiovascular mortality and overall mortality in all age groups. Furthermore, in older community-dwelling elders, moderate alcohol use is associated with fewer falls and greater mobility when compared with persons who do not drink. Less is known about any associations between moderate alcohol intake and the risk for mental illnesses, such as cognitive impairment or affective disorders.

2. Define heavy and moderate alcohol use.

Moderate alcohol use in older persons is an average of 1–2 drinks/day. The typical pattern of drinking for most people is to consume 2 or 3 drinks on the weekend or when dining out. Others may have 1 glass of wine or a nightcap every evening. Although this amount of drinking is typically nonproblematic, patients should be educated about and monitored for the development of any problems indicative of alcohol abuse. **Heavy** alcohol use is > 2 drinks/day.

3. What is alcohol abuse or dependence, and how prevalent is it in late life?

Alcohol abuse is defined by DSM-IV as a maladaptive pattern of drinking that leads to significant impairment in a person's life, including health, legal, or occupational problems or disruption in social or family functioning. **Alcohol dependence** represents a greater severity of impairment as manifested by three or more of the following:
- Tolerance
- Withdrawal symptoms
- Drinking more than intended
- Persistent desire or attempts to cut down
- A great deal of time spent in acquiring or recovering from alcohol
- Important social, occupational, or recreational activities ignored
- Continued use despite adverse problems related to alcohol

Epidemiologic studies have shown that "heavy" drinking is present in 3–9% of people over 65, with the current prevalence of alcohol abuse or dependence in the elderly being between 2–4%. There is about a 5:1 male-to-female ratio for alcohol abuse or dependence.

Alcohol use disorders are much more prevalent in clinics and hospitals. The prevalence of alcohol abuse and dependence among older primary care patients ranges from 4–13% with a lifetime prevalence of 33%. The prevalence for a current diagnosis of alcohol abuse or dependence among older inpatients on medical or surgical units ranges from 5–43%.

4. Did older patients with alcohol problems always begin drinking when they were younger?

No. Patients with an alcohol use disorder can be divided into two categories: those who have had problems most of their lives (early-onset group) and those who started having problems after age 50 (late-onset group). About one-third of older persons who are alcohol-dependent have the onset of their disease in late life. The incidence of alcohol abuse and dependence in late life has been estimated at 0.63 cases/100 person-years. The late-onset group may start problem drinking in relation to life stressors, such as affective disorders, retirement, loss of a spouse, or financial problems, but these are not the entire cause.

5. What are some risk factors that cause a person to start drinking in late life or relapse?

Change in social situation	Demographic factors
Death of spouse	Caucasian
Retirement	Male
Death of friends	Higher income
Increased leisure time	Higher education
Change in financial status	

A family history of alcohol dependence is less common in late-onset alcoholism than early-onset.

6. How can late-onset alcohol use disorders be prevented?

Prevention of excessive alcohol use is enhanced by a good **physician-patient relationship**. Routinely asking a patient about alcohol use, about significant stressors or losses, and about major changes in a patient's life such as retirement or loss of independence are keys to recognizing the onset of many problems, including problems with alcohol use. Recognition of these risk factors is paramount in preventing the escalating use of alcohol. This type of clinical relationship is becoming difficult as less time is spent with patients and as patients transfer care between many physicians.

The **community** can also play a role in preventing alcoholism. Programs at senior centers, churches, or community colleges can provide educational activities as well as social support networks for all elders. Health care providers should routinely inquire about a patient's leisure time management and hobbies and help to support community involvement. An intact social group of non–alcohol-abusing peers is an important aspect to preventing late-onset problem drinking.

7. Do changes in alcohol metabolism and degree of intoxication occur with aging?

The older person is more likely to have a higher blood alcohol level and suffer more acute intoxicating effects, such as trouble with balance, changes in fine motor skills, and cognitive dysfunction. This effect may be more pronounced in older women than in older men but has not been thoroughly studied. This effect represents a change in the volume of distribution of alcohol and not changes in hepatic metabolism. Also, changes in body mass and fat distribution occur with aging that will cause an increase in the blood alcohol level for a given amount of alcohol. Age-associated changes in the blood-brain barrier may make an older person more vulnerable to the intoxicating effects of alcohol. The increased intoxicating effect seen with older people is consistent with findings that the quantity of consumption but not the frequency decreases as people age. The older individual may reduce the amount consumed because less alcohol is necessary to produce a similar effect as when the person was 20 years younger.

8. What is the best way to identify patients with alcohol problems?

The **clinical interview** is the best tool for identifying persons with alcohol-related problems. Alcohol abuse and dependence have been shown to be underdiagnosed among the elderly in hospitals and primary care clinics. Several easily administered screening instruments have both good sensitivity and specificity. The **CAGE** interview is recommended as quick and sensitive. The patient is first asked if they have drunk any alcohol in their life. If the patient answers "yes," they are asked the following four questions:

1. Have you ever had the desire or attempted to **C**ut down on your drinking?
2. Have you ever become **A**nnoyed at someone because they told you that you had a drinking problem?
3. Have you ever felt **G**uilty about your drinking?
4. Have you ever drunk before noon or had an **E**ye-opener?

If the person answers yes to any of these questions, then a detailed alcohol use history is taken, with careful attention to how alcohol use has affected the patient's life. The use of clinic brochures and educating clinic staff about alcohol use problems are also effective ways of recognizing early problems. Prevention is the key to treating late-onset alcoholism.

9. List the medical problems associated with alcohol use.

Alcohol-related medical problems can be one of the best ways of identifying patients with alcohol use disorders, which have been associated with toxic effects on almost every organ system.

Hepatic dysfunction
Gastrointestinal disorders (varices, gastritis, pancreatitis, esophagitis)
Central and peripheral nervous system dysfunction
Anemia (macrocytic)
Myopathy
Cardiomyopathy
Aspiration pneumonia
Malnutrition (specifically thiamine deficiency)
Cancer (hepatic, GI, head and neck)

10. What is the best treatment for acute alcohol withdrawal?

Acute alcohol withdrawal, alcohol withdrawal seizures, and alcohol withdrawal delirium are preventable disorders. Careful history to identify those patients at risk is the key to prevention. In the event that alcohol is not available to a patient, such as after admission to the hospital or when required to stop drinking for tests, proper detoxification can prevent significant morbidity to the patient. Onset of acute confusion or other mental status changes after several days in the hospital should also alert the clinician to the possibility of alcohol withdrawal. The standard treatment for detoxification or for treating withdrawal symptoms is the use of **benzodiazepines** such as oxazepam. The dose of benzodiazepine should be titrated for each individual. The clinician should avoid overmedicating the patient and can use autonomic signs, such as heart rate and blood pressure, to guide the treatment.

11. Discuss the best treatment plan for a patient with an alcohol use disorder.

After you recognize that a patient has an alcohol problem, most patients are best treated in a structured **outpatient addiction program**. Also recognize that for some patients, the stigma associated with being in an addiction program makes them refuse to participate in a program. There is also evidence that the late-onset alcoholic is much less likely to seek treatment, although such individuals do respond to treatment. Some of these patients can be managed as outpatients in a primary care clinic. If a patient does not achieve abstinence or remission of the abuse or dependence, then convincing the patient of the merits of a treatment program becomes a key element in overall care. Although being firm about recommending treatment is important, it is also important for the physician to maintain a relationship with the patient so that you can continue to work with the patient on treating the illness.

Although alcohol use disorders are chronic illnesses and patients are prone to remissions and exacerbations, the long-term outcome for patients can be good. With close attention to drinking, family support, and management of leisure time, patients can change drinking habits. The literature suggests that older patients are as likely as younger patients to respond to treatment. The benefits of abstinence are not only improved quality of life and improved relationships, but also many of the toxic physical effects of alcohol are reversible.

12. Which types of medications should be avoided in patients with alcohol use problems?

Many medications interact with alcohol causing an increase in side effects or toxic effects. Medications that are hepatically metabolized or are active in the CNS should be used with caution in patients who are actively drinking. In patients with an alcohol use disorder that is in remission, it is important to realize that medications such as benzodiazepines and opiates are also addicting and have the potential for abuse or causing a relapse. However, these medications can be used if there is an illness that warrants their use, such as acute pain or anxiety disorders, or for the short-term relief of insomnia. The key to using these medications is the careful monitoring of both the medications and alcohol use.

Medications with potential drug–alcohol interactions include:

H$_2$ blockers	β-blockers	Antihypertensives
Aspirin	NSAIDs	Nitroglycerin
Warfarin	Acetaminophen	Certain antibiotics
Benzodiazepines	Oral hypoglycemics	

13. Should naltrexone or disulfiram (Antabuse) be prescribed?

Medications that reduce a person's craving for alcohol or cause adverse effects after drinking have been demonstrated effective only in the context of an addiction program. They should not be used as the sole method of treatment.

14. How can the clinician respect patient confidentiality while involving the family in treatment?

The family may be one of the best allies in identifying and treating patients with addiction problems. Patients have the right to refuse any discussions with family, and consent from the patient should be obtained before discussing issues about substance use with family members. Care providers should educate patients, however, about eliciting the assistance of family members. As with any chronic condition, emotional support from family members and close friends is an important predictor of treatment response. Patients and physicians should also realize that family members are usually aware of a patient's alcohol use, and refusal to allow family members to help is often a way for a patient to obstruct treatment consciously or unconsciously.

BIBLIOGRAPHY

1. Curtis J, Millman E, Joseph M, et al: Prevalence rates for alcoholism, associated depression and dementia on the Harlem Hospital Medicine and Surgery Services. Adv in Alcohol Subst Abuse 6:45–65, 1986.
2. Frances A: Diagnostic and Statistical Manual of Mental Disorders, 4th ed. Washington, DC, American Psychiatric Press, 1994.
3. LaCroix AZ, Guralnik JM, Berkman LF, et al: Maintaining mobility in late life. Am J Epidemiol 137:858–869, 1993.
4. Liberto J, Oslin D, Ruskin P: Alcoholism in older persons: A review of the literature. Hosp Commun Psychiatry 43:975–984, 1992.
5. Nelson DE, Sattin RW, Langlois JA, et al: Alcohol as a risk factor for fall injury events among elderly persons living in the community. J Am Geriat Soc 40:658–661, 1992.
6. Nelson HD, Nevitt MC, Scott JC, et al: Smoking, alcohol, and neuromuscular and physical function of older women. JAMA 272:1825–1831, 1994.
7. O'Loughlin JL, Robitaille Y, Boivin J-F, Suissa S: Incidence of and risk factors for falls and injurious falls among the community-dwelling elderly. Am J Epidemiol 137:342–354, 1993.
8. Oslin DW, Liberto JG: Substance abuse in the elderly. In O'Brien C (ed.): Psychiatry. Philadelphia, J.B. Lippincott, 1995.

18. TOBACCO USE AMONG THE ELDERLY

Charles Spencer, M.D., Ph.D.

1. What is the prevalence of tobacco use among older adults?

Tobacco use is the leading preventable cause of death in the United States. The total number of smokers in the U.S. in 1991 was 46.3 million. Of these, 16.5% were 65–74 years old and 8.4% were 75 years or older. Most elderly tobacco users began at age 15–25 years and thus have a smoking history greater than 50 pack years. To discourage tobacco use, patients must be convinced that cessation increases longevity and improves quality of life.

Percentage of Adults Who Were Current Cigarette Smokers: United States National Health Interview Survey, 1990, 1991

AGE	MEN (%)		WOMEN (%)		TOTAL	
	1990	1991	1990	1991	1990	1991
18–24	26.6	23.5	22.5	22.4	24.5	22.9
25–44	32.9	32.9	26.6	28.0	29.7	30.4
45–64	29.3	29.3	24.8	24.6	27.0	26.9
65–74	18.3	18.2	15.6	15.1	16.8	16.5
> 75	7.6	9.2	5.8	7.9	6.5	8.4

2. How prevalent is the use of smokeless tobacco among the elderly?

Smokeless tobacco use in 1991 was higher among people 18–24 years of age or 75 years or older. For women the use was highest (2.3%) among those 75 years or older. Men 75 years or older accounted for the second highest age group (5.8%). Women favored snuff chewing tobacco, whereas among men snuff and chewing tobacco were equally distributed. The rural region of the South had the highest prevalence of use of smokeless tobacco.

3. What are the health costs and financial burdens associated with tobacco use?

Tobacco use directly and negatively affects both health and financial status. The financial burden for society of smoking has been recognized for a long time. However, only recently has the social burden of second-hand smoking been addressed. Health care expenditures have been estimated to be in excess of $65 billion in 1985 for the cost of smoking. These costs include extra expenditures for medical insurance, absenteeism from work, and injuries from fires due to cigarette smoking.

In 1989 the most common causes of death among the elderly were similar to those attributable to smoking-related diseases: coronary heart disease, cancer, cerebral vascular accidents, and chronic obstructive lung disease. Tobacco use substantially increases the relative risk of vascular diseases, such as strokes, heart attacks, sudden death, and ischemic peripheral vascular disease. In 1991 tobacco usage was associated with 85% of the 143,000 deaths due to lung cancer. The relative risk for cancer of the oral cavity, pharynx, esophagus, stomach, and bladder is increased by tobacco use. Pulmonary illnesses, such as bronchitis, pneumonia, emphysema, and obstructive lung disease, are strongly related to tobacco usage.

The alkaline constituents of smokeless tobacco are more readily absorbed through the oral and esophageal mucosa, whereas the more acidic cigarette smoke favors absorption through the bronchial airways. The acid-base balance and the method of use may contribute to the higher occurrence of oral lesions with smokeless tobacco.

Passive smoking has been related to heart disease and lung cancer in nonsmokers. Passive smoking also affects the birth weight of infants. The effects of tobacco use by grandparents or other older adults living with young children, infants, or pregnant women may be inferred to be detrimental, but they have not been investigated.

Osteoporosis and cataracts, diseases with particular significance to the well-being of the elderly, are exacerbated by smoking.

Dental health and denture condition are significantly impaired by tobacco use in the elderly. Reluctance to leave elderly tobacco users alone because of the increased risk of fires and burns also contributes to the health and financial burden.

Estimated Smoking-attributable Mortality. Relative Risk Attributable to Smoking (Current) Compared with Non-smokers, 1990

	RELATIVE RISK	
	CURRENT SMOKER, MALE	CURRENT SMOKER, FEMALE
Disease (> 35 yr)		
Cancer		
Lip, oral cavity and pharynx	27.5	5.6
Esophagus	7.6	10.3
Larynx	10.5	17.8
Trachea, lung and bronchus	22.4	11.9
Cardiovascular		
Hypertension	1.9	1.7
Ischemic heart		
35–64	2.8	3.0
> 65	1.6	1.6
Strokes		
35–64	3.7	4.8
> 65	1.9	3.0
Atherosclerosis	4.1	3.0
Respiratory		
Pneumonia, influenza	2.0	2.2
Bronchitis, emphysema	9.7	10.5
Chronic obstructive lung	9.7	10.5

4. Is cessation of tobacco use beneficial in older adults?

Tobacco cessation is beneficial for both the young and the elderly. The health risk of cigarette smoking can be eliminated only by quitting; switching to lower "tar" and nicotine cigarettes is not a safe alternative. Fewer tobacco users survive to be elderly compared with people who have never used tobacco. Life expectancy is approximately 18 years shorter for a 30-year-old smoker. Cessation of smoking at any age increases longevity and has the potential to increase quality of life. For example, 65-year-old, one-pack-a-day smokers who quit can expect to increase their life expectancy by 2–3 years.

5. What characteristics distinguish the older smoker from a younger smoker?

Most older smokers were heavier smokers, smoked brands with higher nicotine content, had social contacts who also were smokers, did not believe that quitting would improve health (47%), and were the least likely to report that they wanted to stop smoking completely.

6. What is the best cessation strategy for older adults?

Because older smokers are heavier users of tobacco and often have a long smoking history, a multipronged approach is recommended to assist cessation. The physical addiction, psychological dependence, and habitual tendencies from tobacco use need to be addressed.

Nicotine substitutes in the form of gum or patch have been advocated. Both approaches require a motivated individual to avoid concurrent tobacco use. Consideration of asymptomatic ischemic heart and peripheral vascular diseases is essential before prescribing nicotine replacement therapy in the elderly. Serious adverse events, including stroke and myocardial infarction, have been reported with high dosages of nicotine substitutes in the elderly. Nervousness, irritability, sleep disturbance, and difficulty with concentration are common symptoms among the elderly and need to be interpreted cautiously by caregivers familiar with the patient.

Older smokers are less likely (14.7%) to succeed when they attempt to stop. Successful adults are usually younger (49.4% are 25–44 years old), more educated (42.2% have > 13 years of education) and less likely to use assisted methods of cessation. However, if older smokers succeed in stopping tobacco usage, they are less likely to relapse (5.7%).

The importance of physician input in smoking cessation is underscored by evidence that 70% of successful and relapse patients in all age groups were urged to stop by a physician.

7. Do withdrawal symptoms differ among the elderly?

Care providers need to be aware of atypical withdrawal symptoms among the elderly. Increased day-time naps and complaints of dyspepsia and rheumatism may be the equivalent of more typical withdrawal symptoms, such as headaches, sleep problems, and nausea.

8. What are the short-term benefits of smoking cessation?

Short-term benefits among the elderly are illustrated by anecdotal reports of less staining of dentures, improvement in breath odor, and fewer holes in clothes. The association of increased weight with cessation of tobacco may be beneficial among frail, elderly smokers.

9. What are the most effective ways of prescribing nicotine substitutes?

An estimate of tobacco dependence should be obtained before prescribing nicotine substitutes. Unstable cardiovascular diseases are a contraindication to the use of substitutes. The medication should be used cautiously in patients with uncontrolled thyroid disease, uncontrolled hypertension, peptic ulcers, severe renal impairment, severe liver disease, and uncontrolled diabetes. The patch should be avoided in patients with active skin problems. Nicotine substitutes should be used only after tobacco use has stopped

Nicotine substitutes should be used with adjuvant behavior modification therapy. Nicotine chewing gums should be chewed only when there is an urge to smoke or on a schedule; the gum is not to be chewed continuously. Nicotine gums may soon be available over the counter without a prescription. The patches are used daily, with tapering dosage every 4–8 weeks. Behavior support should continue after nicotine substitutes are stopped.

10. Do behavior modification techniques work in the elderly?

Behavior therapy in concert with nicotine substitutes has had mixed results. The consensus is that behavior therapy does not increase the cessation rate. Subset analysis on such groups as older smokers, heavier smokers, educated smokers, and single vs. married smokers needs to be studied.

11. Is the recommendation to quit smoking ever unwarranted?

The recommendation to quit smoking is never unwarranted. Smoking cessation benefits both the individual and society. However, one can respect the individual's choice, especially in the hospice patient who is terminally ill.

BIBLIOGRAPHY

1. Bartecchi CE, MacKenzie TD, Schrier RW: The human costs of tobacco use (Pt 1). N Engl J Med 330: 907–912, 1994.
2. Burns D: Cigarettes and cigarette smoking. Clin Chest Med 12:631–642, 1991.
3. Cox J: Smoking cessation in the elderly patient. Clin Chest Med 14:423–428, 1993.
4. Fiore MC (ed): Cigarette smoking. Med Clin North Am 76(2), 1982 [special issue].
5. Fiore MC, Norotny TE, Pierce JP, et al: Methods used to quit smoking in the United States: Do cessation programs help? JAMA 263:2760–2765, 1990.

6. Giovino GA, Schooley MW, Zhu BP, et al: Surveillance for selected tobacco use behaviors, United States, 1900–1994. MMWR 43 (No SS–3):1–43, 1994.

7. Henningfield JE: Drug therapy: Nicotine medications for smoking cessation. N Engl J Med 333: 1196–1203, 1995.

8. Jorenby DE, Smith SS, Fiore MC, et al. Varying nicotine patch dose and type of smoking cessation counseling. JAMA 274:1347–1352, 1995.

9. Nelson DE, Kirkendill RS, Lawton RL, et al: Surveillance for smoking-attributable mortality and years of potential life lost, by state–United States, 1990. MMWR 43 (No SS-1):1–8, 1994.

10. Spangler JG, Salisbury PL: Smokeless tobacco: Epidemiology, health effects and cessation strategies. Am Fam Physician 52:1421–1430, 1995.

11. U.S. Department of Health and Human Services: The Health Consequences of Smoking. Nicotine Addiction. A Report of the Surgeon General. (DHHS Publication No. [CDC] 99–8496). Washington, DC, U.S. Department of Health and Human Services, 1988.

19. SENSORY CHANGES

Eugenia L. Siegler, M.D.

1. What major changes does the eye undergo with aging?

Presbyopia, the loss of accommodative ability, is the best known of the age-associated ocular changes. This is due to hardening of the lens nucleus (nuclear sclerosis) and ciliary muscle atrophy. It begins at approximately age 40 and progresses; by the 60s, little, if any, ability to accommodate remains.

The eye undergoes other changes with age, as well. The retina receives less light as we age, because of increased light absorption by the lens, cornea, and vitreous. Pupils do not dilate as much when the environment darkens, which also reduces the amount of light that reaches the retina. Increasing opacity of the lens and other parts of the eye leads to reduction of contrast by scattering the light. At the retinal level, most elderly lose rods and, to a lesser extent, cones, as well as retinal ganglion cells. These changes can lead to some reduction in visual acuity and/or functional peripheral vision, but the common ophthalmologic diseases have a far greater impact (see Question 3).

2. What is the relationship between visual impairment and age?

Visual loss, thought to lead to functional consequences, is usually defined as < 20/40 in the better eye. In the Baltimore Eye Survey, prevalence of visual loss was approximately 2% in whites and 8% in African-Americans in the 60–69-year age group; in those age 80 and older, the prevalence was 35% in whites and 40% in African-Americans. In a study conducted by the same group in nursing homes, the prevalence of poor vision was found to be almost 36% (of those participating in the study, 57% were white and 43% were African-American). Blindness, defined as visual acuity ≤ 20/200 in the better eye, appears to be far more prevalent in nursing homes than in the community. For example, the prevalences in those aged 70–79 (11.3% in whites and 18% in African-Americans) were 18.8- and 6.2-fold higher than in the corresponding community.

Significant numbers of community-dwelling and institutionalized elderly have refractive errors for which correction could improve vision. Improving vision (through refraction, cataract surgery, or other methods) leads to improved quality of life; the worse the initial vision, the greater the increase in quality of life with an improvement in vision. Individuals with visual impairments may also benefit from low-vision clinics, which can provide both counseling and adaptive devices.

3. Name the four most common ophthalmologic diseases in the elderly.

The Framingham eye study documented the prevalences of these four diseases, and all increased with age. These four are also the most common causes of blindness in community-dwelling elderly. In the nursing home, cataracts, corneal opacity, age-related macular degeneration, and open-angle glaucoma are the most common.

Condition	Prevalence in Those Aged 75–85
Cataract	46%
Age-related macular degeneration	28%
Open-angle glaucoma	7.2%
Diabetic retinopathy	7%

4. What are the potential adverse reactions of medications used to treat open-angle glaucoma?

Both oral and instilled glaucoma medications have significant side effects. Systemic side effects of the drops can be reduced by having the patient occlude the lacrimal puncta for 5 minutes while and after drops are instilled. It is also useful to check bottles to see if the preparation contains sulfites, which may cause allergic reactions.

Common Drugs for Glaucoma and Their Side Effects

CLASS	MECHANISM	PRODUCTS (BRANDNAME)	SIDE EFFECTS
Beta-blockers	Decrease aqueous production	Timolol (Timoptic) Betaxolol (Betoptic) Levobunolol (Betagan)	Bronchospasm, bradycardia, hypotension, slowed conduction, worsened CHF, confusion
Miotics Direct para-sympathetic	Increase aqueous outflow	Pilocarpine (Pilocar, Isopto Carpine, OcuCarpine) Carbachol (IsoptoCarbachol)	GI, bronchospasm, bradycardia, confusion, poor night vision (Worse with cholinesterase inhibitors.)
Cholinesterase inhibitors		Demecarium (Humorsol) Echothiophate (Phospholine) Isoflurophate (Floropryl) Physostigmine (Isoptoeserine)	
Sympathetic agonists	Increase aqueous outflow	Dipivefrin (Propine) Epinephrine (Epifrin, Glaucon)	Dipivefrin is quite safe. Epinephrine can be very cardiotoxic.
Carbonic anhydrase inhibitors	Decrease aqueous production	Acetazolamide (Diamox) Methazolamide (Neptazane) Dichlorphenamide (Daranide)	GI, CNS, aplastic anemia, renal stones, acidosis, altered drug excretion

CHF = congestive heart failure.

5. How does the sense of taste change in the elderly?

Ageusia is the loss of the sense of taste. The sensation of a bad taste in the mouth is called **dysgeusia**. Weiffenbach and Bartoshuk describe a test to distinguish between peripheral (e.g., occurring in the mouth) and central dysgeusias. The patient should first try to rinse the taste away. If it does go away, even only briefly, the origin of the dysgeusia is probably oral. The clinician can then administer a local anesthetic to the mouth. If the dysgeusia gets stronger, the origin is probably in the CNS and referral to a neurologist is indicated. These disorders can include temporal lobe tumors and damage to the chorda tympani.

Although thresholds for both detection of a substance and correct identification (recognition) increase with age beginning about age 60, these changes are of questionable clinical significance. Therefore, most people do not perceive a significant decline in taste with age. Many conditions, such as Bell's palsy, head trauma, chorda tympani damage from upper respiratory and ear infections, cancer, depression, hepatic and renal disease, zinc deficiency, hypothyroidism, and diabetes mellitus, can affect the sense of taste. Laryngectory and local radiation therapy can also alter taste sensation.

6. Can drugs affect the sense of taste?

Of the scores of drugs that can change the sense of taste, the following are commonly used by the elderly:

Antibiotics
  Ampicillin
  Tetracyclines
  Metronidazole
Antihypertensives
  ACE inhibitors
  Calcium channel blockers
  Ethacrynic acid

CNS active agents
  Carbamazepine
  Levodopa
  Lithium
  Phenytoin
Anti-gout medications
  Allopurinol
  Colchicine

7. How does the sense of smell change in the elderly?

Anosmia is the loss of the sense of smell. Those who complain of a persistent bad smell have a **parosmia**. The sense of smell (olfaction) declines far more dramatically with age than does the sense of taste. Some smell-like characteristics, such as pungency, are sensed by the trigeminal nerve and appear not to decline as much as true olfaction. The age-related decline in ability to recognize odors does have clinical significance; for example, elderly may have difficulty detecting that food is no longer edible or that natural gas is escaping from the stove.

Anosmia also has a major impact on quality of life. Much of the sensory stimulus that is perceived as taste, is actually smell. A patient with anosmia can taste the sweetness of ice cream but, without visual cues of color, will not be able to determine the flavor. Such a chemosensory loss may have enormous impact on a patient's appetite or enjoyment of food. Unfortunately, little can be done to treat loss of smell and taste, except for discontinuation of medications that might be contributing to loss of smell. Counseling is another important option.

8. What diseases or conditions often seen in the elderly can affect the sense of smell?

Alzheimer's disease	Rhinitis
Parkinson's disease	Sinusitis
Head trauma	Asthma
Renal and liver disease	Viral infections
Hypothyroidism	Laryngectomy
Diabetes mellitus	

9. What medications?

Calcium channel blockers, antithyroid agents, opiates, and amphetamines.

10. What are the most common causes of hearing loss in the elderly?

Approximately 40% of elderly individuals have some form of chronic hearing impairment, defined as the inability to hear a pure tone softer than 40 dB at more than one frequency in one or both ears. The most common cause of bilateral hearing loss in the elderly is **presbycusis**, which is a sensorineural loss marked by difficulty hearing high frequency tones and by impaired speech comprehension. Patients with presbycusis may also complain of **recruitment**, the perception that a sound has become dramatically louder despite only a modest increase in volume. Other causes of hearing loss in the elderly include cerumen plugs, otosclerosis, ototoxicity, Meniere's disease, and acoustic neuromas.

11. How can a primary care provider screen for hearing loss?

There are two basic kinds of screens.

1. **Measure the extent of hearing loss with a series of sounds or words:** One such tool is the Audioscope (Welch-Allyn, Inc., Skaneateles Falls, NY). The Audioscope resembles an otoscope and tests the patient's ability to hear pure tones. It emits a series of tones ranging from 500–4000 Hz into the ear. Standard pure-tone audiometers have been used for years but are less convenient to use. The Audioscope also enables visual inspection of the ear canal at the time of the test. The test can be deferred or canceled if excessive cerumen or pathology is found.

2. **Question the patient about the impact of hearing loss.** The Hearing Handicap Inventory for the Elderly–Screening Version (HHIE-S) consists of 10 questions that the patient answers either in response to a questioner or on a self-administered form. It measures the impact of hearing loss on social functioning. Scored on a 40-point scale, the test is considered positive for a severe handicap if the patient scores > 24 points. Another verbal handicap screen, the Self-Assessment of Communication (SAC), has also performed well in studies.

Despite their different approaches, these two types of screens have similar test characteristics. Sensitivities and specificities range from roughly 60–90% depending on the test cutoff points that are used. Unfortunately, compliance with advice at time of screening is poor, with only 15% of patients found to have a hearing impairment going on to buy a hearing aid. (See also chapter 11.)

12. What kinds of devices can be used to improve hearing?

There are a wide variety of amplification devices. **Hearing aids** amplify and modify sound and deliver it directly to the canal. Since the early 1980s the most popular type has been worn in the ear. The version worn behind the ear is also popular and may be more easily manipulated by patients with visual impairments or arthritis. Hearing aids can be unilateral or bilateral and can be analog, digital, or hybrid. Despite the high prevalence of hearing loss, approximately 85% of hearing-impaired elderly lack hearing aids.

Assistive listening devices (ALD) are used to connect the hearing-impaired individual directly to the source of the sound. They are usually found in special settings, such as theaters and places of worship. Another kind of ALD, a personal amplifier, can be purchased from electronics stores. Individuals speak directly into the amplifier, which transmits sound to the patient via earphones. These small devices are useful for those who cannot manipulate hearing aids or who need to communicate one-on-one in noisy areas.

A **cochlear implant**, which is a 22-channel electrode that is surgically implanted in the ear, may be helpful for severely hearing-impaired individuals.

13. What techniques can you employ to communicate with those with hearing loss?

Speak clearly and slowly with a normal tone of voice. The hearing-impaired person may hear better if seated or standing against a wall. When the hearing-impaired person does not understand you, rephrase, don't repeat. Avoid competing noises by eliminating television, radio, and other background noises. Keep groups small so that the hearing-impaired individual can follow the conversation. Allow the hearing-impaired person to take advantage of visual cues: make sure your face can be easily seen, and use gestures when appropriate.

14. Do other sensory changes occur in the elderly?

Healthy elderly can show a number of subtle abnormalities on thorough physical examination. Kaye et al., in a cross-sectional study comparing healthy, community-dwelling elderly aged 64–75 (young old) to those aged > 84 (oldest old), documented a high prevalence of many abnormalities in the oldest old, especially in gait, balance, and sensory function (vibration, proprioception, and stereognosis). They then used discriminant analysis to demonstrate that the oldest old performed more poorly than the young old in tests of olfaction, visual pursuit, one-leg standing with eyes closed, and heel-toe walking. Loss of vibratory sense also appeared to be important. These are "usual" aging changes. Elderly with comorbidities can be expected to have additional sensory changes.

BIBLIOGRAPHY

1. Ad Hoc Committee on Hearing Screening in Adults: Considerations in screening adults/older persons for handicapping hearing impairments. ASHA Aug:81–87, 1992.
2. Kaye JA, Oken BS, Howieson DB, et al: Neurologic evaluation of the optimally healthy oldest old. Arch Neurol 51:1205–1211, 1994.
3. Kini MM, Leibowitz HM, Colton T, et al: Prevalence of senile cataract, diabetic retinopathy, senile macular degeneration, and open-angle glaucoma in the Framingham eye study. Am J Ophthalmol 85:28–34, 1978.
4. Lavizzo-Mourey RJ, Siegler EL: Hearing impairment in the elderly. J Gen Intern Med 7:191–197, 1992.
5. Owsley C, Ball K: Assessing visual function in the older driver. Clin Geriatr Med 9:389–401, 1993.
6. Schiffman S: Changes in taste and smell: Drug interactions and food preferences. Nutr Rev 52(II):S11–S14, 1994.
7. Tielsch JM, Javitt JC, Coleman A, et al: The prevalence of blindness and visual impairment among nursing home residents in Baltimore. N Engl J Med 332:1205–1209, 1995.
8. Tielsch JM, Sommer A, Witt K, et al (Baltimore Eye Survey Research Group): Blindness and visual impairment in an American urban population. Arch Ophthalmol 108:286–290, 1990.
9. Weiffenbach JM, Bartoshuk LM: Taste and smell. Clin Geriatr Med 8:543–555, 1992.

20. HYPERTENSION IN THE ELDERLY

Mary Ann Forciea, M.D.

1. What levels of blood pressure are diagnostic of hypertension in the elderly?

Two varieties of hypertension are seen in older patients: (1) **essential hypertension** (also called systolic-diastolic hypertension),where systolic blood pressure (BP) is > 160 mm Hg and diastolic BP is > 95, and (2) **isolated systolic hypertension**, where systolic BP is > 160 mm Hg and diastolic BP is < 90. Both forms can have "borderline" conditions in which systolic BP readings are between 140–160 mm Hg. **Secondary** hypertension is an elevation in BP caused by another disease process, such as pheochromocytoma or renal artery stenosis. These disorders are rare in office practice.

2. How common is hypertension in the elderly?

A large community survey of 906 people aged 71–96 years revealed the following prevalence of hypertension:

Normotensive	39.4%	Isolated systolic hypertension	13.2%
Borderline isolated	28.6%	Diastolic hypertension	9.5%
systolic hypertension		Hypertensive by mixed criteria	9.3%

The prevalence of hypertension varies with race and age. Essential hypertension is seen in patients over 65 years of age in approximately 15% of whites and 25% of blacks. Isolated systolic hypertension is seen in 10% of patients > 70 and 20% of patients > 80.

3. Is the etiology of hypertension different in older patients?

Changes in peripheral vascular resistance are central to the development of both essential and isolated systolic hypertension in older patients. Resistance may increase due to occlusion of a blood vessel lumen (as with atherosclerotic change) and/or changes in vascular smooth muscle. Decreases occur in β-adrenergic smooth muscle dilatation during normal aging, but α-adrenergic-mediated vasoconstriction is largely unchanged. This alteration in balance of adrenergic-mediated vessel wall tone leads to a heightened tendency to vasoconstriction and to increased peripheral vascular resistance.

A second mechanism for elevated BP is an expanded extracellular volume, which may develop especially in black and elderly hypertensives. Both groups of patients exhibit low plasma renin levels and high sensitivity to dietary sodium.

4. Are the complications of hypertension different in older patients?

Cardiovascular disease is strongly linked to hypertension at all ages, including late life.

- The incidence of **left ventricular hypertrophy** (LVH) correlates highly with systolic BP in older patients. The presence of LVH continues to predict for arrhythmias.
- Both essential and isolated systolic hypertension correlate with future vascular events. In a longitudinal study of community-living adults, 70% of **strokes** in elderly women and 42% of strokes in older men were directly attributed to hypertension.
- Another large study of community-dwelling men has shown continued risk of **end-stage renal disease** with hypertension throughout all age ranges.

5. Can the complications of hypertension in elderly patients be avoided with treatment?

Several large studies have documented that cardiovascular mortality and morbidity can be reduced with treatment of hypertension, even in late life. When compared to outcomes in patients of all ages treated with placebo, patients > 60 years old show the same percentage reduction in events as patients < 50. Because the number of events is much larger in older patients, the reduction in absolute numbers of events in older patients is larger. Applegate has summarized the effects of treatment as follows:

Essential hypertension
Mild (diastolic BP 90–105mm Hg): reduction of 5–8 events/1000 patient-years of treatment
Moderate (diastolic BP 105–115mm Hg): reduction of 20–30 events/1000 patient-years of treatment

Isolated systolic hypertension
31% reduction in cardiovascular events
35% reduction in stroke
Reduction of 50 events/1000 patient-years of treatment

Studies have yet to document a benefit on renal function with treatment of hypertension in patients > 70, but there is little reason to believe that a reduction in BP would be less beneficial in older patients.

6. Explain how blood pressure is measured in the elderly patient.

Measurement of BP in older patients must be performed with special care to avoid artifactual elevation. The standard of measurement is described using a sphygmomanometer connected to a column of mercury (Hg). Aneroid manometers can be used but must be calibrated against a mercury standard every 6 months. Measurement techniques are based on the detection of vibrations produced by the arterial wall under pressure (**Korotkoff sounds**).

The arm is the usual site of measurement. The cuff used must be positioned correctly and be large enough that the air bladder compresses an adequate area of the brachial artery. The distal margin of the cuff should be at least 3 cm proximal to the antecubital fossa, with the midline of the bladder (usually marked on the cuff) over the palpable artery. The cuff should extend to at least the midpoint of the biceps. Use of a cuff that is too small can result in readings that are 10–15 mm Hg higher than the actual BP.

The cuff is inflated to a level of Hg that is 30 mm over that at which the brachial pulse disappears. The valve is opened, and the level of Hg is allowed to fall slowly. The bell of the stethoscope is placed lightly over the artery. The level of Hg at which the first sounds appear is the **systolic** BP. The sounds will remain loud for a considerable time. The level at which the sounds disappear is the **diastolic** BP. In many patients, a "muffling" of the sound appears shortly before the sounds disappear completely. When this phenomenon appears, the point of muffling should also be recorded (e.g., 140/85/80).

The listener should continue observations to the point of 0 mm Hg. In some patients, the sounds will reappear. The silent period is called an **auscultatory gap**. The point of permanent disappearance of sound is most reflective of the true diastolic BP. In rare conditions, such as thyrotoxicosis and aortic insufficiency, the sounds may continue to 0. In that event, the point of muffling is the most acccurate assessment of the diastolic pressure.

Measurement with the patient in the seated position with the back supported is again the standard. On an initial visit, BP should be measured in both arms. Atherosclerotic obstruction to flow in an arm may result in a lower BP reading. In patients with such a differential, the higher reading is the more accurate reflection of systemic pressure. An initial visit should also include readings in seated and standing positions, because of the frequency of orthostatic hypotension in elderly patients.

Many patients purchase home BP monitors. These machines vary in quality. Patients should bring the machines with them to their next office visit so that the machines can be calibrated against a mercury sphygmomanometer and so that the reproducibility of the home machine can be checked. In addition, the technique used to measure BP can be checked for adequacy.

7. What is white coat hypertension?

BP should be measured with the patient relaxed and comfortable. "White coat hypertension" is a condition of transient hypertension created by the anxiety of the office encounter.

Hypertension should not be diagnosed in the mild or moderate stages on a single office visit. Pressures should be repeated on 2 or 3 visits before consideration of treatment. Severe BP elevations (diastolic readings of >110) should be treated immediately.

In some situations the patient's arms may be inaccessible. Pressure can be taken in the thigh, using an especially large cuff. Ideally, the patient lies prone. The cuff is wrapped so that it extends a few centimeters proximal to the popliteal fossa. Pressure is measured over the popliteal artery.

8. What is pseudohypertension?

Pseudohypertension is a condition of falsely elevated BP readings caused by calcification of the arteries. The condition can be suspected if mild BP elevation is seen, if no end-organ damage of hypertension is found, and/or if patients rapidly develop symptoms of volume depletion or hypotension on medications. The diagnosis is confirmed with **Osler's maneuver:** the cuff is inflated above the disappearance of sounds, and the brachial artery is palpated. If the artery is easily felt, the diagnosis is confirmed. Such patients should be maintained at modestly higher BP levels before treatment is considered.

9. Which parts of the history and physical exam are most important in hypertensive patients?

Hypertension discovered in the office is notoriously free of symptoms in older as well as younger patients. Inquiry should be made into prior diagnoses of "high blood pressure." The presence of other risk factors for cardiovascular disease, such as smoking, should be determined. A careful listing of prescription and over-the-counter medications should be made both to determine whether medications may be elevating BP and to guard against medication interactions. Baseline determinations of mood, sexual functioning, and sleep habits should be made, since changes in these symptoms are often considered side effects of medication. Social situations such as poverty which might limit compliance should be ascertained.

The physical examination confirms the diagnosis of hypertension. BP determinations are accomplished as described previously (see Question 6). Examination of the eye grounds can document the presence of retinal disease. Stages are:

1—Ratio of diameter of arterioles to veins is < 2:3 or 3:4 ("arteriolar narrowing")
2—Focal spasm of arterioles
3—Hemorrhages and exudates
4—Papilledema

Evidence of left ventricular hypertrophy should be sought. The characteristics of the cardiac apex should be noted, both in size and force of impulse. Because patients with hypertension are at risk for abdominal aortic aneurysm, careful palpation of the abdomen should always be done. The neurologic examination should look for signs associated with stroke.

Secondary hypertension should be suspected in patients who develop new or sudden-onset hypertension with a diastolic BP > 105 mm Hg, who have persistent elevations of diastolic pressures > 100 mm Hg despite treatment regimens, or who develop accelerated elevations in readings. Such patients should be referred for specialty evaluations.

10. Which laboratory tests are important in the initial evaluation of a hypertensive patient?

All new patients should have measurements of complete blood counts, serum sodium, potassium, bicarbonate, chloride, glucose, blood urea nitrogen, creatinine, uric acid, and calcium. Cholesterol screening should be performed (see also Chapter 11), as should an electrocardiogram. The role of routine chest x-ray remains controversial. One strategy is to do a baseline film, with subsequent films obtained only if clinically indicated.

11. What are the goals of treatment?

Treatment goals for most older patients should be systolic pressures of 135–140 mm Hg and diastolic pressures of approximately 85 mm Hg. It is important to remember that overtreatment of hypertension can be dangerous: hypotension may result in falls.

12. How should hypertension be treated?

Options for the traditional treatment of hypertension include **weight reduction** for those patients above ideal body weight, **dietary sodium restriction, exercise**, and **medications**. These treatments are often prescribed in combination. Applegate has described a program of weight loss, exercise, and sodium restriction that resulted in reductions of systolic BP of 6 mm Hg and diastolic BP of 5 mm Hg in older patients with mild hypertension.

Weight loss and **dietary sodium restriction** programs can often be best taught in consultation with a registered dietician (available through most hospitals). In the elderly, some patients become so concerned with diet that malnutrition may result; dietary patterns should be regularly reviewed at office visits.

Exercise programs are highly acceptable to most elderly patients. To affect BP, the exercise regimen should be performed for approximately 30 minutes three times weekly. Initiation of the program should be gradual, with careful warm-up and cool-down periods. The benefits of regular exercise can extend beyond effects of BP (see also Chapter 15).

Alternative therapies for hypertension such as meditation and acupuncture have generated interest in some patients, but no studies have been done that demonstrate their efficacy in older patients. In patients with moderate or severe hypertension, patients should be encouraged to accept traditional therapy while pursuing nontraditional cures.

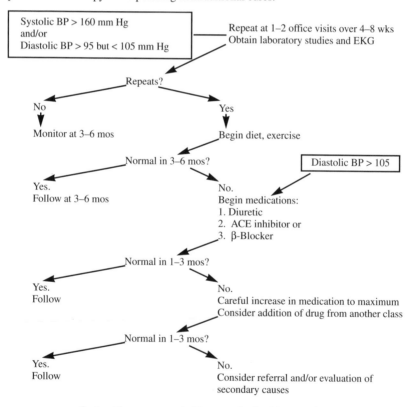

Protocol for management of hypertension in older outpatients.

13. When is drug therapy used?

Drug therapy is initiated when elevated BPs are noted on multiple visits, are in the moderate to severe levels, and/or when nonpharmacologic methods (such as diet and exercise) have not brought BP levels into the desired range.

Commonly Used Antihypertensive Medications

CLASS	DAILY DOSE	COST*
Diuretic		
Thiazides		
Hydrochlorothiazide (HCTZ)	12.5–50 mg	$ 1.04
Chlorthalidone	12.5–50 mg	$ 2.27
Loop diuretics		
Furosemide	20–320 mg	$ 1.73
Combinations		
HCTZ 25/triampterene	37.5, 1 tablet	$ 9.38
β-Adrenergic blockers		
Propranolol		
Regular	40–240 mg in 2 doses	$ 4.10
ER	80–240 mg in 1 dose	$23.18
Atenolol	25–50 mg in 1 or 2 doses	$20.26
ACE inhibitors		
Enalapril	2.5–40 mg in 1 or 2 doses	$19.09
Captopril	12.5–150 mg in 2 or 3 doses	$19.35
Calcium channel blockers		
Diltiazem ER (Cardizem CD)	120–360 mg in 1 dose	$31.32
Verapamil ER (Calan SR)	120–480 mg in 1 or 2 doses	$26.72

* Of lowest dose per 30 days, using average wholesale price.
ER = extended release.

14. Discuss the use of diuretics.

Diuretics were among the first classes of drugs shown to be effective in the treatment of hypertension, and they remain effective and in widespread use today. The efficacy of proximal-tubule diuretics, such as the thiazide group, in the reduction of BP in the elderly has been well documented. Thiazide diuretics can be ineffective in patients whose serum creatinine is > 1.5 mg/dl. Thiazide diuretics have been associated with hypokalemia, decreased glucose tolerance, impotence, and detrimental changes in serum lipids. These side effects may be transient or produce minimal change when compared to the drug's efficacy in lowering BP. Patients with serious or persistent alterations in lipids or glucose should be evaluated for change to another class of agents.

15. What are the drawbacks of β-blockers?

β-Adrenergic blockers are the next most widely used class of antihypertensive medications in general use. In the elderly and in African-American patients, in whom volume overload is a frequent contributor to hypertension, β-blockers may be less effective than they are in younger patients. In addition, traditional β-blockers have been avoided in patients with congestive heart failure and asthma, both of which are relatively common in the elderly. Depression and orthostatic hypotension are frequent complications and can limit the usefulness of this group in older patients.

16. Are any precautions necessary when using the ACE inhibitors?

Angiotensin-converting enzyme (ACE) inhibitors are effective and generally safe if used carefully. In diabetic patients, this class of agent has been shown to preserve renal function. Side effects include nonproductive cough in approximately 10% of elderly patients, hyperkalemia in patients with impaired renal function, and actual deterioration in renal function in those patients with impaired renal blood flow. Patients with high renin levels (as in volume depletion or congestive heart failure) may also develop abrupt and severe hypotension in response to ACE inhibition. Clearly, this class of antihypertensive must be initiated with caution in older patients.

17. Discuss the use of calcium channel blockers.

Calcium channel blockers have been widely used in the treatment of coronary artery disease. They cause vasodilatation and decreases in peripheral vascular resistance, which have made them attractive in the treatment of hypertension. Certain members of the class (e.g., nifedipine and isradipine) are associated with increases in heart rate. Verapamil and diltiazem are not associated with tachycardia but may slow conduction in the heart. Recent studies have demonstrated an increased rate of death in patients using the short-acting preparation of nifedipine. Data on the death rate in patients using the sustained-release forms of nifedipine are not yet available. For patients with hypertension as an isolated problem (e.g., no angina), a choice of antihypertensive agent from another class may be preferable.

18. When can antihypertensive medications be safely withdrawn?

Many experts now believe that careful withdrawal of antihypertensive medications can be attempted if:

1. The original level of BP was in the mild to moderate range
2. The patient's BP has been in good control for a sustained period (at least 12 months).

Monitored withdrawal of medication may be most successful in those patients who have been successful in weight loss, dietary modification, and exercise.

BIBLIOGRAPHY

1. Allman RM: Basic evaluation of older persons with hypertension. Clin Geriatr Med 5:717–732, 1989.
2. Applegate WB: High blood pressure treatment in the elderly. Clin Geriatr Med 8:103–117, 1992.
3. DeGowan EL, DeGowan RL: Bedside Diagnostic Examination. London, Macmillan, 1969, pp 379–382.
4. Drugs for hypertension. Med Lett 37:45–50, 1995.
5. Klag MJ, Whelton PK, Randall BL, et al: Blood pressure and end-stage renal disease in men. N Eng J Med 334:13–18, 1996.
6. Pahor M, Guralnik JM, Corti MC, et al: Long-term survival and use of antihypertensive medications in older persons. J Am Geriatr Soc 43:1191–1197, 1995.

21. DENTAL CARE

Roy S. Feldman, D.D.S., D.M.Sc., and Mary Ann Forciea, M.D.

1. Why is oral health particularly important for the elderly?

The mouth and oral cavity serve a variety of critical functions in people of all ages:

- Entry of food into the gastrointestinal tract
- Implementation of speech and communication (verbal and nonverbal)
- Maintenance of identity and self-esteem with facial appearance

In addition, examination of the mouth and oral cavity can provide critical information about the presence of systemic disease.

Elderly patients are at a much higher risk than younger patients for tooth loss, dental caries, gingival and periodontal disease, and oral cancers. This increased risk is due not only to increased "wear-and-tear" on the teeth and gingiva over a lifetime, but also to lower standards for dental care and less access to care during the youth and maturity of patients who now find themselves to be elderly.

2. How should the primary care provider ask patients about their oral health?

The following is a synopsis of screening questions useful in the history. Occasionally family caregivers may have to provide supplementary information.

- Do you have pain in your teeth, gums, or tongue?
- Do you experience bleeding from your gums?
- Is your mouth continually dry?
- Do you have sores in your mouth or on your tongue?
- Do you have loose, missing, or broken teeth?
- Do you have difficulty biting, chewing, or swallowing?
- Do you think you have halitosis?
- Do you have an altered sense of taste?
- If you wear dentures, do you have problems with any of the following:

  Fit?   Sores on palate or gums under dentures?
  Stability during chewing?   Impaction of food under dentures?
- How do you take care of your oral hygiene?

3. What constitutes a reasonable screening examination of the oral cavity for the primary care provider?

Primary care providers should always ask patients to remove prostheses before the examination. Tongue blades and gauze pads may be used to assist in exposing the structures of the oral cavity for examination. Palpation with gloved fingers is necessary to probe for induration. Examination with a flashlight increases the yield of discovered lesions. The following structures and associated lesions should receive special attention:

Structure	Lesion
Extraoral	
Skeletal structure	Misalignment of jaw, symmetry
Neck	Lymph node enlargement or pain, salivary gland size and consistency
Ears	Sensitivity to pain, congestion behind tympanic membrane
Temporomandibular joint	Tenderness, crepitus
Paranasal sinuses	Pain, reduced transillumination
Breath	Halitosis

Intraoral
Lips and mouth	Ulcers, swelling, redness, cracking lesions
Buccal mucosa	Tenderness, discoloration, induration
Tongue (dorsal and ventral)	Color, coating lesions, tremor
Palate	Symmetry, discolorations, lesions
Oropharynx	Color, masses, exudates, gag reflex
Gingiva	Color, bleeding, hypertrophy, exudates, food impaction
Teeth	Caries, root exposure
Prostheses	Fractures, retention, stability

4. When is a referral to a dentist appropriate?

Ettinger has developed the following useful list:

General	**Tooth-related**	**Denture-related**
Unexplained pain	Visible decay	Loose
Infection unresponsive to treatment	Loose or mobile teeth	Missing denture teeth
Persistent problems with mastication	Persistent bleeding	Palatal or gingival
Persistent halitosis		lesion under
Visible or palpable lesions		dentures

5. How should good oral hygiene be maintained?

Many older patients retain many of their own teeth. Brushing regularly with a toothpaste containing fluoride remains critical, even late in life. Dental floss should continue to be used to remove plaque and food from between teeth. Fluorides, present for decades in dentifrices, gels, and pastes, are now available in rinses, which may be excellent additions to the daily routine of people at risk for root surface caries. Acidulated sodium fluoride and stannous fluoride may be applied either within prostheses that are constructed as overdentures and maintain roots of teeth for support or to exposed roots with finger, brush, or cotton swab. Additional products are marketed without flavoring as mild dentifrices for sore and sensitive mouths and gums.

Geriatric patients should use mouth rinses with caution. Many contain relatively high alcohol concentrations (up to 25%), and most have been derived from the dental equivalent of herbal therapy, often at levels capable of promoting sensitivity and irritation in frail mouths. Chlorhexidine is most frequently prescribed at monthly intervals but should not be scheduled as a maintenance therapy for periodontal disease. Oral care is required on a regular basis, including plaque control and elimination of etiologic factors by prophylaxis (tooth-cleaning), scaling (scraping of calculus from tooth roots, often below the gingiva), and root planing (smoothing of the root to facilitate plaque removal). Extensive data document the efficacy of these therapies in controlling disease.

6. How should patients care for their dentures?

Dentures should be cleansed daily, much like the natural dentition. Perhaps twice a day, the dentures may be washed or scrubbed with any cleaning solution, even toothpaste. Most importantly, dentures must be cleaned on both surfaces. Removing the denture at night is advised, because the mouth is most comfortable when the dentures are not worn overnight. A soak is not necessary; 100% humidity (e.g., wrapped in a wet paper towel) is sufficient. If a soak is chosen, the solution may include a commercial cleanser, dilute vinegar, or even bleach at 1:10 dilution.

7. What methods of control may be useful in geriatric periodontal patients?

Control of periodontitis by mechanical (removal of etiologic agents by scaling) and antimicrobial therapies is effective at slowing or arresting progression of tissue loss about the teeth. Localized drug delivery systems may hold the key to maintenance therapy in geriatric patients. The combination of mechanical therapy and plastic fibers containing the tetracyclines, to which many periodontal pathogenic bacteria are susceptible, has proved more successful than conventional therapies or fibers alone. Fibers alone, even in the absence of supportive care, have significantly reduced disease recurrence after treatment and may offer a promising alternative to personnel-intensive mechanical therapy, which is often difficult to achieve in long-term care populations. The use of chlorhexidine mouthwash (Peridex or Dental-Guard) for antimicrobial effect in the management of gingivitis may well assist antifungal therapy.

Gingival inflammation, postoperative healing, and oral ulcerative diseases may benefit from some antimicrobials. However, no chemical agents have been shown to benefit periodontitis, which is an infection within periodontal tissues and presumably beyond the therapeutic efficacy of mouthwashes and rinses. Attempts to infuse inflamed tissues with these agents have failed to demonstrate efficacy in clinical trials.

8. When should oral candidiasis be suspected?
Oral candidiasis is frequently detected as a white pseudomembranous slough that is easily wiped off the mucosa to reveal an erythematous base. Pain may be a feature, leading to the term **denture-sore mouth**. Oral candidal infection does not lead to the formation of pockets of infection around teeth roots or result in loosening of the teeth.

9. List the risk factors for oral candidiasis.

Nutritional deficiencies	Immune deficiencies (e.g., AIDS, malignancy)
Antibiotic therapy	Ill-fitting or worn dental prostheses
Chemotherapy	Xerostomia
Steroid therapy	

10. What are the common clinical manifestations of oral candidiasis?
• Acute atrophic candidiasis (antibiotic-sore mouth)
• Angular cheilitis (perlèche)
• Chronic atrophic candidiasis (denture-sore mouth)
• Pseudomembranous candidiasis (thrush)

11. Are pharmacotherapeutic agents helpful in managing candidal infection?
Therapy directed at the candidal infection, either local and topical or systemic, also requires decontamination of dental prostheses, which otherwise will reseed the oral cavity. Dental prostheses are washed, scrubbed, and maintained in either commercial antifungal agents or dilute bleach or vinegar solutions. The dentures are then rinsed before they are replaced into the mouth.

12. What is xerostomia? How is it treated?
Xerostomia ("dry mouth") may be a sign or symptom as well as a clinical diagnosis of decreased or absent salivary production and secretion. Salivary glycoproteins, prominent in two distinct molecular weights, may be responsible for symptoms of dryness when salivary production is apparently normal. Conversely, clinicians are familiar with elders who fail to recognize severe salivary deficiency. Other symptoms that help to identify the cause include dysphagia, dysgeusia, burning mouth or tongue, and difficulty in phonation. Observation of diminished salivary flow rate or complaints of chronic dry mouth sensation are not sufficient diagnostic criteria; rather, combinations of these factors provide clinically important indications.

Xerostomia affects the ability to chew, presumably at the inception of the swallow. Accordingly, patients may avoid certain foods, especially chewy and crunchy foods, in favor of drier, sticky, and presumably sweeter alternatives. This pattern may lead to or perpetuate nutritional imbalances as well as dental pathology.

Pharmacologic aids in the management of xerostomia include salivary substitutes and salivary stimulants. Salivary substitutes may aid mastication in that the mucosa may allow the food bolus to be positioned for occlusion and prevent sequestration of stagnant food in the cheek, a condition that mimics the rodent buccal cheek pouch. An added benefit is the inclusion of fluoride in some substitutes. Unfortunately, salivary stimulation with sugared candies is a frequent self-medication favored by elders, many of whom have exposed cervical (root) areas of the teeth. In this fragile and sensitive environment, such a practice precipitates caries. Salivary stimulation may be successful as long as residual salivary gland tissue remains after radiation therapy, infection, or surgical ablation. Of interest is the recent introduction of systemic pilocarpine to the armamentarium.

Simple stimulation by chewing gums or sugarless lemon drops is an appropriate first-line prescription. Unflavored stimulants are currently marketed for patients with hypersensitivity to flavoring because of mucositis or ulcerations. The prevalence of xerostomia among certain patient populations may compromise nutrition, medication compliance, social function, and activities of daily living. A successful secretogogue may become the standard of care. Although we do not know the prevalence of xerostomia in different populations, we are well aware of the sequelae of dental caries, pain, and loss of function.

13. Can anything be done about halitosis?

Halitosis is probably not strongly associated with xerostomia, but underlying periodontal disease, poor oral hygiene, or dental abscess may be significant. Such problems may also be associated with the frequency of "morning breath" and the complaint of xerostomia in the morning. Halitosis is the most frequently reported temporal complaint, and the differences in stimulated salivary flow and minor salivary gland output are pronounced between complainers and noncomplainers. Oral hygiene measures, including removal of residual keratin and accretions on the tongue, are best directed at morning accumulations, along with hydration and salivary stimulation.

14. What special considerations about oral health arise in long-term care settings?

Denture adhesives, including powders, creams, and pastes, often pose a major problem in long-term care settings. Although they are least favored on both coasts and have little acceptance in the dental community, they are more commonly used in the central regions of the United States. Moreover, denture wearers seem to use adhesives without correlation to denture quality or fit. Many patients believe that adhesives increase retention or resistance to lateral displacement and thus improve denture function.

Because patients usually apply adhesive when fitting prostheses in the morning, cleaning the mouth may best be scheduled either early in the day or during the evening shift. Because the tasks to be performed in the morning frequently overshadow oral care, the evening may be more appropriate in some environments; there is little advantage to one time over another. Nursing staff may be trained to dislodge retentive dentures by placing the broad side of a finger against the lateral border of the denture and applying pressure medially and downward to break the vacuum seal by which the adhesive increases retention. The adhesive should be removed at each cleaning.

Dental prostheses should be removed each evening to allow healing of the oral mucosa, which is prone to ulceration; unlike skin, the oral mucosa does not keratinize. Dentures worn around the clock are associated with increased atrophy of the maxillary and mandibular ridges; thus, dentures should be removed to retard loss of alveolar (bony) ridges.

Dentures should be kept in 100% humidity for the period of sleep. Immersion in liquid is unnecessary unless chemical cleansers or other agents are appropriate. If antifungal therapy is required for an oral infection, the dentures are sanitized overnight. One can add to the overnight water a commercial cleanser, vinegar, or dilute bleach solution.

BIBLIOGRAPHY

1. Berkey DB, Shay K: General dental care for the elderly. Clin Geriatr Med 8:579–597, 1992.
2. Ettinger RL: Oral care for the homebound and institutionalized. Clin Geriatr Med 8:659–672, 1992.
3. Feldman RS, Kapur KK, Alman JE, Chauncey HH: Aging and mastication: Changes in performance and in the swallowing threshold with natural dentition. J Am Geriatr Soc 28:97–103, 1980.
4. Loesche WJ, Bromberg J, Terpenning MS, et al: Xerostomia, xerogenic medications and food avoidances in selected geriatric groups. J Am Geriatr Soc 43:401–407, 1995.
5. Schmidt A, Lemback H, Feldman RS: Dental health factors in long term care environments. In Ellen RP (ed): Periodontal Care for Older Adults. Toronto, Canadian Scholars' Press, 1991, pp 48–59.
6. Williams RC: Periodontal disease. N Engl J Med 322:373–377, 1990.

IV: Conditions Requiring Special Consideration in Older Adults

22. PREVENTING ADVERSE DRUG REACTIONS

Daniel E. Everitt, M.D.

1. Why are elderly patients more susceptible to adverse drug reactions?

Thirty percent of elderly outpatients have suffered from adverse drug reactions (ADRs) in some studies. ADRs may play a role in causing up to 10% of hospital admissions for elderly patients. On average, elderly patients use 30% of all medications, although they account for only about 12% of the total population. However, age is only one factor that may increase the risk of ADRs; indeed, about 25% of persons over age 65 may not routinely take any medications in a given year. Age is clearly associated with both chronic and acute illness, and these illnesses are associated with the use of multiple drugs. This multiple drug use (polypharmacy) increases the likelihood of unwanted drug interactions, and multiple health providers who may consult on various illnesses make it more likely that the prescribing physician is not fully aware of all medications taken by the patient. Age-related decreases in organ function reserve and impaired homeostatic mechanisms combine with chronic illnesses to make frail elderly patients much more vulnerable to unwanted drug effects.

2. When should an ADR be suspected?

It is a relatively straightforward task to watch for ADRs that are common and well understood, such as bleeding complications associated with anticoagulation or dyspepsia or gastritis related to nonsteroidal anti-inflammatory agents (NSAIDs). However, any time an elderly patient has an unexpected change in function, an ADR should be considered and should prompt a careful evaluation of drug therapy and a workup for potential infectious, metabolic, or environmental precipitants of the change. A functional change may involve the physical, cognitive, affective, or virtually any domain of function. A deterioration of cognition (delirium) in a patient with mild Alzheimer's disease may well be caused by a hypnotic or antihistamine bought over-the-counter. Similarly, a gait disorder caused by parkinsonism may be precipitated by an antipsychotic drug.

A drug chronically taken may also lead to a change in function if a new drug or changing physiology increases the drug's plasma concentration or sensitivity to the drug's effect. For example, phenytoin-induced ataxia may be prompted by addition of one of the many drugs that may increase phenytoin levels. Any time a new medication is prescribed to a patient, a careful review should be made of concomitant drugs, with attention paid to potential interactions or synergies that may lead to an ADR.

3. When should non-drug therapy be considered?

Many acute and chronic illnesses require drug therapy for optimal management. However, non-drug approaches should always be considered, as adverse reactions are a possibility whenever drugs are involved. Too often, physicians feel a pressure to close an ambulatory visit with the writing of a prescription. Often, we misjudge a patient's concern about symptoms as a desire for a medication when in reality the concern is for reassurance or merely attention.

The jump to prescribe should never be a substitute for a careful workup and a potentially more beneficial non-drug approach. This consideration is particularly important for patients with symptoms or behavior that may warrant a psychotropic drug. A patient with insomnia may be using caffeine or other stimulants late in the day, have unrealistic expectations of the sleep cycle, or have an inadequately treated medical illness that would be better served by careful evaluation and education rather than by the quick prescribing of a sedating hypnotic. Patients with dementia-related behavior disorders may respond better and avoid serious ADRs when environmental modifications are made rather than when antipsychotic/neuroleptic drugs are given. Consideration should always be given to discontinuation of a drug that is not having the intended effect, is poorly tolerated, or is not taken as prescribed.

4. How do the elderly differ in their metabolism and elimination of drugs?
   The route a drug takes may be divided simplistically into 5 steps:
   1. Ingestion and absorption
   2. Distribution within the body
   3. Effect at receptors and ultimate physiologic effect
   4. Metabolic transformation
   5. Final elimination
   The most important aspect of **ingestion** involves compliance (see Question 17). Aging in general does not have a significant impact on the **absorption** of oral drugs. The **distribution** of a drug in the body depends to a large degree on whether it is more lipid- or water-soluble. Aging is associated with a reduction in lean body mass and an increase in fat tissue; drugs that are extensively fat-soluble, such as many psychotropic drugs, are distributed more widely in elderly patients and thus may be eliminated more slowly. Distribution also includes binding to plasma proteins. While age alone is not usually associated with changes in the concentration of plasma proteins, disease states, such as renal failure or hypoalbuminemia, cause a larger fraction of the total drug to be unbound and active (and thus available for either intended or unwanted activity).
   Many drugs are **metabolized** by hepatic enzymes. The phase I or preparatory processes, which involve many of the P450 microsomal enzymes, generally are less active in older age. Consequently, drugs largely eliminated by these enzyme systems often are eliminated more slowly and are prone to accumulate with repeated dosing. The kidneys are the most important route of **elimination** for some common drugs. Normal aging is associated with a 10% decrease in renal function for each decade over age 40, and thus the clearance of these drugs decreases with aging.

5. What is the difference between pharmacokinetics and pharmacodynamics? How do they relate to aging?
   Pharmacokinetics refers to "what the body does to the drug." It describes the time course and characteristics of the rise and fall of drug plasma concentrations. The half-life (t1/2) describes the amount of time it takes for the drug concentration to fall by one-half after uptake into the body. The volume of distribution (Vd) describes the theoretical volume of tissue or body fluids that serves as a reservoir for the drug and clearance (Cl) characterizes the number of milliliters of plasma per unit of time that is cleared (by whatever mechanism) of a drug. These pharmacokinetic parameters bear straightforward arithmetic relationships. The half-life of a drug is proportional to the volume of distribution of the drug divided by the clearance. Thus, if the volume of distribution of a drug increases with age and the clearance decreases, the half-life may increase substantially.
   Pharmacodynamics describes "what the drug does to the body." Ultimately, it is the pharmacodynamic effect that allows a drug either to be effective or to have an unwanted or adverse effect. In some cases the intended pharmacodynamic effect may yield an unwanted effect. For example, the desired sedating effect of a hypnotic may lead to oversedation and deterioration of cognitive or physical function. Aging and disease may each alter the pharmacokinetics and pharmacodynamics of a drug which may make ADRs more likely.

6. How can knowledge of a drug's pharmacokinetics help prevent ADR's?
   A drug's pharmacokinetic profile tells on average how long a drug takes to reach maximum concentration, how quickly it is eliminated (half-life), how the concentration accumulates on

repeated dosing, and when steady-state concentrations will be reached. For a drug given as a single dose, such as a hypnotic or analgesic, the time to the maximum concentration and the half-life are important factors to determining the intended effect. Drugs with delayed maximum concentrations and long half-lives should be avoided as hypnotics; a patient should have the desired effect at the appropriate time and not later the next day when sedation would clearly be unwanted. While once-a-day drugs may enhance compliance, long half-life drugs should be avoided in general in the elderly. The up- and down-titration of doses is quicker and safer for shorter half-life drugs.

It is important to keep in mind the simple formula that it takes about 5 half-lives of a drug, given on repeated dosing, to reach steady-state plasma concentrations. If a new drug is initiated or a dose increased, concentrations will be close to steady-state in about 5 half-lives. Thus, if a digoxin dose is increased from 0.125 to 0.25 mg/day in an older patient, with a 48-hour digoxin half-life a new steady-state will not be reached for at least 10 days.

This principle has important implications for the monitoring of drug levels and surveillance for wanted and unwanted drug effects. For example, if a patient chronically takes a benzodiazepine with a long half-life of up to 100 hours, steady-state will not be reached for weeks. This patient may be discharged from a short acute hospital stay on such a hypnotic with no adverse effects and then be nearly obtunded 3 weeks later on the same dose. Indeed, the kinetic profile is the most significant characteristic that differentiates drugs in some categories, and this profile should be considered carefully in prescribing for older patients.

7. What age-related pharmacodynamic differences contribute to ADRs?

Pharmacodynamic differences in drug effect associated with aging are much less understood and studied than pharmacokinetic differences. Older patients are generally more sensitive to the doses or plasma levels of a number of medications considered appropriate for younger patients, such as sedatives and narcotic analgesics. Lower doses of these drugs may give the desired effect, whereas "usual" doses may give unwanted sedation and associated cognitive deficits or gait instability. Similarly, many older patients may have adequate therapeutic response to relatively low doses and serum concentrations of some other drugs, including digoxin, theophylline, phenytoin, and most psychotropic drugs, and serum concentrations appropriate for the young may cause toxicity in the elderly. There are only rare drugs, such as the beta-adrenergic blockers and beta-agonists, for which older patients have less sensitivity.

Age- and disease-related decreases in organ functional reserve may increase an older patient's vulnerability to adverse pharmacodynamic effects. A mildly nephrotoxic drug may have disastrous consequences in an elderly patient with impaired renal function at baseline. NSAIDs may substantially worsen renal function in elderly patients who are volume-contracted on diuretics and who have mild underlying renal failure. Similarly, a patient with a mild dementia may decompensate when exposed to drugs with mild anticholinergic or sedating effects. Thus, any prescription should include a careful assessment of the drug's pharmacodynamic properties in combination with an understanding of the patient's physiologic vulnerabilities.

8. Which classes of drugs are most likely to cause ADRs?

Any drug may cause an ADR, and drugs used with a high prevalence in an elderly population are most often implicated in ADRs. Surveys of older persons living in the community show that analgesic and cardiovascular medications are used by at least over one-third of men and over one-half of women. Gastrointestinal agents, CNS agents, and endocrine/metabolic drugs are reportedly used by about 10% of older persons. It is important to note that 30–65% of older persons report using over-the-counter (OTC) analgesics and 11–25% report using OTC gastrointestinal drugs. Studies of hospitalized elderly find that analgesics, sedatives, and antipsychotics account for nearly 50% of preventable ADRs in this setting. Those with preventable ADRs related to psychotropic drugs are, in general, found to be taking multiple psychoactive drugs concurrently, and long half-life sedatives more commonly cause problems. Excessive doses of haloperidol and other antipsychotics and drug overdoses in patients with renal failure are frequently implicated. In both the community and nursing homes, psychotropic drugs are also commonly associated with ADRs. Other drugs commonly associated with ADRs include digoxin, furosemide, potassium, phenytoin, warfarin, and NSAIDs.

Common Culprits for Adverse Drug Effects

DRUG CATEGORY	EXAMPLE	TYPE OF ADR
Sedatives	Benzodiazepines	Delirium
	Chloral hydrate	Worsening of dementia
	Diphenhydramine (OTC and prescribed)	Urinary incontinence
	Sedating analgesics	Postural instability
	Antipsychotics	Aspiration
Anticholinergics	Antihistamines (often OTC)	Delirium
	Antidepressants	Worsening of dementia
	Some cardiovascular	Angle-closure glaucoma
	Bladder relaxants	Urinary retention
	Antidepressants	Worsening of bladder outlet obstruction
	Antipsychotics	Worsened "overflow" incontinence
Dopamine-blocking agents	Antipsychotics	Extrapyramidal motor system effects
	Metoclopramide	Postural instability, falls, decreased
	Prochlorperazine	physical function

9. When and how should drug levels be monitored to help prevent ADRs?

Serum and plasma concentrations, or "drug levels," are typically available for drugs that have low therapeutic-to-toxic ratios and for which the concentrations produced by a given dose are likely to be quite variable. Consequently, such drugs require especially close monitoring in the elderly to avoid ADRs. Drugs that often require monitoring, such as digoxin, phenytoin, phenobarbitol, aminoglycosides, lithium, quinidine, and some antidepressants, frequently interact with other drugs and are commonly implicated in ADRs.

However, assessment of the drug concentration must not replace the careful assessment of the drug's intended and unwanted pharmacodynamic effects. For example, a theophylline level of 12 ng/ml may be subtherapeutic in a young asthmatic patient but may cause anorexia and weight loss in a frail elderly one. Any drug concentration must be interpreted carefully in the context of the individual patient. Additionally, most assays of drug concentrations quantitate total drug, which includes both the protein-bound and active unbound fractions. For a drug that is highly protein-bound, such as phenytoin, a "normal" total concentration in a frail hypoproteinemic patient may belie an increased free fraction, with possible toxicity, that is due to less-avid protein-binding in such a patient. Thus, drug concentration monitoring may serve as a guide to avoid gross overdosage, but it must not substitute for thoughtful evaluation of the individual patient.

10. Which kind of drug interactions are likely to cause the greatest problems?

Drug interactions may be based on pharmacokinetic or pharmacodynamic interactions. It is well known that quinidine may increase digoxin levels, high doses of H_2-receptor antagonists may increase theophylline levels, and a number of highly protein-bound drugs may displace warfarin from plasma proteins and lead to adverse effects. These pharmacokinetic interactions are important, but pharmacodynamic interactions may have equally dangerous consequences and are more often overlooked. Common problems include patients taking multiple drugs with sedating or anticholinergic properties. Many OTC drugs contain antihistamines that are both sedating and anticholinergic, and these drugs are often overlooked in the medication history. The additive effects of drugs with these properties taken concurrently can profoundly impair cognitive or physical function. Any review of the medication list of an older patient should include a count of the number of drugs with sedating or anticholinergic action. Similarly, more than one drug with effects on the extrapyramidal motor system should be avoided; two antipsychotic drugs or an antipsychotic drug with metoclopramide or prochlorperazine should virtually never be used in combination.

11. How can knowledge of a drug's route of elimination be helpful in preventing ADRs?

Most drugs are eliminated by a combination of **hepatic** biotransformation and **renal** excretion. Normal aging is associated with diminished renal function, and mild to moderate renal failure is common. Thus, for drugs excreted renally, the clearance is decreased, half-life is increased, and repeat dosing leads to higher steady-state concentrations and potential toxicity. This consideration is especially important when dosing and monitoring digoxin, the aminoglycosides, and lithium. Many other drugs should have dosages adjusted for renal failure, and the product labeling always notes whether this is the case.

12. How is creatinine clearance used to estimate potential renal impairment?

Because muscle mass tends to decrease with age, the serum creatinine concentration should decrease with age if renal function remains constant. It is often helpful to calculate creatinine clearance (CrCl), using age, weight, and serum creatinine levels, to give a ballpark estimation of potential renal impairment. One of the useful formulas is the Cockroft-Gault equation:

$$\text{Calculated CrCl} = \frac{(140 - \text{age in yrs}) \times \text{serum Cr}}{\text{weight (in kg) x 72}} \times 0.85 \text{ (if female)}$$

By this equation, the calculated CrCl of an 80-year-old, 45-kg woman with a serum creatinine of 1.0 mg/dl is 32 ml/min. Knowledge of this moderate renal failure, despite a "normal" serum creatinine of 1.0 mg/dl, is important when considering the appropriate maintenance dose of drugs that undergo substantial renal excretion.

13. How can a drug adversely affect physical function?

Several categories of drugs may cause movement or gait disorders which impair physical function by action on the CNS. Any sedative may impair attention, concentration and coordination and may literally tip the older patient over the edge if postural stability is already impaired. Other drugs that block central dopaminergic function may cause the debilitating movement disorders such as parkinsonism, dystonia, tardive dyskinesia, or akathisia. Drugs with this action include the antipsychotic/neuroleptics and metoclopramide. Among antipsychotics, haloperidol has the most potent central extrapyramidal effects, although any of these drugs may have marked motor system effects. Prochlorperazine, used for chronic dizziness or nausea, has been associated with a number of cases of parkinsonism.

14. How can I know if a drug is having the intended effect?

It is frequently difficult to determine if a drug is effective in a given patient. However, it is crucial for the prescriber to be sure that each drug in a regimen provides benefit, as even an inert drug would have the adverse effect of diminishing compliance with concomitant effective drugs. Thus, a clear endpoint must be identified for each drug, and this must be evaluated at regular intervals. If there is no beneficial effect on the endpoint, consideration should be given to increasing the dose, discontinuing the drug, or switching to alternate therapy.

This approach may be particularly important for drugs used to treat depression, behavior disorders, parkinsonism, GI symptoms, and pulmonary disease. Endpoints for these diseases may be difficult to identify and quantify, but many of the therapies are prone to have adverse effects and thus any risk must be outweighed by benefit. The endpoint should be a measure of function that is truly relevant to the particular patient in context. Thus, an emphysematous patient's ability to take walks with a spouse may be a far more important measure of bronchodilator effectiveness than quantitative pulmonary function test results. Similarly, a frail depressed elderly patient may not complain of typical affective symptoms, but the monitoring of appetite and weight gain may be more relevant.

15. When is it safe to withdraw a drug?

It is easy to be uncomfortable with a long medication list for an elderly patient, but it is often difficult to be confident that drugs may be safely withdrawn. Yet because compliance worsens markedly and adverse effects increase with an increasing number of medications, it is important to simplify medication regimens. It may be obvious but often overlooked that a drug may be safely "withdrawn" if the patient does not take it or takes it very erratically. It is also both safe and important to discontinue a drug that does not clearly have a beneficial effect on a defined endpoint. In many cases a simplified, reduced regimen will enhance compliance and lead to better effectiveness. The finely tuned 5-drug antihypertensive, antianginal regimen that is inconsistently taken may be far less effective than a simple once-a-day 2-drug regimen. However, in some cases, careful monitoring of a carefully defined endpoint may be necessary to be sure that a condition does not decompensate with drug reduction or withdrawal.

16. Which drugs are most likely to produce problems on withdrawal?

One survey of adverse events related to drug withdrawal found that the greatest number of these events were associated with the withdrawal of digoxin, furosemide, H_2-receptor blocking agents, and psychotropic drugs. However, these drugs are among the most commonly overused and are often prescribed or maintained without clear indication.

17. How can I get my elderly patients to comply better with their drug regimens?

While age itself appears not to contribute to better or worse drug compliance, a larger number of drugs taken concurrently clearly correlates with decreasing compliance. Over 10% of hospital admissions have been attributed to medication noncompliance. Those who comply poorly are more likely to be elderly living alone with no assistance, those with cognitive impairment, and those using two or more drugs. At every visit, an accurate drug history must be probed. Permission should be given for the patient to be honest; a question such as "It must be difficult to take all these medications as prescribed?" may give permission. A direct question may also be asked about the number of doses missed in an average week. Family and visiting nurses may help with medication regimens, and pill boxes with daily compartments may be preloaded.

Once-daily dose forms, if safe, are more likely to be taken as prescribed. The minimum number of drugs should be used to treat a condition, and all drugs should be avoided that do not have a clearly beneficial impact on a defined endpoint. In this respect, "less" is often "more" when intended drug effects are considered. Cost may be an important contributor to compliance for some patients, and attention should be paid to the use of generics and low-cost regimens. Most elderly patients should ask the pharmacist to avoid child-proof bottles that are difficult to open.

Measures to Enhance Compliance

- Understand the patient's drug history in detail
  Use the "brown bag" approach at each ambulatory visit
  Probe for use of over-the-counter drugs and drugs not prescribed for the patient
- Give permission for the patient to relate exactly how drugs are taken
- Probe for the patient's opinion about problems and adverse effects
- Educate the patient on the relative importance of each medication
- Use family, visiting nurses, and home health aids as allies
- Simplify drug regimens and encourage easy-open bottles
- Pay attention to cost if this is a concern to the patient

BIBLIOGRAPHY

1. Bates DW, Cullen DJ, Laird N, et al: Incidence of adverse drug events and potential adverse drug events: Implications for prevention. JAMA 274:29–34, 1995.
2. Beers MH, Ouslander JG, Fingold SF, et al: Inappropriate medication prescribing in skilled nursing facilities. Ann Intern Med 117:682–689, 1992.
3. Bressler R, Katz MD (eds): Geriatric Pharmacology. New York, McGraw-Hill, 1993, p 689.

4. Chrischilles EA, Foley DJ, Wallace RB, et al: Use of medications by persons 65 and over: Data from the established populations for epidemiologic studies of the elderly. J Gerontol 47: M137–M144, 1992.
5. Everitt DE, Avorn J, Baker MW: Clinical decision-making in the evaluation and treatment of insomnia. Am J Med 89:357–362, 1990.
6. Gerety MB, Cornell JE, Plichta DT, Eimer M: Adverse events related to drugs and drug withdrawal in nursing home residents. J Am Geriatr Soc 41:1326–1332, 1993.
7. Montamat SC, Cusak B: Overcoming problems with polypharmacy and drug misuse in the elderly. Clin Geriatr Med 8:143–158, 1992.

23. FALLS

Elizabeth Capezuti, Ph.D., R.N.

1. How frequently do falls occur in the elderly?

Regardless of living arrangements, accidents are the sixth leading cause of death in the elderly, with falls being the most frequently reported type of accident. Approximately 30–40% of community-residing older adults and 30–60% of nursing home residents fall each year.

2. How do falls affect the morbidity and mortality of older persons?

- \> 90% of hip fractures are associated with falls, with the great majority of fractures occurring in persons over age 70.
- Persons with hip fractures have a 12–22% higher mortality rate than those without hip fractures when matched by age and/or gender.
- Survivors of hip fracture are frequently institutionalized for short-term rehab or long-term placement due to permanent disability or coexisting mental or physical problems.
- Of those who return home, many suffer substantial functional deficits requiring assistance by others or mobility aids.
- Treatment and related cared due to fall-related injuries account for a disproportionately high use and expenditure of health care resources in the elderly.
- Fractures, other than of the hip or pelvis, account for about 2–3% of fall-related injuries.
- Serious soft-tissue injuries requiring medical intervention and resulting in impaired functional status occur in approximately 10% of falls.
- Approximately 9500 deaths of older Americans are associated with falls each year.
- 20% of fatal falls occur in nursing home residents.

3. What are the psychological consequences of falling?

A fall may immobilize an older person, who then fears that her or his next fall will result in a hip fracture and eventual institutionalization. For many older persons, fear of falling results in excess disability, with fear leading to dependence and immobility, followed by functional deficits and the greater likelihood of falls.

4. Why should the clinician ask directly about falls? How often?

Because of the fears many elders harbor regarding institutionalization, clinicians should ask specifically about falls and should not expect the older person to provide this information as a chief complaint. Direct questioning regarding falls should occur at least annually.

5. How many falls would signal the clinician to perform a falls workup?

One fall does not mean that the person is at risk for subsequent falls; it may simply be an isolated event without indicating risk of falling in the future. Recurrent falls (typically defined as ≥ 2 falls in a 6-month period), however, often necessitate a workup to determine the presence of treatable causes.

6. What are the usual causes of falls?

The frequency of falling in older adults is related to the accumulated effect of multiple disorders superimposed on age-related changes. These multiple disorders, or risk factors, have been studied extensively to predict fall risk. Although risk factors have been categorized in several ways, they can be broadly grouped into intrinsic and extrinsic factors. **Intrinsic factors** are those characteristics inherent to the individual and include presence of chronic disease, age-related physical and mental changes, acute health problems or acute exacerbations of disease, and the concomitant effects of medication usage. **Extrinsic factors** include environmental hazards as well as activity-related factors.

7. **Give examples of intrinsic risk factors for falling.**

Demographics
Older age
Female sex
White race
History
Cane/walker use
Recurrent falls
Chronic illnesses
Stroke
Parkinson's disease
Other neuromuscular disease
Arthritis
Diabetes
Heart disease and hypertension
Acute illnesses
Infection
Myocardial infarction

History *(cont.)*
Medications
Polypharmacy
Long-acting hypnotics-anxiolytics
Tricyclic antidepressants
Antipsychotics
Antiparkinsonism drugs
Other cardiac, diuretic,
or antihypertensive drugs
Physical findings (deficits)
Orthostatic hypotension
Vision
Walking speed
Lower and upper extremity strength
Lower extremity sensory perception

8. **Discuss the chronic and acute illnesses that affect fall risk.**

Multiple chronic illnesses can directly affect mobility status, especially arthritis, cardiovascular insufficiency, and diabetes, as well as most neuromuscular diseases such as Parkinson's disease and stroke. Problems with balance manifested by dizziness or vertigo may indicate seizure disorder, hypothyroidism, or inner ear dysfunction. The associated weakness accompanying some acute illnesses (infection, myocardial infarction) and acute exacerbations of chronic disease (congestive heart failure, diabetes, hypertension) can increase the older individual's tendency to fall. Moreover, the sudden onset of repeated falls is considered a sign of underlying acute pathology. Therefore, when an older person presents with new-onset repeated falls, acute illness must be ruled out.

9. **What points should the clinician focus on in obtaining a history of falls?**

Many patients attribute their falls to "just tripping," but the clinician should attempt to ascertain if the fall is due to an environmental factor and/or if other precipitating causes are present. Ask if the fall occurred after a position change, which may indicate orthostatic hypotension, carotid sinus hypersensitivity, or cervical disc spondylosis. A thorough review of the musculoskeletal and neurologic systems will reveal most intrinsic risk factors as well as identify problems for further inquiry; for example, if there is a history of dizziness or vertigo, you should focus on the cardiovascular, visual, auditory-labyrinthine, and proprioceptive systems. Within these systems, symptoms of orthostatic hypotension (positional dizziness), macular disequilibrium, acute labyrinthitis (vertigo with nausea and headache), Meniere's disease (vertigo with tinnitus and hearing loss), benign paroxysmal vertigo (positional vertigo with nystagmus), and peripheral neuropathy should be ascertained.

These conditions are often referred to by patients by a wide variety of terms, such as "falling out" and even "fall," which may have a different meaning from the medical definition of fall. The clinician should clarify with the patient what he or she means when describing conditions.

10. **Which drugs may have side effects related to falls?**

Polypharmacy and increased fall risk have been linked in a number of studies. However, examination of specific medications, their individual side effects, and potential drug interactions is needed. Often, it is helpful to ask an older person to bring in all their current and past prescribed medications as well as those purchased over-the-counter. This step helps to identify medication misuse. Classes of drugs that have been strongly correlated with fall/fracture risk and therefore need to be reviewed include long-acting hypnotics-anxiolytics (including benzodiazepines), tricyclic antidepressants, and antipsychotics. Also, overzealous pharmacologic treatment of cardiac and respiratory disease can adversely affect the vestibular system, impair balance, and create side effects such as severe orthostatic hypotension, all of which lead to greater fall risk.

Drugs That May Affect Fall Risk

Hypnotics-anxiolytics (including benzodiazepines) Chlordiazepoxide HCl Chloral hydrate Diazepam Ethchlorvynol Quazepam Temazepam	Tricyclic antidepressants Amitriptyline Amoxapine Doxepin Imipramine HCl Nortriptyline HCl Protriptyline HCl	Antipsychotics Haloperidol Risperidone Trifluoperazine

11. What are environmental or extrinsic risk factors for falling?

Most falls occur when older person are performing their usual activities, such as rising from a chair or walking. Beds and chairs that are too low, soft, on wheels, or on uneven or slippery surfaces can lead to problems. Hazards implicated in patient's homes include inappropriately placed furniture or objects, scatter rugs, carpeted stairs, and lighting that is too dim or causes glare. Some of these problems can be identified by direct interview. Also, observe the patient's footwear. Loose-fitting and/or badly worn shoes, as well as slippers, have been identified to increase fall risk.

Extrinsic Risk Factors or Environmental Home Hazards

Ground surfaces	**Lighting**
Throw rugs or loose carpets	Glare from unshielded windows or lamps
Slippery floors	or highly polished floors
Low-lying objects on the floor,	Absence of night lights
e.g., cords and wires	**Bathroom**
Stairs with rugs or in poor repair	Low toilet seats and/or no secure grab bars
Furniture	Absence of nonslip surfaces
Clutter	**Other**
Unstable or low-lying furniture	Poorly maintained walking aids and equipment
Low chairs without armrest support or seat back	Improper shoes (not slip-resistant, high-heeled,
Beds/cabinets that are too high or too low	too large)

12. How is an environmental assessment done?

If there are questions regarding the safety of the home environment after interviewing the older person in the office, nurses and physical/occupational therapists in home-care agencies can provide in-home evaluations for potential hazards and offer suggestions such as the installation of grab bars for the tub and toilet.

13. What areas of the physical exam are important in a falls evaluation?

A thorough head and neck, musculoskeletal, neurologic, and foot examination will help reveal areas of dysfunction and weakness that can contribute to fall risk and may be amenable to treatment. The sensory exam should include evaluation of vibratory sense of both upper and lower extremities (marker of peripheral neuropathy), vision (acuity and fields), and hearing. Testing of motor functioning should focus on assessment of joint range of motion (flexibility) and muscle strength. If joint range of motion is limited, document the angle of motion, preferably with a goniometer. Particular areas of muscle strength to evaluate include the hip abduction, adduction, and extension, knees extension (quadriceps) and flexion (hamstring), and ankle plantar and dorsiflexion.

Observe the person walking, checking for posture and balance. In testing for balance, check for unsteadiness in the following tasks: standing on one leg unsupported (unipedal stance), turning (360°), and after a gentle push or "tap" on the sternum. Specific aspects of an ataxia gait associated with fall risk include increased trunk sway, inability to walk in a straight line (path deviation), and inability to increase walking pace. In evaluating gait, note if the person becomes short of breath or complains of chest pain or palpitations. If so, perform a thorough cardiovascular and chest examination, including changes in vital signs with exercise.

14. Which functional or performance-based tests can be used to assess fall risk?

The physical examination should be supplemented with performance-based tests to improve accuracy in assessing fall risk. Observe the person standing and sitting down, rising from supine to sitting position, lifting a book and reaching to put it on a shelf, picking up a small object from the floor, and climbing stairs. Performance tests of position changes should also include blood pressure and pulse for objective measurement of orthostatic hypotension. (See also Chapter 42.)

15. How do you evaluate a woman's risk for osteoporosis?

Recent evidence indicates that screening for osteoporosis in older women can provide more accurate information when balancing the risk of fracture and of endometrial and breast cancer against the benefits of cardiovascular protection provided by hormonal replacement therapy. Bone mineral density (BMD), especially measured in the proximal femur, is the primary diagnostic tool for identifying those at high risk for osteoporosis and fracture. Single-photon and single-energy x-ray absorptiometry have been used for several decades, but dual-energy x-ray absorptiometry demonstrates high accuracy and precision of BMD in preferred peripheral sites (lumbar spine and proximal femur) while using an extremely low amount of radiation.

16. Discuss pharmacologic treatment of osteoporosis for older women.

Prevention of bone loss is preferred and is accomplished by initiating hormonal replacement therapy (HRT) perimenopausally; however, HRT cannot be given indefinitely. Research shows that women between ages 65–90 who were never treated with HRT have continued bone loss, especially in the hip. Older women who have never received HRT and are at high risk for cardiovascular disease but not breast cancer are ideal candidates for HRT therapy. Although there is a known increased risk of endometrial cancer with the long-term use of unopposed estrogen (i.e., not in combination with progesterone), it remains uncertain whether estrogen plus progesterone has the same cardioprotective effect as unopposed estrogen. Calcium and vitamin D supplementation, calcitonin, and several biphosphonates have been demonstrated to reduce bone reabsorption. Recently, aminobiphosphonates plus calcium have demonstrated promising results in increasing bone density in postmenopausal women.

17. How can exercise improve function and reduce fall risk?

In a large, multicenter research initiative known as FICSIT (Frailty and Injuries: Cooperative Studies of Intervention Techniques), exercise has been found to improve functional status and reduce the risk of falls and injurious falls. Various modalities have been found to be useful, including resistance training to increase muscle strength and exercises that improve endurance, flexibility, and balance.

Sedentary lifestyle, especially immobilization, is associated with increased risk of osteoporosis. Although weight-bearing activity (walking, cycling, dancing, swimming) in those with established osteoporosis may only result in minor gains in skeletal mass, it is believed that the effect of exercise on muscle strength, gait, and confidence reduces risk of fracture. This type of exercise improves cardiovascular function which may be a contributing factor for fall risk and/or sedentary lifestyle.

18. When is a rehab/exercise referral necessary?

Individuals with deficits in gait/balance skills should be evaluated for their potential to improve with a structured exercise program. Evaluation of cardiac risk, including exercise stress testing, depends on significant findings in the history, including cardiac dysrhythmia, severe congestive heart failure, angina, exercise-related chest pain or myocardial infarct, diabetes mellitus, hypertension, elevated cholesterol levels, and current cigarette smoking. Patients with exercise-induced angina, intermittent claudication, chronic obstructive lung disease, degenerative joint disease, orthopedic problems, and neurologic abnormalities require both professional evaluation and supervised exercise programs.

19. What types of supervised rehab/exercise programs are available for referral?

An exercise program should be tailored to the needs of the older person by a knowledgeable exercise professional, such as a physical therapist, occupational therapist, or physiatrist. Many cardiac rehabilitation programs and health clubs with a physical therapy department provide gait and balance evaluations as well as prescribe exercise regimens. Many also provide supervised exercise programs for those with specific health problems. Programs that employ exercise physiologists, physical therapists, occupational therapists, and/or rehabilitation nurses working collaboratively with physiatrists, sports medicine specialists, and/or cardiologists are ideal.

20. What is the role of physical restraints in institutionalized elders?

Despite the assumed safety of nursing home environments, falls remain an important clinical problem and present a complicated dilemma for nursing homes and other institutions caring for the elderly. Research has described a syndrome called "spiraling immobility," a virtual "catch-22" in which an older person perceived to be at risk of falling is restrained to prevent falling and is then unable to ambulate again, independently or safely, due to the immobilizing consequences of physical restraint. All restraints, especially vest restraints and geri-chairs (chairs with fixed tray tables), have been correlated with the negative sequelae of immobility as well as reports of restraint-related injury and death. Current federal nursing home regulations discourage the use of such devices. Reducing mobility through the use of physical restraints has been demonstrated to be counterproductive. Interventions including regular ambulation and other exercises that increase strength, balance, and coordination have been shown to be the most effective measures in preventing falls.

21. Are physical restraints useful in preventing falls in the hospitalized elder?

No. Despite growing empirical evidence that the use of physical restraints produces more problems than it solves, American physicians and nurses continue to believe that these restraints are an effective strategy for preventing falls and injuries in elders. In addition, there is a perception that failure to restrain puts nurses and facilities at risk for legal liability. However, as the courts are being educated regarding the negative effects of physical restraint, settlement and court decisions in fall-related injury cases have begun to shift. Moreover, suits are being won against nursing homes and hospitals for using physical restraints that lead to adverse consequences of enforced immobility or restraint-related deaths. Recent JCAHO (Joint Commission for Accreditation of Healthcare Organizations) guidelines restrict use of physical restraints to limited situations.

22. What can be recommended for a nonambulatory older person at risk of falling?

Falls in nonambulatory persons usually occur as a result of sliding or slipping out of chairs or transferring unassisted from chair to bed. If the person falls because they are attempting to get out of an uncomfortable chair, then several seating "alternatives" are available. Wedge cushions or recliner chairs may prevent such unassisted ambulation while assuring comfort. For elders who wish to be mobile despite their inability to ambulate, interventions which improve wheelchair skills along with more user-friendly wheelchairs have been found to increase mobility. Belts serve to remind the nursing home resident to seek assistance when attempting to ambulate. Physical and occupational therapists can provide guidance in prescribing these interventions.

BIBLIOGRAPHY

1. Grisso JA, Kelsey JL, Strom BL, et al: Risk factors for falls as a cause of hip fracture in women. N Engl J Med 324:1326–1330, 1991.
2. Marcus R, Feldman D, Kelsey J: Osteoporosis. San Diego, Academic Press, 1996.
3. Northridge ME, Nevitt MC, Kelsey JL, et al: Home hazards and falls in the elderly: The role of health and functional status. Am J Public Health 85:509–515, 1995.
4. Province MA, Hadley EC, Hornbrook MC, et al: The effects of exercise on falls in elderly patients: A preplanned meta-analysis of the FICSIT trials. JAMA 273:1341–1347, 1995.
5. Rubenstein LZ, Josephson KR, Robbins AS: Falls in nursing homes. Ann Intern Med 121:442–451, 1994.
6. Tinetti ME, Ginter SF: Identifying mobility dysfunctions in elderly patients—standard neuromuscular examination or direct assessment? JAMA 259:1190–1193, 1988.
7. Tinetti ME, Liu WL, Ginter SF: Mechanical restraints use and fall-related injuries among residents of skilled nursing facilities. Ann Intern Med 116:369–374, 1992.
8. Tinetti ME, Speechley M, Ginter SF: Risk factors for falls among elderly persons living in the community. N Engl J Med 319:170, 1988.

24. DEPRESSION

Ira Katz, M.D., Ph.D., and David Miller, M.D.

1. What is the difference between depression and normal sadness?

Depressive illnesses in older people, like those in younger adults, can occur without obvious causes or precipitants. More often, however, late-life depression occurs in the context of medical illness, psychosocial stress, and loss, and so most depressions make sense empathetically and intuitively. Unfortunately, this often leads to the view that depression is a "natural" state of aging rather than a medical symptom requiring evaluation.

Despite these misconceptions, the distinction between depressive illness and normal sadness is straightforward. Depressive illnesses are persistent, lasting for several weeks or longer. Depressive illnesses can be disabling, interfering with social, instrumental, or self-care activities either by themselves or by amplifying the disability associated with medical illness. Although the relationships between depression and disability can be complex and bidirectional, patients who have persistent depression coexisting with functional impairments require medical evaluation.

2. What subtypes of depression are relevant in late life?

Major depressive disorder is characterized by episodes in which the following symptoms persist:

Persistent depressed mood
Markedly decreased interest or pleasure
   in usual activities
Decreased appetite and weight loss
Increased appetite and weight gain
   (more rarely)
Insomnia
Hypersomnia
Psychomotor agitation or retardation
Fatigue or loss of energy
Feelings of worthlessness or excessive guilt
Decreased ability to think or concentrate
Suicidal thoughts, wishes, plan, or intent

According to the *Diagnostic and Statistical Manual for Mental Disorders* (DSM-IV), the diagnosis of a **major depressive episode** can be made when patients have depressed mood and/or loss of interests or pleasure and a total of five of the above symptoms to a significant degree for a period of at least 2 weeks.

Major depression can occur as a *single* episode or as part of a *recurring* pattern of episodes. Depressions occurring in the elderly can be of *early-onset*, in which the late-life depression occurs as a recurrence of an illness that began in younger adulthood; or *late onset*, in which illness began initially at an older age. Recurrent depression can be *bipolar*, where both depressive and manic or hypomanic episodes occur; or *unipolar*, in which only depressions occur. This distinction between unipolar and bipolar is important because antidepressant treatment of bipolar patients may precipitate manic or hypomanic episodes. Depressions can also be associated with *psychotic* features (hallucinations or delusions). Psychotic depressions do not, as a rule, respond to antidepressants alone and instead require both antidepressants and antipsychotic medications or electroconvulsive therapy.

Although less severe, other types of depressions are also clinically significant. **Dysthymic disorder** is a condition in which lower levels of depressive symptoms exist chronically for a period of 2 years or more. **Minor depressions** include those in which symptoms of depression and anxiety coexist and those in which more severe depressive symptoms occur briefly but recurrently.

3. How is depression related to other medical illness?

The NIH consensus conference on the Diagnosis and Treatment of Late-Life Depression noted that the hallmark of depression in the elderly was its association with medical illness. Late-onset depressions, in general, emerged in the context of chronic medical or neurologic illness, and a growing body of epidemiologic research demonstrates an increased prevalence of major depression in medical care settings. Major depression occurs in approximately 2–4% of healthy elderly in the community, 10–12% of elderly medical inpatients, and 20–25% of cognitively intact nursing home residents. In addition, as many as 30–50% of patients in medical care settings have clinically significant minor depressions. Clinicians should systematically determine whether comorbid depression is present in all elderly patients with significant medical illness whom they see. Conversely, all elderly individuals who present to mental health care settings for evaluation of depression should be evaluated for significant medical illnesses.

4. How do you treat depression that occurs as part of a medical illness?

When depression complicates significant **acute medical illnesses**, patients require support. Specific treatment is necessary when depression is severe or when it interferes with medical management. For more moderate depressions, continued monitoring of affective symptoms during the course of recovery from the medical illness is necessary. Treatment for depression should be instituted when the depression persists despite improvement in medical status.

When depression occurs in medically stable patients with **chronic illness**, systems should be reviewed to identify possible medical causes of the affective symptoms. Common causes include unrecognized acute illnesses (e.g., heart failure, urinary tract infections), side effects of medications (e.g., reserpine, alpha-methyldopa), electrolyte abnormalities (e.g., hyponatremia, hypercalcemia), thyroid dysfunction, and vitamin B12 or folate deficiency. A review of systems is also necessary to identify medical conditions that could complicate treatment; for example, before use of tricyclic antidepressants, patients must be evaluated for disorders of cardiac conduction, prostate hypertrophy, or glaucoma.

5. How can you tell if a particular symptom is due to medical illness or to depression?

A rather extensive literature in the field of consultation-liaison psychiatry has focused on the possibility that medical symptoms can obscure the diagnosis of major depression. Some symptoms, such as fatigue, can be due to medical illnesses (e.g., heart failure) or to depression. Experienced clinicians can evaluate the etiology of symptoms and "factor" them into their medical and depressive components. Even with truly ambiguous symptoms, utilizing an inclusive approach to diagnosis based on all observed symptoms, regardless of their apparent etiology, can still be helpful. Despite the theoretical difficulties, current approaches to diagnosis have, in fact, been validated in patients suffering from many of the comorbid medical disorders that are common in late life. Controlled clinical trials have demonstrated that depressions diagnosed in patients with medical illnesses as diverse as stroke, parkinsonism, cancer, ischemic heart disease, chronic obstructive pulmonary disease, and arthritis still respond to treatment.

6. What is depressive pseudodementia?

Classically, most textbooks in geriatric psychiatry emphasized the difficulties in identifying patients in whom major depression caused significant cognitive impairment and in distinguishing between these potentially treatable cases of "pseudodementia" and irreversible dementias such as Alzheimer's disease. The use of the term pseudodementia has been criticized by some investigators who note that severe depression can cause real cognitive impairment. The name **dementia syndrome of depression** has been proposed to emphasize that although these conditions are treatable, there is nothing "pseudo" about the disability resulting from severe depression.

More significantly, Reifler and colleagues noted that patients with coexisting depression and cognitive impairment could have either one disease or two. Patients could have a pure depressive disorder associated with cognitive impairment (pseudodementia), in which case, treatment of depression could restore normal levels of functioning. Alternatively, they could have an irreversible dementia with a superimposed depressive disorder. In these cases, treatment of depression could reverse only a component of the patient's disability. In either case, recognition, diagnosis, and treatment of depression could be of benefit to the patient.

7. What is the long-term prognosis for patients having depression with pseudodementia?

Recent research has been reevaluating the long-term prognosis of patients with depression associated with cognitive impairment that is alleviated through treatment. Two generations ago, there were concerns that all depressions with onset in late-life were prodromes of dementia. A generation ago, systematic follow-up studies on patients hospitalized for depression demonstrated that depression and dementia were, in fact, separable disorders and that the long-term outcome of most patients with late-life depression did not include cognitive deterioration. New research in this area, however, suggests that patients with depression associated with reversible cognitive impairment are at increased risk for developing dementia over the subsequent few years. At present, these findings should not be taken to reflect nihilism about outcomes for these patients, but rather, the importance of long-term follow-up and treatment.

8. What are the problems associated with untreated depression?

Untreated or undertreated depression is associated with both psychiatric and general medical consequences. Psychiatric morbidity includes chronicity with its associated psychosocial disability, risks of alcohol or substance abuse in attempts at self-treatment, and suicide. The most compelling case for the importance of the recognition of depression by primary care physicians comes from the finding that 75% of older people who kill themselves saw their physicians within 30 days of their deaths.

Suicide can occur not only when depression is missed but at any time during the treatment course of a depressive episode. Closer surveillance is indicated if the patient expresses suicidal thoughts, intent, and/or describes a plan. There is a transient increased suicide risk in the early stages of treatment, as patients gain the energy and capacity to act on their earlier plans.

Medical morbidity associated with depression includes increased disability, protein-calorie undernutrition, increased pain complaints, and greater sensitivity to subjective side effects of medications. There are also increases in utilization of general medical care services (inpatient and outpatient) and in caregiver burden. Finally, there is an increase in mortality, even after controlling for the increased severity of medical illnesses in patients with depression.

9. When should patients receive antidepressant medications?

The efficacy of antidepressant medications has been established for the treatment of patients with major depression. Thus, clinicians should inquire about the presence of the DSM-IV diagnostic symptoms. Significantly (and counterintuitively), evaluating a patient's need for antidepressant medication requires knowledge about symptoms but not about the presence or absence of reasons for the depression.

In addition to their well-established use in the treatment of major depression, antidepressants may also be of value in patients with dysthymia or minor depression, who either do not respond to psychosocial treatment or are not amenable to it.

10. When should older patients receive psychotherapy?

Structured psychotherapies, such as cognitive-behavioral therapy, interpersonal therapy, or brief dynamic therapies, may be the treatments of choice for dysthymia or minor depression. They may also be a first-line treatment for milder major depression; however, if these patients do not experience a significant amelioration of their symptoms within several weeks, use of antidepressants should be reconsidered.

In general, depression in the elderly frequently has associated functional and social difficulties. Among these are loss of or changed roles, lack of social support, chronic medical illnesses, hopelessness, disability, and bereavement. Therefore, psychotherapy can be extremely useful as an adjunct to pharmacotherapy in patients with major depression of moderate severity.

11. What are first- and second-line agents used in the pharmacotherapy of depression?

Selective serotonin reuptake inhibitors (SSRIs—e.g., fluoxetine, sertraline, paroxetine): Given their tolerable side effect profile and safety in overdose, these agents are appropriate first-line treatments for depression in ambulatory elderly, especially those seen by primary care providers. They have fewer anticholinergic and cardiac side effects but may cause nausea, diarrhea, somnolence, and headache. Their once-daily dosing and tolerability may enhance compliance. However, their efficacy and safety in those who are very old, frail, or medically ill has not been established. In these patients, SSRIs may cause lethargy, anorexia, and SIADH (syndrome of inappropriate secretion of antidiuretic hormone). Additional problems may include drug interactions, extrapyramidal symptoms, bradycardia, and sexual dysfunction.

Tricyclic antidepressants (TCAs): The secondary amine TCAs nortriptyline and desipramine are preferred for use in the elderly. Their efficacy in the elderly, including patients with significant medical comorbidity, has been well-established. Moreover, these agents are less likely to produce orthostasis (which can lead to falls and fractures), excessive sedation, anticholinergic symptoms, or cardiac toxicity than the tertiary amine TCAs (e.g., amitriptyline or imipramine). The secondary amine TCAs can be used safely in patients who do not have cardiac conduction problems, acute narrow-angle glaucoma, and prostatic hypertrophy with urinary retention. With these agents, plasma level–response correlations have been established, and therapeutic blood levels (80–120 ng/ml for nortriptyline and > 125 ng/ml for desipramine) can be utilized to individualize doses for the individual patient.

Other agents: Among the newer antidepressants, buspirone, venlafaxine, and nefazadone may all be of value in treating older patients. Among the older medications, the TCA doxepin and the monoamine oxidase inhibitors have been demonstrated to be effective in the elderly. The use of the monoamine oxidase inhibitors, however, is complicated by the need to avoid potentially serious drug-drug or drug-food interactions.

12. How do you select an appropriate medication?

Before an antidepressant is chosen one must consider the risks and benefits for that particular patient. Factors to be mindful of are concurrent medical conditions and medications, substance abuse problems (e.g., alcohol abuse), and the likelihood of overdose, either by suicide attempt or secondary to cognitive problems. Several basic principles can be outlined:

- For ambulatory outpatients with major depression that is mild-to-moderate in severity, the first-line use of SSRIs or other well-tolerated agents is reasonable.
- For patients with more severe depression, early use of the better-established TCAs should be considered.
- In patients who are frail or with specific medical conditions that could complicate use of these agents, hospitalization may be necessary to optimize safety during the institution of treatment.
- Regardless of which medications are used initially, it is necessary to monitor patients to evaluate both therapeutic responses and to identify side effects.
- If patients do not show early signs of response within 4–6 weeks, it is important to consider modifying the treatment plan.

13. How long should treatment be continued?

Treatment of depression can be divided into three phases:

Acute phase (goal: to achieve symptom remission)—The median time to recover from the acute phase of an index episode of depression is 12 weeks (longer than for younger patients). Discerning whether a patient is responding can only reliably be done after 4–6 weeks.

Continuation phase (goal: to stabilize patients during a period when they are highly vulnerable to relapse)—All patients recovering from an episode of depression are vulnerable to relapse during the first 6–9 months after symptoms remission. All patients should remain in continuation-phase treatment for this period of time.

Maintenance phase (goal: to prevent recurrence)—At the completion of the continuation phase, patients and their physicians must decide whether treatment should be discontinued (by slowly tapering antidepressant doses) or whether the patient should remain on long-term maintenance treatment to decrease the probability of recurrences. If treatment is discontinued, the patient and family should be educated and informed about the need for continued monitoring to facilitate the early identification of recurrences. If the patient has had > 2 episodes of depression, or if the initial episodes were particularly severe or lengthy, long-term (possibly lifetime) maintenance therapy should be considered.

14. When should electroconvulsive therapy (ECT) be considered?

The indications for ECT in both younger and older patients include severe major depression and mania. Older patients with severe depression often present with psychotic symptoms and suicidality (occasionally taking the form of food refusal). They may respond to SSRIs less consistently and may be less able to tolerate the anticholinergic and cardiac side effects of the TCAs. Therefore, the elderly are more likely to require ECT. They actually account for a disproportionate percentage of those who get ECT (receiving > 30% of all ECTs despite representing < 10% of all hospitalized psychiatric patients).

ECT is safe and effective, even when there are physical comorbidities or dementia. It should be considered the treatment of choice when a rapid response is needed for severely depressed patients. It should also be considered in patients who have previously not responded to adequate trials of antidepressant treatment.

15. What can be done when patients don't respond to treatment?

Between 20–30% of patients fail to respond satisfactorily to initial treatment with an antidepressant medication. Possible explanations include improper diagnosis, inadequate treatment, and failure to identify and treat concurrent general medical and psychiatric disorders.

Obstacles to administering adequate treatment include:
• Poor compliance by both patient and family (who may fail to understand the illness, its course, and/or the importance of compliance)
• Side effects
• Hidden self-medication (e.g., alcohol)
• Adverse psychosocial factors (which may diminish the desire to comply)
• Medical comorbidities (which can interfere with antidepressant response or attainment of adequate dosages)

Steps the clinician can take to enhance compliance include creating an alliance with and providing education about depression to the patient and family, being mindful of side effects so as to decrease them when they occur, and maintaining a supportive attitude.

Once satisfied on all counts that the initial trial was adequate, one can either augment the present medication or switch to another agent (from another class of antidepressant). Adjuvant treatments include:
• Lithium (a response should be seen within a few days to few weeks; blood levels indicating therapeutic levels are not clear)
• Thyroid hormone
• Psychostimulants

The anticonvulsants carbamazepine and valproic acid have been used both as primary and adjuvant agents for treatment-resistant depression. Sometimes, multiple antidepressants are used simultaneously. Combined treatment, however, carries the risk of adverse interactions and may require dose adjustment (e.g., SSRIs can increase TCA blood levels, and thus TCA doses may need to be reduced to avoid toxicity). If a patient fails two separate trials of antidepressant medication, ECT should be considered.

16. What are the most important points about late-life depression for primary care doctors?

1. The diagnosis of late-life depression is as valid as that of other significant medical disorders.

2. Major depression in the elderly is a significant disorder associated with both psychiatric and medical morbidity, increased utilization of general health care services, and increased mortality.

3. Late-life depression is a treatable disorder.

BIBLIOGRAPHY

1. Alexopoulos GS, Meyers GS, Young RC, et al: The course of geriatric depression with "reversible dementia": A controlled study. Am J Psychiatry 150:1693–1699, 1993.
2. Conwell Y: Suicide in elderly patients. In Schneider LS, Reynolds CF, Lebowitz BD, Friedhoff AJ (eds):
   Diagnosis and Treatment of Depression in Late Life. Washington D.C., American Psychiatric Press,
   1994, pp 397–418.
3. Jones BN, Reifler BV: Depression coexisting with dementia: Evaluation and treatment. Med Clin North
   Am 78:823–840, 1994.
4. Katz IR: Drug treatment of depression in the frail elderly: Discussion of the NIH consensus development
   conference on the diagnosis and treatment of depression in late life. Psychopharmacol Bull 29(1):
   101–108, 1993.
5. Katz IR, Streim J, Parmelee P: Prevention of depression, recurrences, and complications in late life. Prev
   Med 23:743–750, 1994.
6. Reynolds CF, Alexopoulos G, Katz IR, Mulsant BH: Treatment of geriatric mood disorders. In Rush AJ,
   ed: Current Review of Mood Disorder, In press.
7. Schneider LS, Reynolds CF, Lebowitz BD, Friedhoff AJ (eds): Diagnosis and Treatment of Depression in
   Late Life: Results of the NIH Consensus Development Conference. American Psychiatric Press,
   Washington, D.C., 1994.

25. EARLY DETECTION OF ELDER ABUSE, NEGLECT, AND EXPLOITATION

Elizabeth Capezuti, Ph.D., R.N.

1. What constitutes elder abuse and neglect?

- **Physical abuse** is the infliction of bodily injury and can be manifested by lacerations, fractures, soft-tissue trauma, burns, or bruises.
- **Sexual abuse** is any form of intimate sexual activity without consent. This includes sexual activity with those unable to give adequate consent, such as those with dementia or the older mentally retarded person.
- **Emotional or psychological abuse** is the infliction of mental anguish, such as intimidation by yelling, insulting, threatening, or silence.
- **Financial exploitation** is the misuse of an older person's funds or assets without his or her explicit knowledge or consent. It may take many forms, such as the withdrawal of small amounts of money from banking accounts or the overcharging for grocery shopping or housekeeping by persons providing these services.
- **Caregiver neglect** is the malicious neglect by a caregiver of an older person's needs, whether for retaliation, disinterest, or financial incentives. Examples include inadequate provision of nutrition and the misuse of medications, such as oversedation with tranquilizers.
- **Self-neglect** is disregard of one's personal well-being and home environment.

2. How common is elder mistreatment?

One to 2 million older Americans are mistreated annually. To date, there has been only one population-based survey conducted, which found a prevalence of 32/1000 older persons.

3. What causes elder abuse?

Physical abuse and financial exploitation are usually due to the psychopathology of the perpetrator and have little to do with the older person's characteristics. Perpetrators (family members or nonrelatives) are more likely to abuse alcohol or drugs, to be mentally ill, and/or to be financially dependent on the older person.

Neglect of an older individual due to lack of information or resources, usually referred to as "passive neglect," is not considered mistreatment. It is often seen when the caregivers have their own physical or mental handicaps. Adult children may be developmentally disabled or mentally ill or may be elderly themselves and, as a result, unable to provide sufficient care. Passive caregiver neglect may be rectified by providing education and community supports.

Active caregiver neglect, which implies malicious intent, has not been demonstrated to be due to the stress and burdens of providing care to an older person. These caregivers also are likely to have substance abuse issues, have serious untreated mental illness, or be financially dependent on the older person. Caregivers who are socially isolated and lack social supports (family, friends, or community-based services) or those with a history of violence, such as spousal abuse, have also been implicated.

Victims and perpetrators of any type of mistreatment are found in all socioeconomic groups.

4. What leads to self-neglect?

The exact cause of self-neglect is often difficult to determine. In some cases, there appears to be a mental health problem, such as chronic schizophrenia, depression, or dementia. In other cases, the older person demonstrates no deficits in cognitive functioning but is fearful of "outsiders." These older persons might be reclusive, suspicious, and territorial. The key to successful intervention with this type of elder is to establish a trusting relationship that allows the older person to feel in control. This is usually best handled by case managers in private or county social service agencies, who can provide long-term follow-up.

5. Discuss the role of mental status assessment in the evaluation of elder mistreatment.

Mental status assessment, especially cognitive functioning, is an essential component of the evaluation; it is necessary to determine if the person is able to make a decision to remain in an abusive relationship with a perpetrator or remain in a self-neglecting situation. Accusations of abuse should be assessed within the context of other psychiatric symptoms, such as delusions and hallucinations, which may or may not lend credence to the allegations. Displays of paranoia or anxiety in the presence of the suspected perpetrator may be related to fear, thus leading to inquiries of other family members or friends to provide further information about the relationship. The older person presenting with new onset of disorientation, confusion, or extreme lethargy may be the victim of oversedation. Depression can be the cause of self-neglect or may indicate resignation to an abusive situation.

6. What are the physical findings of physical abuse?

Physical abuse should be considered when investigating the underlying cause of any injury. Identification of physical abuse, however, is often complicated by normal age changes that may mimic trauma. In senile purpura, even gentle handing of an older person's skin may result in bruising because of capillary fragility. Bilateral **bruises** of the upper arms, however, are more likely to result from forcibly holding, grabbing, or shaking a person. **Fractures, dislocations, and sprains** need to be explored within the context of other suspicious signs and symptoms of abuse. **Imprint injuries** (bruises that retain the shape of the object, such as a belt buckle, hand, or iron) are strong physical indicators of abuse. A person physically restrained may have **rope burns** or marks on the ankles or wrists. **Burns** in an unusual location, such as cigarette burns on the back, are highly significant. **Spotty absence of hair**, contrary to the typical temporal pattern of balding in aging men, can be due to vigorous hair-pulling.

7. List the chief indicators of neglect.
- Malnutrition
- Dehydration
- Pressure ulcers
- Contractures
- Oversedation
- Poor hygiene
- Urine burn excoriations
- Manifestations of inadequately treated medical problems, i.e., unfilled prescriptions and recurrent urinary tract infections

One indicator alone cannot confirm a diagnosis of mistreatment, but a suspicious history with a recurrent presentation of signs should raise the clinician's suspicions of mistreatment. Many signs of neglect can also be attributed to common age-related health problems. For example, malnutrition may be explained as the older person's lack of appetite, just as poor personal hygiene may be attributed to one's refusal to be bathed. Therefore, care must be exercised not to be overly accusatory and threaten your relationship with the caregiver.

8. What should be emphasized in interviewing possible victims and perpetrators of mistreatment?

The interview should proceed from the least threatening questions to a more directed inquiry. The history of a presenting physical injury needs to be evaluated for **inconsistencies** and questions asked:

Could the injury actually have occurred in the manner in which the suspected abuser or victim has explained?

Is the individual bed bound and seeking treatment for several fractures?

Did the person "fall down the stairs" and present with bilateral upper arm bruising?

If possible, interview the victim separate from the caregiver. However, do not always expect to get a different story than the suspected abuser's story, as the victim may have been coached or threatened before being brought in for treatment.

When evaluating an injury or signs of deteriorating health (e.g., malnutrition, dehydration, multiple pressure sores), the **index of suspicion** is raised when the elderly individual is taken to an emergency department or family physician located far from home. This occurs when the family or caregiver believes the staff in the local emergency department or the physician has become suspicious of the home situation. It is also suspect when someone other than the primary caregiver brings the person to the physician's office or emergency department and knows little of the older person's health status, medications, and so forth. The inability to answer questions may be a way to block the physician's probing of the cause of an injury or of inadequate care. Any individual who is brought in for treatment late in the illness process or who repeatedly needs treatment despite a previously well-thought-out discharge plan should be evaluated for needed in-home supports or breakdown of a current home care system.

9. What type of situations should alert the clinician to the possibility of financial exploitation?

If a cognitively intact individual is unaware of his or her own financial situation or there is an apparent discrepancy between financial resources and lifestyle, the clinician may want to probe further or to refer to a social worker. In the latter instance, it is important to be aware that lifestyle preferences and income may be incongruent, particularly as some individuals may not be willing to spend money on necessary services. On the other hand, some individuals in the early stages of dementia will often lose the ability to manage their money. Without intervention in these situations, bills may go unpaid, social security checks uncashed, and available money squandered.

10. What are available resources for intervention?

Currently, every state has an Adult Protective Services (APS) system, which, in addition to investigating suspected cases (usually with a home visit), provides special services for the victims of mistreatment. Provisions for emergency shelter, home care, food, and transportation, as well as legal counsel and evaluations by health care providers, may be provided, depending on each state's funding of APS services. The amount of involuntary intervention by protective service workers also depends on individual state laws.

Geriatric and geropsychiatric programs in hospitals and outpatient offices are familiar with the problems of elder mistreatment. If such specialized services are not available, hospital social work departments, local area agencies on aging, and visiting nurses associations can provide coordination and referral services.

Many police departments and district attorney's offices have special domestic violence units to handle cases of abuse or neglect.

11. Are physicians mandated to report suspected elder mistreatment?

In 42 states, physicians are required to report suspected elder mistreatment to APS systems. With few exceptions, the mistreatment need only be suspected, not fully substantiated. Many mandatory and voluntary reporting statutes grant immunity from civil and criminal liability to those who report in good faith. States without mandatory reporting laws (as of 1993) include, Colorado, Illinois, New York, New Jersey, North Dakota, Pennsylvania, South Dakota, and Wisconsin. The primary functions of physicians in suspected cases that are being referred to APS is to document the physical findings and to provide a judgment about the older person's decision-making capacity.

The Joint Commission on the Accreditation of Health Care Organizations requires hospital emergency departments to provide personnel training in the detection and management of the problem. Moreover, emergency departments must develop protocols to deal with cases of mistreatment that address the collection of evidence, the documentation of examinations, and the treatment provided. A current list of community agencies for referral for services should also be readily available. These agencies can provide both immediate and long-term support for victims of elder mistreatment.

12. How does institutional mistreatment differ from mistreatment that occurs in the community?

The various types and manifestations of mistreatment are the same, but the location and responsibility of the perpetrator are chief differences. Institutional mistreatment can occur in hospitals, nursing homes, or board-and-care facilities. The perpetrator may be an individual staff member who physically or sexually abuses a patient, or the perpetrator may be an institutional milieu that discourages the appropriate provision of care. For example, the patients may be physically restrained instead of ambulated because of inadequate staffing levels, thus leading to problems associated with immobility such as contractures and pressure ulcers.

Reporting of suspicions of institutional mistreatment should be made to the state ombudsman. The Older Americans Act of 1976 mandated that each state establish ombudsman programs to investigate allegations of mistreatment in nursing homes.

BIBLIOGRAPHY

1. AMA Council on Scientific Affairs: Elder abuse and neglect. JAMA 257:966–971, 1987.
2. Aravanis SC, Adelman RD, Breckman P, et al: Diagnostic and treatment guidelines on elder abuse and neglect. Arch Fam Med 2:317–388, 1993.
3. Clark-Daniels CL, Daniels RS, Baumhover LA: Abuse and neglect of the elderly: Are emergency department personnel aware of mandatory reporting laws? Ann Emerg Med 19:970–977, 1990.
4. Fulmer TF, Ashley J: Clinical indicators of elder neglect. Appl Nurs Res 2:161–167, 1989.
5. Jones JS: Elder abuse and neglect: Responding to a national problem. Ann Emerg Med 23:845–848, 1994.
6. Lachs MS, Pillemer K: Abuse and neglect of elderly persons. N Engl J Med 332:437–443, 1995.

26. AGING AND COGNITIVE FUNCTIONING

Ruben C. Gur, Ph.D., Paul J. Moberg, Ph.D., and Raquel E. Gur, M.D., Ph.D.

1. What is the pattern of cognitive decline in normal aging?

As you might suspect, most cognitive abilities decline with age, once adulthood is reached, just like physical abilities. However, not all "mental muscles" "shrivel" at the same rate, and it is important to weigh the negative effects of reduced mental abilities against the positive impact of experience. Thus, even though psychological test performance may decline with age, for particular real-life tasks the relevant experience of an individual may be much more important than the score on a cognitive test. For example, a test may show decline in verbal fluency, but an experienced lawyer would perhaps be better able to select the more effective, if fewer, words compared with younger and more likely fluent counterparts.

Numerous specific changes in cognitive performance are exhibited by persons with dementia. Such changes differ both in magnitude and extent from those seen in the normal aging process. Abilities more commonly affected in dementia include verbal and nonverbal memory, perceptual-organizational abilities, communication skills, and psychomotor performance. The nature, extent, and rate of decline depend on the cause, the person's educational attainment, activity level, and general health status. It is important to remember that about 80% of people living into very old age never experience a significant memory loss or other symptoms of dementia. A slight forgetfulness is common as we age, but it is usually not enough to interfere with our functioning. Pablo Picasso, Margaret Mead, and Duke Ellington were productive well past their 75th birthdays, suggesting that successful aging is both possible and probable.

2. How is cognition assessed?

To understand which cognitive activities decline more than others, we need to divide cognition into components or domains. Recently it has become customary to evaluate the following clusters of cognitive abilities:

Executive functions: the ability to plan, to abstract principles from examples of a set, to shift sets, and to keep ongoing operations in "working memory."

Attention and vigilance: the ability to select relevant stimuli for further processing and response and to concentrate on specific tasks for extended periods.

Learning and memory: the ability to acquire new information and to retrieve it on demand. This ability seems to differ—and perhaps follow specific rules—for verbally encoded and spatial information.

Intellectual functions: analytic abilities, fund of information and vocabulary, and effectiveness of processing complex information. These abilities also seem to differ for verbal and spatial functions.

Sensorimotor functions: the acuity of the senses and the speed and accuracy of motor responses.

Of these domains of behavior, there is evidence for age-related decline in attentional processing, memory (both verbal and spatial), intellectual functions (primarily spatial), and the sensorimotor domain, particularly motor speed. On the other hand, executive functions seem relatively preserved.

3. Can the effects of age on cognition be separated from the effects of illness?

A difficulty in answering the question of domain-specific cognitive decline is the need to separate normal aging effects from the effects of age-related disorders likely to influence cognitive dysfunction. As we age, we are more likely to experience accidents in which we lose consciousness, our arteries harden, and we may experience subclinical ischemic episodes that could nonetheless affect specific cognitive abilities. Other brain disorders are also more prevalent in older age. One way to address this methodologic problem is to screen research subjects carefully for any disorder that may affect cognition. In addition, it is helpful to examine the effects of aging within the younger age range, where it is less likely that age-related disorders have occurred. Obviously the effects of age will be smaller in this population, but the effects observed would point to the cognitive systems most vulnerable to the normal aging process. One should also bear in mind that some functions may show little if any decline initially and steeper decline after a certain age.

4. Are there sex-related differences in this decline?

This issue has been relatively less investigated, because for a long time such differences were ignored and frequently only men were studied. However, there seems to be evidence that the rate of decline with age is faster for men than for women.

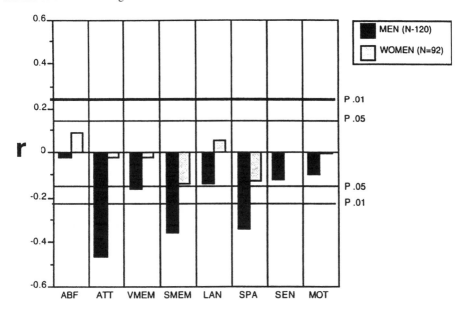

Rates of cognitive decline in men and women. ABF = abstract function; ATT = attention; VMEM = verbal memory; SMEM = spatial memory; LAN = language; SPA = spatial function; SEN = sensory perception; MOT = motor function.

5. What causes age-related changes in cognitive functioning?

Most likely the cognitive decline associated with aging is linked to brain function, and indeed there is evidence for both anatomic and physiologic brain changes with normal aging. Brain volume is reduced with normal aging, and the reduction in the volume of brain tissue is accompanied by an increase in the volume of the cerebrospinal fluid (CSF). This was demonstrated initially by direct postmortem measurements of brains, using the old Archimedes method of measuring the volume of displaced liquid into which the brain is immersed. More recently, computed tomography (CT) and magnetic resonance imaging (MRI) have been used to measure brain volume. These methods are based on computerized "segmentation" of tissue into brain and CSF, which give different image intensities. Such studies confirm the results of postmortem measurements and also suggest sex differences in the rate at which tissue is lost with normal aging. Men show a steeper loss of tissue and increase in CSF than women. Indeed, the decline in the frontal and temporal regions is so pronounced in men compared with women that, whereas young men have larger volumes than young women (commensurate with their overall larger bodies), the volumes in elderly men and elderly women are identical.

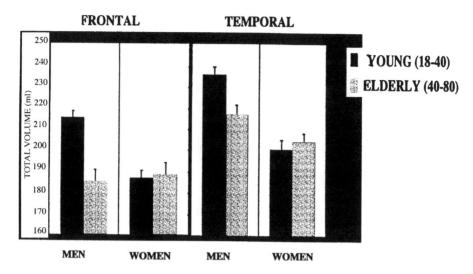

Loss of temporal and frontal brain tissue in men and women.

6. How is the pattern different in the dementias?

As noted earlier, changes in brain structure and function are inevitable with the aging process. For example, speed of response tends to slow, and mild forgetfulness is usually present as a person gets older. While some level of cognitive decline is expected with age, at what point does it become abnormal? The basic question is whether a person exhibits cognitive changes above and beyond those expected for his or her age. Research with healthy aged individuals provides a benchmark of mental abilities for people of various ages and educational and occupational backgrounds as well as gender. Such abnormality is typically assessed against this benchmark. For example, an elderly person with a dementing illness may remember only 50% of what is said to them, whereas a healthy person matched in age, gender, and education may remember 80% or more. In addition, the person with dementia shows other deficits of a substantial scope and magnitude in addition to "forgetfulness." Deficits in problem-solving, language, and visual-perceptual abilities are often present. The stigma attached to cognitive decline is not applied to age-associated physical ailments. Older adults suffering from heart disease are not labeled as abnormal, but this term is applied to those suffering from "dementia." Yet just as the definition of aging can include heart disease, so can it include dementia. Many names have been given to the symptoms of memory loss and loss of cognitive abilities in older adults. Terms such as *senility, hardening of the arteries,* and *organic brain syndrome* have been commonly used. *Alzheimer's disease, multi-infarct disease,* and *senile dementia* are terms often used by health care professionals. The word *dementia* means a loss or impairment of mental abilities; it does not mean "crazy": It comes from two Latin words which translate into *away* and *mind*. Dementia is a term chosen by health care professionals to describe a group of symptoms expressed by various disease states. The question is whether dementia is the inevitable end-point of the normal aging process if one lives long enough. While the evidence for either outcome is not entirely clear, the prevailing thought is that the degenerative organic brain state known as dementia is not part of normal aging. Many types of illnesses are associated with dementia, including Alzheimer's disease, multi-infarct disease, Parkinson's disease, Pick's disease, and progressive supranuclear palsy. The most common causes of dementia in elderly persons are Alzheimer's disease and multi-infarct disease.

Dementia knows no social or racial lines: rich and poor, wise and simple alike can be victims. Many brilliant and famous people have suffered from dementing illnesses, and it is likely that we all know someone with such cognitive impairment. Many elderly people live in the community with mild levels of dementia. Typically they can function if environmental supports (e.g., a caring wife, husband, family members) are available. This impairment becomes clinically meaningful when it impairs the person's level of day-to-day functioning. Although we may all be irritated by occasional forgetfulness, it does not prevent us from performing our daily duties and activities.

7. How do the medicines that older people take affect cognitive function?

The concept that medicine can alter a person's cognitive processes is generally well-accepted by most investigators. Aging brings changes in the way that medicine is broken down and used by the body. For example, studies have shown that age-related changes in the gastrointestinal system, increases in body fat, cardiovascular alterations, reduction in blood flow in the brain, reductions in liver and kidney function, and changes in tissue response to hormones interact with medicines and their effect on the patient. In addition, age has a definite impact on the person's ability to adapt to internal or external stressors. For example, elderly people tend to recover more slowly from the adverse side effects of many medications. This issue becomes more complicated if the older adult is also taking more than one medicine. The disorders for which elderly people most commonly receive medication are depression, anxiety, and apprehension; cognitive and memory impairment; sleep disturbances; and behavior disorders. Drugs with anticholinergic properties (e.g., antidepressants, antihistamines, antimotion sickness medications) are the most likely to cause cognitive side effects. Whereas younger people may experience minimal cognitive effects, such effects are magnified in the elderly by physiological changes. The cognitive effects of drugs used to treat most medical conditions have not, however, been studied systematically.

The greater sensitivity to drug effects in elderly persons also makes the ingestion of "social drugs" problematic and can clearly increase the frequency of negative drug reactions. It is a common practice for patients with diabetes to change their diet to help control the illness. In contrast, it is not unusual to see patients arrive at a precise combination of medicines and dosages through close consultation with their physician—and yet ingest 10–20 cups of coffee a day! Caffeine, nicotine, and other chemicals in common day-to-day beverages and foods can also interact with medicine (or act on their own) to produce adverse cognitive and physiologic effects. Coffee and cola drinks are not the only culprits in such "social drug" consumption. Tea, chocolate, cocoa, cigarettes, and alcohol must also be listed. In addition, seemingly harmless over-the-counter medications (e.g., cold capsules, sleeping medicines, pain relievers) can also interact with prescribed medications. Perhaps the claim of homeopathic physicians that they successfully treat patients with a minimal dosage of drugs can be explained by their close attention to diet and its direct relationship to the taking of prescribed drugs.

In general, many medicines can have an impact on cognitive processes, especially when the increased vulnerability of the brain and associated physical systems is considered. However, such concerns are often secondary to the cognitive effects of the illnesses for which such medications are prescribed. For example, untreated hypertension or diabetes has a greater adverse effect on cognitive function than the medicines used to treat either condition. The best way to minimize the cognitive impact of medicines is to ask questions. Physicians should be able to answer questions about the effect of medications on cognitive status and how different medicines interact.

BIBLIOGRAPHY

1. Birren JE, Fisher LM: Aging and speed of behavior: Possible consequences for psychological functioning. Ann Rev Psychol, 46:329–353, 1995.
2. Salzman C, Shader RI, Van Der Kolk BA: Clinical psychopharmacology and the elderly patient. N Y State J Med 76, 71–77, 1976.
3. Salthouse TA: Adult Cognition: An Experimental Psychology of Human Aging. New York, Springer-Verlag, 1982.
4. Cowell PE, Turetsky BT, et al: Sex differences in aging of the human frontal and temporal lobe. J Neurosc 14:4748–4755, 1994.

27. PARKINSON'S DISEASE

Howard Hurtig, M.D.

1. Who is Parkinson's disease named after?

James Parkinson is credited with the first detailed description in 1817 of the illness that now bears his name.

2. How is Parkinson's disease different from Parkinson syndrome?

Parkinson syndrome, or parkinsonism, is an umbrella term that applies to a recognizable cluster of neurologic symptoms (fatigue, tremor, slowed mobility, difficulty walking) and signs (bradykinesia, stooped posture, shuffling gait, cogwheel rigidity, rest tremor). Most symptoms of parkinsonism appear in middle-aged adults and increase in frequency with the advance of old age. Approximately 1% of people in the developed world over age 60 have some form of parkinsonism, although it is prevalent everywhere it has been sought.

Any combination of signs and symptoms of parkinsonism can occur, most often emerging gradually, or even imperceptibly. Not all components of the symptom complex are present in every patient. Rest tremor is often the only early symptom, but because it is distinctively different from other types of tremor, it is usually recognizable as parkinsonian. Rarely, self-recognition of the signs of parkinsonism is abrupt; for example, in the form of tremor starting in the aftermath of physical or psychological trauma.

Eighty to 90% of people who develop the cardinal symptoms and signs of parkinsonism will have *idiopathic* parkinsonism or **Parkinson's disease**. A clinical diagnosis of Parkinson's disease can be made confidently if at least 3 major signs are identified. Parkinson's disease is a *clinical* diagnosis, reached after other causes of parkinsonism have been excluded by a careful history, thorough physical examination, and a few specific laboratory tests.

Criteria for Diagnosis of Parkinson's Disease*

Unilateral onset and persistent asymmetry	Levodopa-induced dyskinesias
Rest tremor	Levodopa response for $\geq$ 5 yrs
Progressive disability	Clinical course of $\geq$ 10 yrs
Excellent response to levodopa	

* Three or more required for diagnosis of definite Parkinson's disease.
From United Kingdom Parkinson's Disease Society Brain Bank.

3. What are the pathologic findings associated with Parkinson's disease?

The disease is confined to the upper brainstem, where a particular collection of pigmented (melanin) neurons in the substantia nigra undergo progressive degeneration from an unkown cause. The **Lewy body**, an intracytoplasmic inclusion body found at autopsy in the few nigral neurons that survive the process of progressive degeneration, is the histologic signature of Parkinson's disease.

Nigral neurons, when healthy, are the main source of the brain's supply of catecholamine and the neurotransmitter **dopamine**. Dopamine is transported from the brainstem rostrally via the **nigrostriatal** anatomic pathway, beginning in the subtantia nigra and ending at the corpus striatum (caudate and putamen) adjacent to the lateral ventricles. The assemblage of neurons in this brain region is known collectively as the **basal ganglia**. Dopamine plays a major role in the normal physiologic circuitry that connects the basal ganglia to the cerebral cortex and is a major contributor to the complex neurotransmission responsible for programming and executing voluntary movement. Dopamine replacement therapy with the dopamine precursor **levodopa** often alleviates many of Parkinson's disease's most disabling symptoms.

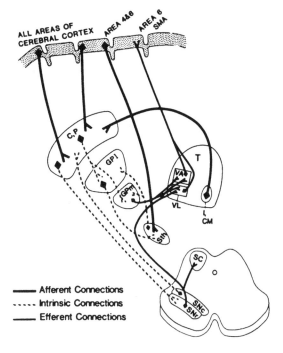

Major afferent, efferent, and internuclear pathways of the basal ganglia. C,P = caudate nucleus and putamen (striatum), GP = globus pallidus (l = lateral, m = medial), SN = substantia nigra (c = compacta, r = reticulata), Sth = subthalamic nucleus, T = thalamus (nuclei: VA = ventral anterior, VL = ventrolateral, CM = centromedian, I = other intralaminar nuclei), SMA = supplementary motor area of cortex, SC = superior colliculus. (From Riley DE, Lang AE: Movement Disorders. In Bradley WG, et al (eds): Neurology in Clinical Practice. Boston, Butterworth-Heinemann, 1996, with permission.)

⸺ Afferent Connections
---- Intrinsic Connections
⸺ Efferent Connections

4. Name the major and minor signs and symptoms of parkinsonism.

Signs of Parkinsonism

MAJOR	MINOR
Rest tremor (4–6 Hz)	Masked facies
Bradykinesia	Micrographia
Muscular rigidity with cogwheeling	Fatigue
Postural instability	Drooling
	Hypophonia

5. Which other neurologic disorders have parkinsonism as a major clinical feature?

Parkinson-plus syndromes—Approximately 10% of people with parkinsonism have pathology in anatomic sites other than the pigmented neurons of the substantia nigra. Degenerative disorders such as progressive supranuclear palsy (PSP), striatonigral degeneration, and parkinsonism with autonomic failure (Shy-Drager syndrome) often resemble Parkinson's disease early in the course, except that patients with these Parkinson-plus syndromes are less likely to have tremor and more likely to have postural instability and significant gait problems at the beginning. The generic term **multisystems atrophy** has become a popular label for degenerative disorders that affect more than one motor system in the same person. Moreover, levodopa usually gives little or no benefit to Parkinson-plus patients, and as a result, the rate of progression is often faster.

Cerebrovascular disease—In the elderly with vascular risk factors, especially hypertension, parkinsonism can evolve as a result of multifocal ischemia and be almost indistinguishable from Parkinson's disease. Early onset of gait instability, presence of frontal release signs, prominent cognitive loss, little or no tremor, and an MRI scan showing multiple infarcts are a few features that help to characterize vascular parkinsonism as a distinct entity.

6. Can medications cause parkinsonism?

Any neuroleptic drug used for any length of time can produce signs of parkinsonism and other movement disorders in older patients. It is important to remember that metoclopramide (Reglan) is a neuroleptic with the same potential for causing parkinsonism as the more potent drugs, such as chlorpromazine and haloperidol. Neuroleptics cause Parkinson symptoms by the same mechanism that they relieve the symptoms of psychosis; they block postsynaptic dopamine receptors in the basal ganglia and mesolimbic cerebral cortex. Reserpine, once a standard antihypertensive, is still used occasionally, often in a combination drug. Reserpine causes parkinsonism by depleting the presynaptic stores of catecholamines, including dopamine. It has no effect on dopamine receptors.

7. What disorders of the nervous system are commonly confused with parkinsonism?

1. **Senile gait** is a disorder of locomotion among older people that resembles the shuffle of parkinsonism, but it can be so severe that walking is impossible due to the inability to initiate or sustain the rhythmic sequence of movements basic to normal walking. This condition has been called **lower-body parkinsonism** because the usual other symptoms of parkinsonism found above the waist are missing. Senile gait overlaps with the mincing steps of older persons who have a background of multiple small strokes and with "gait ignition failure," transient freezing that occurs with initiation of walking.

2. **Essential tremor** (ET) is another common idiopathic movement disorder that is usually familial (autosomal dominant) and increases in frequency with aging. It is the mirror image of parkinsonian rest tremor; i.e., it is activated by voluntary movement and subsides at rest. A careful neurologic examination is the key to separating ET from parkinson's disease. Handwriting is often a clue: micrographic and tight in Parkinson's (usually not shaky), shaky and large in ET.

3. **Stroke** is sometimes blamed for conditions that are actually Parkinson's. Since parkinsonism often starts unilaterally, a flexed and rigid arm or leg can look as if it was caused by a stroke (especially if tremor is absent). Yet, examination shows the telltale signs of unilateral parkinsonism (cogwheel rigidity, bradykinesia of fingers and toes) and the absence of findings typically seen in stroke-related neurologic deficits: strength and sensation are normal, reflexes symmetrical, and Babinski signs absent.

8. What is the relationship between Alzheimer's disease and Parkinson's disease?

Alzheimer's dementia (AD) is by far the most common neurologic disorder of the aging population in the western world. Mild parkinsonism occurs in 20–30% of patients with AD, a reflection of the frequent autopsy finding of a moderate decrease in the number of neurons in the substantia nigra of Alzheimer-affected brains. This interesting overlap between AD and Parkinson's disease is also evident in the higher-than-chance occurrence (20–30%) of dementia in a cross-section of elderly patients with Parkinson's disease, a significant number of whom have Alzheimer's pathology at autopsy.

A clinical diagnosis of AD with parkinsonism versus Parkinson's disease with dementia is a common chicken-and-egg dilemma in neurology. It is often unscrambled by identifying the symptom complex that came first as the primary disorder. Under such circumstances, the clinicopathologic correlation is strong. The high rate of coexistence of AD and Parkinson's disease suggests a common but as-yet-unidentified pathogenetic mechanism that gives rise to neurofibrillary degeneration of vulnerable cell groups in particular but different locations in the brain.

9. Describe an appropriate diagnostic workup for someone with parkinsonism.

In reality, the diagnosis of classic Parkinson's disease is purely clinical and no tests are needed. However, when diagnostic criteria are not met confidently, many doctors choose to do a **brain imaging study**, especially an MRI scan. MRI or CT scans show no definitive abnormalities in Parkinson's disease and only occasionally are helpful in patients with the atypical forms of parkinsonism. Rarely, **severe hydrocephalus** can cause parkinsonism, and only a CT or MRI can show the large ventricles. A ventriculoperitoneal shunt will improve neurologic function in these cases.

Blood and urine tests for **copper** are mandatory in the workup of parkinsonism in anyone under 40 to exclude **Wilson's disease**, an inherited disorder of copper metabolism. Parkinsonism in children and young adults also can be part of the phenotype in certain other hereditary conditions, such as the autosomal dominant **Machado-Joseph disease** (MJD).

A strongly positive response to **levodopa** is usually the best indicator that Parkinson's disease is the right diagnosis. As a rule, a weak or absent response suggests one of the atypical parkinsonian states, although a significant response to levodopa may occur early in the course of any patient with any form of parkinsonism.

10. Does parkinsonism affect other organ systems?

Gastrointestinal tract	Respiratory system
Slowed motility	Hypoventilation
Constipation	Laryngeal stridor
Pseudo-obstruction or megacolon (rarely)	Visual system
Obstipation and impactions	Visual blurring
Urinary tract	Diplopia
Increased frequency	
Urgency	
Incontinence	

11. What causes Parkinson's disease?

This is the question that tantalizes everyone. While there is enough circumstantial evidence to permit experts to formulate a unified working causal hypothesis, the mystery of causation for the most part has not been deciphered. The evidence falls into 3 broad categories with many points of convergence and intersection:

1. Although it has been known for most of this century that approximately 10–15% of patients with Parkinson's disease have a positive family history of parkinsonism, autosomal dominant pedigrees with autopsy proof of Parkinson's disease (Lewy bodies) have been rare. Moreover, studies of identical twins have shown a relatively low rate of concordance when one twin has Parkinson's disease. Yet, the occurrence of these autosomal dominant families and the more common, nonspecific familial aggregations of Parkinson's disease gives some weight to the belief that an abnormal gene with variable penetrance and expressivity is fundamentally responsible for *all* cases of Parkinson's disease.

2. Numerous epidemiologic studies have suggested, albeit weakly, that a host of environmental insults, including past head injury, chronic exposure to pesticides (or other toxins), and rural living, might be risk factors for later development of Parkinson's disease.

3. Neurons die slowly as the brain ages, and neural tissue does not regenerate. Consequently, advancing age contributes to the loss of chemical transmitters manufactured by those dying neurons, and the result in susceptible individuals (i.e., those genetically predisposed or environmentally exposed) is age-related neurologic illness, such as Parkinson's disease and Alzheimer's.

12. What is neuroprotection or neuroprotective therapy?

The basis of neuroprotection is the belief that neural degeneration can be slowed or halted by using agents that stabilize cells and keep them from dying. The discovery that the drug **deprenyl**, an inhibitor of the B form of monoamine oxidase, could block the formation of MPP+ from MPTP (MPP+ is a highly neurotoxic, oxidized byproduct of the recreational drug MPTP that produces severe parkinsonism) and thereby prevent its toxicity led to the hypothesis that deprenyl could slow progression of the disability of Parkinson's disease by preventing the formation of membrane-damaging oxygen free radicals that result from the oxidation of dopamine. A double-blind, randomized clinical trial of deprenyl in patients with early Parkinson's disease showed that deprenyl delayed the need for levodopa therapy by almost a year when compared with placebo. Unfortunately, solid proof that deprenyl actually does protect neurons has been elusive. Many neurologists now prescribe deprenyl in early Parkinson's disease for its putative neuroprotective effect.

The recent discovery of a variety of **growth factors** in the human nervous system has created the possibility of an entirely new form of clinically viable neuroprotection. These biologically active substances naturally promote growth and membrane stability of all cells during development.

13. Which drugs are most effective in treating Parkinson's disease?

Drugs for Treatment of Parkinson's Disease

DRUG	MECHANISM OF ACTION	RELATIVE POTENCY	SIDE EFFECTS
Levodopa/carbidopa (Sinemet)	Activates DA receptors	++++	Nausea Dyskinesia Psychosis Hypotension Constipation
Dopamine agonists (Parlodel, Pergolide)	Activates DA receptors	++	Nausea Hypotension Leg edema Psychosis
Amantadine (Symmetrel)	Releases DA from vesicles	+	Psychosis Leg edema Livedo reticularis
Anticholinergics (Artane, Cogentin, Kemadrin)	Blocks ACh receptors	+	Memory loss Blurred vision Psychosis Prostatism Dry mouth
Deprenyl (Eldepryl)	MAO inhibitor—blocks reuptake of DA ?Neuroprotection	+	Psychosis Hypotension

DA = dopamine; ACh = acetylcholine; MAO = monoamine oxidase.

Four important axioms underlie the application of any of these drugs to the treatment of Parkinson's disease:
1. Never start treatment with > 1 drug.
2. Start with the lowest practical dose and increase slowly—there's never a need to rush.
3. Never make > 1 change at a time when raising or lowering doses, unless the patient is in crisis.
4. Polypharmacy is not necessarily a bad thing. Many neurologists introduce second and third drugs early in the treatment if the primary one (usually levodopa) is not giving adequate benefit.

14. Why is levodopa given with carbidopa?

Levodopa, after almost 30 years since its introduction as a dramatic new treatment for Parkinson's disease, remains the best drug with the best therapeutic margin (fewest side effects in relation to benefit), despite its complicated pharmacology. Levodopa, a precursor of dopamine, is biochemically inert (i.e., not a neurotransmitter), but it easily crosses the blood-brain barrier (BBB) to get into the brain where it is converted to dopamine by the enzyme dopa-decarboxylase (DD). The active transmitter dopamine, on the other hand, is excluded from the brain when used systemically because its molecular structure does not permit it to cross the BBB. The problem is that levodopa is rapidly decarboxylated to dopamine peripherally by DD in the gut and liver before it reaches the brain; thus it is rendered useless for clinical purposes unless given in large amounts to saturate the converting enzyme, in which case intolerable nausea usually occurs. The solution to this therapeutic "catch 22" came in the early 1970s with the development of the DD inhibitor, **carbidopa**. When carbidopa is given in combination with levodopa (Sinemet), it reduces by 80% the amount of levodopa required to have a clinical effect, eliminates most of the side effects associated with using pure levodopa, and makes levodopa accessible to a much larger population of patients.

15. Do all patients with parkinsonism and all symptoms of parkinsonism respond to treatment?

No, unfortunately. The cardinal symptoms of early disease—rest tremor, rigidity and brady-kinesia—usually respond well but not necessarily at the same time. Tremor tends to lag behind the other two but eventually follows. Only 50% of all responders will grade the response as very good or excellent. A completely negative response to levodopa/carbidopa usually portends an un-favorable prognosis as well as a diagnosis of one of the Parkinson-plus disorders.

The most vexing of all symptoms of parkinsonism is postural instability (PI). Most drugs, in-cluding Sinemet, have little or no effect on PI, although occasional significant improvements in equilibrium make the effort of trying the various available dopaminergic medications worth-while. The relatively poor response of PI to dopamine replacement therapy compared with many of the other symptoms of parkinsonism suggests a nondopaminergic pathophysiology.

16. What are the important adjunctive drugs used in treating secondary problems in Parkinson's disease?

Adjunctive Drugs Used in Parkinson's Disease

DRUG	INDICATION	DRUG	INDICATION

Antidepressants
  Tricyclics
  SSRIs
	Depression	Cisapride
		Clozapine
			Constipation
			Drug-induced psychosis

		Fludrocortisone	Orthostatic hypotension

Anxiolytics
  Benzodiazepines
	Anxiety, panic	Hypnotics
		  Benzodiazepines
			Insomnia

Carbidopa	Sinemet-induced nausea	Diphenhydramine	

SSRI = Selective serotonin reuptake inhibitor.

17. What drugs can interfere with the anti-Parkinson drugs (APDs)?

Drugs That Can Aggravate Parkinsonism

DRUG	HOW USED	ADVERSE PHARM EFFECT
Alpha methyldopa	Antihypertensive	Depletes presynaptic catecholamines
Amiodarone	Antiarrhythmic	Unknown
Amoxapine	Antidepressant	Blocks reuptake of NE and serotonin, blocks DA receptors
Diltiazem	Calcium channel blocker	Unknown
Lithium	Antipsychotic, bipolar disease	Unknown
MAO Inhibitors*	Antidepressants	Blocks reuptake of DA and NE
Meperidine	Analgesic	?
Metoclopramide	GI promotility	Blocks DA receptors
Neuroleptics (except clozapine)	Antipsychotic, schizophrenia	Blocks DA receptors
Papaverine	Vasodilator	?Blocks DA receptors
Reserpine	Antihypertensive	Depletes presynaptic catecholamines

* MAO (monoamine oxidase) inhibitors of subtypes A and B—to be distinguished from Deprenyl, which in-hibits only type B. But MAO inhibitors can cause severe hypertension when used in combination with Sinemet, and thus they should never be used in combination. DA = dopamine; NE = norepinephrine.

The table lists the drugs that anyone with Parkinson's disease should either avoid or at least know about when using APDs. Neuroleptics (major tranquilizers and metoclopramide) head the list because they block dopamine receptors in the striatum and can produce severe "extrapyramidal" (parkinsonian) side effects in patients with or without Parkinson's disease. The introduction of clozapine, an "atypical" neuroleptic which does not produce extrapyramidal side effects, allows control of psychosis in patients with Parkinson's disease, especially when these symptoms are caused by the APDs.

Recently a warning was issued concerning the simultaneous use of deprenyl and the antidepressants that inhibit serotonin uptake (the selective serotonin reuptake inhibitors and the tricyclics) because of the rare occurrence of an acute serotonin crisis (hypertension, sweating, agitation, psychosis).

18. Can nonpharmacologic treatments help?

The most important are physical, occupational, and speech therapy. Each has a place and a time and they can be repeated without fear of overdosing. **Physical exercise** is good for conditioning and for stretching stiff, underutilized muscles. Working with a good therapist can restore confidence and stability to a deteriorating patient, especially when drug options are limited in the more advanced stages of disease.

Good **nutrition** also keeps the body strong. Most patients are aware that large protein meals may block or truncate the response to a dose of Sinemet taken near mealtime. Transport of the large neutral amino acids in the blood following breakdown of ingested protein employs the same carrier system that delivers absorbed levodopa to the brain.

Acupuncture may relieve pain and even depression associated with parkinsonism. Despite centuries of use, its mechanism of action in the nervous system remains unknown.

19. What surgical procedures are available for the treatment of Parkinson's disease?

Neurosurgical treatment of Parkinson's disease falls into two broad categories:

Ablative procedures destroy small, precisely targeted groups of cells in strategic locations within the basal ganglia. The medial globus pallidus and the ventral-lateral thalamus are specific anatomic targets in the two most common operations, because pathologically hyperactive neurons in these regions contribute to the severity of bradykinesia, rigidity, and rest tremor. **Pallidotomy** virtually disappeared after the introduction of levodopa in the late 1960s, but it is making a comeback now that it has been shown to relieve some of the more serious motor problems related to chronic levodopa usage (particularly dyskinesias). Sophisticated computerized imaging has allowed target localization to become more precise. **Thalamotomy** has been used specifically to control medically intractable parkinsonian tremor. The other symptoms of Parkinson's disease are alleviated much less by it than by pallidotomy. Preliminary observations suggest that **electrical stimulation** of sites in the basal ganglia that are currently being surgically ablated may become a safer alternative with equivalent results.

Restorative procedures include transplantation with fetal mesencephalon and implantation of various genetically engineered cell lines or devices that deliver dopamine directly into neuron-rich striatal tissue. **Fetal tissue transplantation** is being done in only a few places in the world. Its usefulness is still uncertain after a decade of experimental use with humans and primates. Ethical and logistical concerns will probably restrict its application. Other implantation techniques, using genetically altered viral vectors or cultured cells that deliver dopamine and growth factors, are being developed in experimental animals.

20. Can pain and altered sensation be part of the symptom complex of Parkinson's disease?

Yes, fairly often. It is not uncommon for patients to report stiff, achy joints or numbness and tingling early on before the diagnosis is made. Since Parkinson's disease usually presents as a unilateral or asymmetric clinical disorder, pain and sensory symptoms tend to occur on the side of greater motor involvement. Effective treatment alleviates pain in parallel with the relief of rigidity and improved joint mobility. Physical therapy has the potential for contributing significantly to the patient's well-being.

Pain can also occur as a side effect from APD therapy. Levodopa sometimes induces painful dystonic contractions of limb muscles, either at peak dose effect or as the drug's effect is wearing off. Dystonia of the foot on awakening from sleep in the morning is not uncommon and usually clears after the first dose of Sinemet of the day.

21. How common is depression in Parkinson's disease?

Very. Depression occurs throughout the course of Parkinson's disease, and although antidepressants or psychotherapy help, depression tends to recur. Serious and unexplained depression may herald or precede the onset of the motor symptoms by months or years.

Dopamine deficiency in the basal ganglia is the major biochemical abnormality responsible for the motor trouble in Parkinson's disease. Norepinephrine and serotonin are also depleted, but to a lesser extent than dopamine, as a result of a milder loss of neurons in the midbrain. Virtually all of today's antidepressants work in the brain by blocking reuptake of serotonin, norepinephrine, or both at the synapse, so that more of these transmitters are available to stimulate noradrenergic or serotonergic receptors. The major and minor biochemical losses in Parkinson's disease therefore predispose every patient to a combination of motor and mental changes that include depression as a natural expression of the underlying pathology.

22. What cognitive problems occur in Parkinson's disease?

Most patients with Parkinson's disease, even early in the course of illness, have abnormalities of mental processing. These subtle changes, linguistic and mnestic mainly, are usually clinically insignificant. Many patients, however, complain of mental sluggishness and difficulty with the highest levels of cognition, especially if occupational demands are both physically and intellectually taxing. The term **bradyphrenia** has been applied to this state of slowed thinking. Abnormalities of executive function (decision-making) are well-documented in the intermediate stages of disease progression, and may force patients in high-pressure jobs to take early retirement, even when they are still independent in every respect outside the office.

Mental and motor deteriorations tend to occur in parallel as Parkinson's disease progresses. Serious mental disturbances, such as periodic confusion, visual hallucinations, delusions, and agitation with insomnia at night occur much later in the course and are frequently caused or aggravated by the various APDs. Drug-induced delirium is more likely to occur in patients whose cognitive function is already compromised by the underlying illness. Dementia, which affects 20–30% of patients, occurs late in the course in most cases, when motor function is severely impaired, but not always. The dementia of Parkinson's disease has a more complicated effect on social and personal functions than that of Alzheimer's disease because of the additive impact of the motor and mental disabilities. Unlike Alzheimer's dementia, which is classified neuropsychologically as a cortical dementia because of the high frequency of severe language dysfunction in late stages, Parkinson dementia is designated a **subcortical dementia**. Nonlanguage functions, such as memory retrieval, visual-spatial orientation, and frontal lobe executive functions are the most seriously impaired areas of performance.

23. Describe the natural history of Parkinson's disease.

Variability is the single most remarkable feature of the natural history of Parkinson's disease. All patients tend to get worse over many years, but the pace of that progression differs. Few if any features are reliable indicators of prognosis.

Most patients notice a very gradual increase in disability, sometimes over a period of 30 or more years. The timing of the onset of postural instability during the course of illness is also unpredictable, but it usually appears several years after the other symptoms have been treated successfully. When and if it occurs, postural instability signals a major downturn in disability, although steady deterioration does not necessarily follow. Many patients, again unpredictably, remain on the new plateau for variable amounts of time until the next sign of progression occurs.

24. Is chronic levodopa usage harmful?

The possibility that chronic levodopa usage might accelerate progression has been hotly debated without resolution for almost 2 decades. Levodopa, with its potential to generate oxygen free radicals and to downregulate dopamine receptors, reaches a point of diminishing returns with prolonged usage, according to the skeptics. Therefore, the doctor should delay starting it for as long as possible and use the other APDs first. Levodopa promoters, on the other hand, point to the normalization of lifespan for patients with Parkinsonism, compared to shortened lifespans in the era before levodopa, and to the vastly improved quality of life in most users, irrespective of the complications that often occur. Therefore, why not start it as soon as the patient's disability dictates a need for effective treatment?

Irreconcilable positions notwithstanding, one fact is indisputable: Everyone with Parkinson's disease at some point requires levodopa to achieve maximal functional ability, usually around 4 years into the disease. Postponing the use of the best drug for a year or 2 when the disease often runs a 20- or 25-year course does not buy much time. Besides, there is essentially no hard clinical evidence that witholding levodopa for any length of time makes any difference in the long run.

25. How do people who have Parkinson's disease die?

Patients live a relatively normal lifespan now, compared to expectations 30 years ago before levodopa was introduced. Many die in old age or earlier of other causes, before they progress to the point of extreme immobility. The general rate of deterioration is usually slow enough that most patients learn to accommodate, although none too happily, as the next level of compromise is reached.

In some instances, deterioration and progression to endstage disability are unpredictably precipitous after years of stability. The cause of this rare abrupt decline is unknown, but rapid worsening sometimes follows hospitalization (e.g., for surgery, a broken hip, or heart attack) or some other period of forced immobilization associated with an intercurrent illness. Nigral cell loss at postmortem is usually directly proportional to the degree of clinical disability at the time of death. It is likely that an accelerated increase in disability at the end of life reflects the death of the substantia nigra's last few cells. The conversion of levodopa to dopamine in the brain can no longer occur because there are no cells with enough dopa decarboxylase to promote the conversion. The patient's clinical response to Sinemet ceases and voluntary movement becomes impossible. A parallel decline in cognitive function is a common end-stage occurrence. Dementia, especially in very old patients, affects as many as 50% at the very end of life. Pneumonia, urinary tract infections, and pulmonary emboli are often the direct antecedents of death from cardiac arrhythmia or myocardial infarction.

BIBLIOGRAPHY

1. Goetz CG, DeLong MR, Penn RD, Bakay RAE: Neurosurgical horizons in Parkinson's disease. Neurology 43:1–7, 1993.
2. Hoehn MM, Yahr MD: Parkinsonism: Onset, progression and mortality. Neurology 17:427–442,1967.
3. Jankovic J, Tolosa, E (eds): Parkinson's Disease and Movement Disorders, 2nd ed. Baltimore, Williams & Wilkins, 1993.
4. Marsden CD, Fahn S: Akinetic rigid syndromes. In Marsden CD, Fahn S (eds). Movement Disorders 3. Oxford, Butterworth-Heinemann, 1994.
5. Quinn N: Drug treatment of Parkinson's disease. BMJ 310:575–579,1995.

28. RENAL DISEASE

Ray Townsend, M.D.

1. What changes in kidney function occur with aging?

Concentrating ability of the kidney declines with age. As a result, solute loads such as salt and protein are not excreted as quickly or as efficiently. Older patients are at greater risk for hypernatremia and hyperosmolality if they are deprived of adequate water intake. The higher risk of hypernatremia is in part worsened by a reduction in thirst sensation with advancing age. Drugs such as lithium (which impairs thirst and also results in a nephrogenic diabetes insipidus), osmotic diuretics (mannitol and radiology contrast media), and high protein feedings should be used and monitored cautiously in the elderly.

Diluting ability also declines with advancing years, leading to a substantial prevalence of hyponatremia in the elderly. Thiazide diuretics and older antihyperglycemic medications (chlorpropamide) may produce severe hyponatremia in some elderly patients.

2. In older people, does a serum creatinine within the normal range mean that kidney functions are normal?

Not necessarily. After the 40th birthday, there is an average decrease in kidney function of about 1% per year, or roughly 10% per decade. However, the serum creatinine does not increase by 10% per decade; this is due to the fact that at the same time kidney function declines, creatinine production declines proportionately because of a progressive decrease in body muscle mass. Creatinine is produced by a nonenzymatic dehydration of muscle creatine, and the amount of creatinine produced each day is proportional to the size of the muscle mass. Kidney function is generally measured by a creatinine clearance derived from a 24-hour urine collection and a serum creatinine measurement using a standard clearance formula. For example, if a 25-year-old man who is 6'2" tall, weighs 220 pounds, and has an obviously well-developed muscle mass collects a 24-hour urine sample and undergoes a blood test, the lab may report the following: 24-hour urine volume of 2750 ml, urine creatinine concentration of 85 mg/dl, serum creatinine of 1.6 mg/dl. To calculate his creatinine clearance:

1. Determine the amount of creatinine excreted: $[(2750 \text{ ml}/24 \text{ hr}) \times (85 \text{ mg/dl})]/(100 \text{ ml/dl})$ = 2337.5 mg/24 hr.

2. Determine the minute excretion of creatinine (since clearance is expressed in the amount of blood cleared of a substance per minute) by dividing the total excreted by 1440 minutes in a day: $[(2337.5 \text{ mg}/24\text{hr})/(1440 \text{ min}/24\text{hr})] = 1.62 \text{ mg/min}$.

3. To determine the clearance, divide the minute excretion of creatinine by the serum concentration: $[(1.62 \text{ mg/min})/(1.6 \text{ mg/dl})] \times (100 \text{ ml/dl}) = 101.5 \text{ ml/min}$.

An average creatinine clearance is about 100 ml/min. If the young man's 185-pound, 5'10" grandfather performed a similar collection, the following results may be expected: 24-hour volume of 2750 ml, urine creatinine concentration of 45 mg/dl, serum creatinine of 1.4 mg/dl. This would yield a creatinine clearance of:

1. Calculate mg of creatinine excreted in 24 hours:

$$\frac{2750 \text{ ml}/24 \text{ hr} \times 45 \text{ mg/dl}}{100 \text{ ml/dl}} = 1237.5 \text{ mg/24hr}$$

2. Calculate the minute excretion of creatinine:

$$\frac{1237.5 \text{ mg}/24 \text{ hr}}{1440 \text{ min}/24 \text{ hr}} = 0.86 \text{ mg/min}$$

3. Calculate the creatinine clearance:

$$\frac{0.86 \text{ mg/min}}{1.4 \text{ mg/dl}} \times 100 \text{ ml/dl} = 61.4 \text{ ml/min}$$

Despite a lower serum creatinine level, the older patient actually has less kidney function because the daily creatinine production is less. When a 24-hour urine collection is not available or not practical, a useful formula to estimate kidney function—one which takes into account age, weight, and gender (women tend to have proportionately less muscle mass)—is that of Cockcroft and Gault:

$$\text{Creatinine clearance} = \frac{[(140 - \text{age in years}) \times (\text{weight in kg})]}{[(72) \times (\text{serum creatinine in mg/dl})]}$$

The result is multiplied by 0.85 for women. In the example given, if an elderly man is 71 years old, the formula predicts his creatinine clearance as follows:

$$[(140 - 71) \times (185 \text{ lb}/2.2 \text{ lb/kg})/[(72) \times 1.4 \text{ mg/dl})] = 57.6 \text{ ml/min}$$

This result is acceptably close to the 61.4 ml/min actually measured. The (72) in the formula is a constant factor for the units that, after division, result in the final value of ml/min for the calculation. For an elderly woman of the same age and weight, the result would be $57.6 \times 0.85 = 48.9$ ml/min. This formula is particularly useful for dosing guidelines in hospitalized elderly renal patients when there is not enough time to collect a 24-hour urine.

The Cockcroft and Gault formula, however, is not as useful in obese patients. For patients more than 25–30% above ideal body weight, the following formulas of Salazar and Corcoran should be used:

Male creatinine clearance =

$$\frac{(137 - \text{age in yr} \times [(0.285 \times \text{weight in kg}) + (12.1 \times \text{height in meters}^2)]}{(51 \times \text{serum creatinine in mg/dl})}$$

Female creatinine clearance =

$$\frac{(146 - \text{age in yr}) \times [(0.287 \times \text{weight in kg}) + (9.74 \times \text{height in meters}^2)]}{(60 \times \text{serum creatinine in mg/dl})}$$

Try the Cockcroft formula on an 80-year old woman who weighs 110 pounds and has a "normal" creatinine of 1.3 mg/dl (do not forget to multiply by 0.85). Then run the same calculation for the 25-year-old man used as the first example.

3. When should an elderly patient be referred to a nephrologist?

There are no strict guidelines; however, consider referring an older patient to a nephrologist when he or she has:

- Unexplained proteinuria (dipstick $\geq$ ++ or $\geq$ 1.0 gm/24 hr)
- Unexpected or unexplained decline in renal function (increase in serum creatinine by > 20% from baseline and confirmed by rechecking)
- Hematuria (gross or microscopic)
- Late onset of hypertension (> age 55 years)
- Refractory or unexplained electrolyte disorders (e.g., hyponatremia, hypo/hyperkalemia, hypomagnesemia)
- Noncardiac peripheral edema

In general, elderly patients with a creatinine $\geq$ 3.0 mg/dl should be considered for nephrologic evaluation, in part to address unapparent renal problems (such as renal osteodystrophy), in part to establish a relationship for future dialysis or transplant care, and in part to address subtleties of divalent ion metabolism (such as decreases in serum calcium and increases in serum phosphorous), which tend to occur early in renal insufficiency.

4. Which kinds of medications are particularly troublesome in elderly patients with renal disease?

Drug/Class	Clinical Effect
Digoxin	Accumulates more readily due to less renal excretion (digitalis toxicity)
Aminoglycosides	May impair renal function through tubular toxicity

NSAIDs	Sodium retention, loss of blood pressure control; impair kidney function by interfering with renal blood flow
Lithium	Hypernatremia—through impaired thirst and impairment of urinary concentration mechanisms
Thiazides	Hyponatremia—through impaired renal diluting mechanisms and water retention

5. Is there anything special I need to know about proteinuria in older patients?

The main causes of nephrotic syndrome (characterized by 3 or more grams of protein excreted in the urine over 24 hours and usually attended by a low serum albumin, peripheral edema, and increases in triglyceride and/or cholesterol) differ in old and young patients. In the elderly, the most common cause of proteinuria is diabetes mellitus. In the absence of diabetes, membranous glomerulopathy is the most common idiopathic form of nephrotic syndrome in the elderly (about ⅓ of cases), followed by minimal change disease (about ⅕–¼ of cases). The finding of membranous glomerulopathy on a kidney biopsy is an important observation because about 1 of 5 patients has a malignancy associated with membranous glomerulopathy. A thorough history and physical, a chest x-ray, rectal and prostate exam (including a stool for occult blood), and a gynecologic exam with mammography are usually adequate screening procedures for malignancy when membranous glomerulopathy is found.

6. Which kinds of renal disease are more common in the elderly? How do I recognize them?

Obstructive uropathy due to prostate hyperplasia or neoplasia is clearly more common in elderly men as opposed to women or younger men. The history is helpful in that older men may have noticed a decrease in the size or force of the urine stream, hesitancy in starting urine stream, straining, dribbling, and a feeling that the bladder is not empty after voiding. In addition, some elderly men may develop an acute worsening of underlying prostate problems when they take an anticholinergic or antihistaminic drug. A rectal exam confirms prostate enlargement and/or neoplasia.

Cholesterol embolization is a clinically challenging condition to recognize. In older patients it results from atheroma in the arterial circulation. It typically becomes manifest after an arteriogram with or without an angioplasty or after anticoagulant therapy. The clinician may see livedo reticularis, cyanosis, or (ultimately) gangrene in the toes; fever; eosinophilia; a progressive rise in serum creatinine concentration; and a loss of blood pressure control. A skin or renal biopsy showing typical cholesterol clefts in the arterioles confirms the clinical diagnosis.

Ischemic renal disease is characterized by progressive atherosclerotic obliteration of the main renal arteries and their branches, with a loss in kidney volume and function over time. It is increasingly recognized as more older patients undergo arteriographic procedures, and it may be responsible for 10–15% of renal failure leading to dialysis in elderly patients. Important clues are a smoking history, known coronary artery disease, bruits (anywhere, but especially in the flank areas), and an increase in the serum creatinine concentration after the use of an angiotensin-converting enzyme inhibitor, especially in patients who are also on a diuretic. Another clue is repeated episodes of pulmonary edema. Magnetic resonance angiography, Doppler ultrasound, spiral computed tomography and angiography are useful procedures in making the diagnosis.

Clues to Ischemic Renal Disease

HISTORY	PHYSICAL	LABORATORY
Cigarette use	Bruits (anywhere)	Increase in serum creatinine following angiotensin converting enzyme inhibitor therapy (especially with diuretic)
Angina	Pulmonary edema	

7. Is acute renal failure more common in elderly patients? How do I recognize which older patients are at risk for a sudden decline in renal function?

Although intuitively one may think that older patients frequently have a loss of kidney function after surgery or a hypotensive episode, in fact older patients typically do well after elective or emergent surgical procedures. The most common identifiable risk factor that predisposes to acute renal failure (often defined simply as a doubling of the serum creatinine concentration over 1–2 days) is volume depletion, either as a consequence of intentional diuretic usage or as a result of unrecognized osmotic diuresis or diarrhea in patients who receive parenteral or enteral nutrition that is high in protein or who are hyperglycemic. A daily weight (unarguably one of the least expensive in-hospital procedures) can help to identify an older patient who is becoming volume depleted. Other situations that should be kept in mind include:

- Aminoglycoside antibiotic usage—doses that are well tolerated by younger patients are more likely to cause a fall in renal function in elderly patients
- Obstructive uropathy, especially when induced by medications that may impair bladder emptying in older patients
- Usage of the histamine-blocking agent cimetidine or the antibiotic trimethoprim, both of which compete with creatinine for secretion in the proximal tubule of the kidney and may functionally elevate the serum creatinine (not by reducing filtration but by impairing secretion)
- Intravenous contrast usage—the risk of acute renal failure depends on the initial level of kidney function and the presence of other disorders (e.g., diabetes, myeloma, preexisting renal disease from any cause, and volume depletion).

8. What are the main causes of kidney failure leading to dialysis in the elderly?

Diabetes and hypertension, as in younger patients. The incidence of older patients who begin dialysis as a result of ischemic renal disease is also increasing.

9. Should age be a barrier to starting a patient on dialysis?

Age alone is not a barrier to dialysis. In patients with dementia (but not uremic encephalopathy), malignancy, and advanced hepatic failure, however, its use should be carefully reviewed. Initiation of dialysis is not a mandate for its continuance in patients who tolerate dialysis poorly or who fail to thrive. Dialysis, an expensive resource, should be used to maintain life rather than to prolong death. If it is clear that a patient is continuing to fail despite adequate dialysis, a dialogue between the patient and his or her family and the medical team should remain open, and the option to stop dialysis should be a topic of continued discussion.

10. Do elderly patients do poorly on dialysis compared with younger patients?

Elderly patients often do quite well on dialysis. Both hemodialysis and peritoneal dialysis have been used in the care of end-stage renal disease in the elderly, and patient survival is similar between the two dialysis modalities. Compared with younger patients, elderly patients on hemodialysis are at greater risk for hypotension during dialysis, malnutrition, dialysis-associated amyloidosis, gastrointestinal bleeding, depression, subdural hematoma, voluntary withdrawal from the hemodialysis program, and inadequate dialysis (either because of limitations imposed by poor access—i.e., poor blood flow in the arteriovenous connection in the patient—or because of problems such as nausea, muscle cramping, or hypotension during dialysis, which reduce blood flow rates and thus impair efficiency). Elderly patients on peritoneal dialysis may become volume-depleted, develop peritonitis, or experience metabolic consequences such as hyperglycemia and hyperlipidemia (hypetriglyceridemia) from the high glucose concentrations in the peritoneal dialysate.

11. What are the main causes of death in elderly patients on dialysis?

The main causes of death depend in part on the modality used, but in general they are as follows (in descending order):

Hemodialysis	**Peritoneal dialysis**
Heart disease and stroke	Heart disease and stroke
Infection	Peritonitis
Voluntary discontinuation	Other infections

Voluntary discontinuation is not uncommon in hospitalized patients dying from multisystem organ failure; withdrawal of dialysis sets up a terminal event.

12. Should older patients in renal failure be considered for a kidney transplant?

Although roughly 40% of patients with end-stage renal disease (including both dialysis and transplant patients) are > 65 years old, < 3% of patients in this age range receive a kidney transplant. Contributing factors include cadaver-kidney shortage (more potential recipients than donors), poor results with prior immunosuppressive regimens (i.e., past experience with antirejection drugs), and the idea that age alone is a barrier to transplantation. However, with careful patient selection and particular attention to the immunosuppressive regimen (e.g., recognizing that the P450 enzyme system which metabolizes cyclosporine is less active in the elderly and may allow use of a lower dose), elderly patients should not be refused transplantation on the basis of age alone. Transplanted kidneys are lost in the elderly mostly because of patient death (about 50%, with the chief causes being heart disease, infection, and malignancy, in that order). In younger patients, death accounts for only about 15% of graft loss, with acute and chronic rejection accounting for most of the remainder. In evaluating an older patient for transplant, the following procedures are commonly used:

- Exercise stress test with thallium and coronary angiogram for patients with coronary symptoms or diabetes
- Careful evaluation of peripheral pulses, because the transplanted kidney may "steal" blood flow from the leg
- Ultrasound of gallbladder, because cholelithiasis is a problem in the elderly, especially those with diabetes
- Barium enema, although its value is debatable in some patients, is considered useful because of the poor outcome in transplant patients with a colon perforation (usually from underlying diverticular disease) and the possible masking of bowel symptoms when a patient is on immunosuppressive drugs. Many authorities strongly consider a barium enema in patients with polycystic kidney disease.
- Mammography and prostate evaluations

13. What other factors affect the treatment of elderly patients with acute renal failure?

1. Recovery from acute renal failure in the elderly is no different from recovery in younger patients, and the patient's ultimate prognosis, not their age, should weigh heavily in the decision to use renal replacement therapy (dialysis).

2. Maintain a reasonable index of suspicion for ischemic renal disease, which may be responsive to angioplasty or arterial bypass, thus prolonging the renal life span.

3. Recognize that elderly patients are more prone to dialysis-related events such as hypotension and hemodialysis access problems, but these events are usually manageable. Many elderly patients do quite well on dialysis.

4. Do not rule out transplantation in an older patient with failing kidney function on the basis of age alone.

Bear in mind, however, that a transplant evaluation committee is more likely to approve older patients as potential transplant recipients if they appear in good health, with reasonably stable weight, no claudication, and a low index of suspicion for coronary artery and gastrointestinal diseases (gallstones and diverticulosis).

14. How does renal function in the elderly affect prescription of medications?

Elderly patients frequently consume a great number and remarkable variety of medications. Drug interaction, which is difficult to predict in normal patients with healthy kidneys and livers, becomes impossibly difficult in patients with compromised renal function. The following guidelines may be helpful:

1. Start with low doses, titrate slowly, and be willing to consider discontinuing drugs with marginal benefit.

2. Expect normal electrolytes and acid-base metabolism in older patients and look for precipitating drugs and intercurrent illnesses when abnormalities occur.

ACKNOWLEDGMENT

The research reported in this chapter was supported in part by NIH grants DK-07006, DK-45191, and by administrative/educational funds from the DCI RED Fund.

BIBLIOGRAPHY

1. Abrass CK: Glomerulonephritis in the elderly. Am J Med 5:409–418, 1985.
2. Cockcroft DW, Gault MH: Prediction of creatinine clearance from serum creatinine. Nephron 16:31–41, 1976.
3. Ismail N, Hakim R, Helderman JH: In-depth review. Renal replacement therapies in the elderly, Part II: Renal transplantation. Am J Kidney Dis 23:1–15, 1994.
4. Ismail N, Hakim R., Oreopoulos DG, Patrikarea A: In-depth review. Renal replacement therapies in the elderly. Part I: Hemodialysis and chronic peritoneal dialysis. Am J Kidney Dis 22:759–782, 1993.
5. Lye WC, Cheah JS, Sinniah R: Renal cholesterol embolic disease. Case report and review of the literature. Am J Nephrol 13:489–493, 1993.
6. Novick AC: Atherosclerotic ischemic nephropathy. Epidemiology and clinical considerations. Urol Clin North Am 21:195–200, 1994.
7. Salazar D, Corcoran G: Predicting creatinine clearance and renal drug clearance in obese patients from estimated fat-free body mass. Am J Med 84:1053–1060, 1988.

29. LIPID DISORDERS IN THE ELDERLY

Cheng-An Mao, M.D., M.P.H.

1. How are lipids metabolized?

Lipids are bound to carrier proteins and circulated in the human body. These complexes, called lipoproteins, can be separated by density during centrifugation. The degree of density is inversely related to lipid contents. The most important forms are:

Chylomicrons

Contain triglyceride and cholesterol obtained from dietary fat

Low-density lipoprotein cholesterol (LDL-C)

Generated from chylomicrons and VLDL-C by the action of lipoprotein lipases

Contains most of the plasma cholesterol

Contributes to cholesterol plaque formation

Significant risk factor for coronary artery disease (CAD)

Very-low density lipoprotein cholesterol (VLDL-C)

Contains triglyceride and cholesterol synthesized in the liver

Synthesis regulated by hydroxymethyl glutaryl CoA reductase (HMG-CoA reductase)

High-density lipoprotein cholesterol (HDL-C)

Inversely correlated with CAD, which may be because HDL-C removes cholesterol from the peripheral system back to the liver and further prevents cholesterol plaque formation in the vascular system

2. What are the effects of aging on lipids?

Whether or not cholesterol levels are important in the elderly is controversial. Older CAD patients have multiple risk factors affecting cardiovascular risk.

One study indicates that the cholesterol/HDL-C ratio relates significantly to CAD in people above 50 years. HDL-C appears more important in predicting CAD in older persons than LDL-C, which is a vital factor in estimating CAD risks in middle-aged persons. Low HDL-C can predict CAD mortality in persons > 70 years. Elevated total cholesterol (TC) is not associated with CAD mortality in older men but may be a risk factor in older women. Generally speaking, a patient with a TC/HDL-C ratio > 5 may be at an increased risk of CAD. A TC/HDL-C ratio increased by 1 may heighten risk of CAD by 17%.

In both men and women, TC levels increase from adolescence and achieve the plateau in middle-age, then decline slightly after age 70 years. The levels are lower in women than in men until menopause. In addition to TC, LDL-C levels are slightly lower in older persons than in younger persons. HDL-C levels increase slightly in older people and are higher in women than in men. A recent study in older persons has reported central fat deposition, glucose intolerance, obesity (in women), and use of ß-blockers (in men) are associated with decreased HDL-C and increased TC. Higher LDL-C is also seen in obese patients and in those with central fat deposition.

Lipoprotein Lipids in Older Persons, By Age

	MALE		FEMALE	
	> 70 YRS	50–69 YRS	> 70 YRS	50–69 YRS
TC	207	214	228	231
Triglyceride	130	141	132	125
HDL-C	51	48	60	59
LDL-C	143	146	149	152
TC/HDL-C	4.06	4.46	3.8	3.91

Cholesterol values given in mg/dl.

3. In addition to age itself, what other elements influence plasma lipid levels in older patients?

Heredity

Genetic abnormalities causing lower HDL-C or higher LDL-C increase the risk of atherosclerosis.

Some families whose members usually live long lives show high HDL-C levels.

Progeric patients with shorter life expectancies have been described with elevated LDL-C and low HDL-C.

Life style

Weight reduction can lower LDL-C and may raise HDL-C.

Exercise increases HDL-C.

HDL-C levels are shown to rise when a tobacco user quits smoking.

Alcoholism is strongly related to lipid abnormalities.

Disease

Cholesterol and LDL-C levels are elevated in hypothyroidism.

Poorly controlled diabetes can increase triglyceride and cholesterol levels.

Syndrome X is a condition associated with hyperglycemia, hypertension, hypertriglyceridemia, and low HDL-C.

Nephrotic syndrome raises plasma lipid levels.

Liver disease affects plasma lipid levels.

Acute illness, such as infection or myocardial infarctions can increase lipid levels.

Correcting the underlying disease is the treatment of choice.

4. How do drugs and hormones influence plasma lipid levels in elderly patients?

Hormones and Drugs	*Reactions*
Thyroid hormone	↓ TC, ↓ LDL-C
Testosterone	↑ LDL-C, ↓ HDL-C
Estrogen	↓ LDL-C, ↑ HDL-C
Progesterone	May ↑ LDL-C, ↓ HDL-C
Thiazide	↑ LDL-C
β-Blocker	↑ LDL-C
Hypolipidemics	
Bile acid sequestrant	↓ LDL-C
Nicotinic acid	↓ TG, LDL-C and VLDL-C; may ↑ HDL-C
HMG CoA reductase inhibitor	↓ LDL-C, ↓ VLDL-C
Fibric acid	Mildly ↓ LDL-C and TG, ↑ HDL-C
Probucol	↓ LDL-C and HDL-C

TG = triglyceride

5. When should cholesterol levels be measured? How?

Clinical trials have demonstrated that lowering LDL-C and raising HDL-C can stop progression and even cause regression of coronary atherosclerotic lesions in middle-aged persons. It is recommended that serum cholesterol levels be measured at least once every 5 years in all adults 20 years of age and above.

Because cholesterol levels can be influenced by acute illness, measurement should not be performed in acutely ill patients. High cholesterol should not be diagnosed from a single test indicating an elevated level of cholesterol; instead, repeated tests should be conducted after the initial reading to corroborate the results. A lipoprotein analysis is indicated when:

• HDL-C is < 35 mg/dl or TC > 240 mg/dl
• TC between 200–239 mg/dl, HDL-C < 35 mg/dl, or ≥ 2 risk factors.

The risk factors for increased levels are age (male > 45, female > 55), family history of premature CAD, current cigarette smoking, hypertension, low HDL-C (< 35 mg/dl), and diabetes mellitus.

6. How are cholesterol levels measured?

A lipoprotein analysis contains TC, triglyceride, HDL-C, and calculated LDL-C. The blood sample should be collected after a 12 hours' fasting as triglyceride (TG) levels are very sensitive to fat intake. LDL-C is calculated by using the following formula:

$$LDL-C = TC - (HDL-C) - (TG/5)$$

7. Does hyperlipidemia in the elderly need treatment?

Many clinical trials showing the effect of reducing cholesterol on CAD mortality and morbidity were done in middle-aged subjects, but supporters suggest the results may be extrapolated to older persons. They believe lowering LDL-C and increasing HDL-C can stop the progression and may reverse the process of atherogenesis. Opponents are unsure how soon the effect of cholesterol reduction on vascular disease will be seen and question if older patients will live long enough to see the benefits. Costs and side effects are other considerations when using drug therapy.

There is no straightforward answer for treating hyperlipidemia in the elderly. The decision should be justified individually after measuring the benefits and risks. Life expectancy, quality of life, and the patient's general health should be considered. Sometimes, cholesterol-lowering therapy may "do more harm than good," such as if a patient is fragile and with a limited life expectancy of < 5 years. In these situations, it may be preferable to leave hyperlipidemia without treatment. Aggressive cholesterol-lowering therapy can be applied to those who have a reasonable life expectancy (at least 5–10 years) and those who are not frail or do not have terminal conditions such as malignancy, dementia, or severe CAD. Attention to other risk factors can be as important as reduction in cholesterol levels. Life style changes should be attempted before dietary and drug therapy. Smoking cessation has a significant impact on reducing CAD incidence. Treating hypertension and diabetes is essential in CAD prevention.

8. What cholesterol levels should be considered as treatment goals in the elderly?

Currently, there are not enough data to define the goal of cholesterol-lowering treatment in the elderly, especially when using drug therapy. Even though normal LDL-C levels are used as a treatment target for middle-aged patients, LDL-C levels seem to have a less significant impact in the elderly. TC/HDL-C ratio may be an appropriate reading as a follow-up method in treating the elderly. More research is needed before definite recommendations can be given.

9. Discuss the principles of treating hyperlipidemia in the elderly.

All programs for cholesterol reduction should begin with a complete **history** and **physical examination**. Special attention should be given to diseases that may influence cholesterol levels. Correction of underlying hyperglycemia or hypothyroidism may restore lipid levels to normal.

Increasing **exercise** and **dietary modifications** are usually first recommendations. Reducing body fat and increasing the percentage of lean mass modified through exercise can increase HDL-C and decrease chylomicron. Diet control can reduce LDL-C, VLDL-C, and chylomicrons. HDL–C may be decreased by diet control. The goal of dietary modification is to cut the total intake of cholesterol and saturated fat. Total fat content of the diet should be lowered to 30–35% of daily calories supply, and the fat intake should consist of a high polyunsaturated fat/saturated fat ratio, meaning patients should strive to avoid animal fat. Caloric restriction is indicated for those who are overweight. There is always a danger of malnutrition during diet modification for weight reduction in older persons, especially if patients are consuming < 1200 cal/day. The patient's nutritional condition should be regularly assessed.

Drug therapy is usually reserved for those who do not have a good response after at least 3–6–month trial of life style modification and dietary intervention, but cholesterol-lowering drugs should be used cautiously in elderly persons. Costs and side effects need to be considered. Estrogens lower LDL-C and raise HDL-C. Estrogens may be beneficial to older women who have osteoporosis or CAD and need lipid control.

10. Name the five types of hypolipidemic agents.

Cholesterol-lowering drugs consist of bile acid sequestrants, nicotinic acids, HMG-CoA reductase inhibitors, fibric acids, and probucol.

11. How do bile acid sequestrants act on cholesterol levels?

Cholestyramine and colestipol interfere with the absorption of bile acids in the GI tract, lowering LDL-C levels by about 10–25%. Sequestrants are safe and effective in persons with moderately elevated LDL-C. Cholestyramine has been proved to reduce mortality of CAD in middle-aged persons. Sequestrants can be combined with other drugs, such as HMG-CoA reductase inhibitors, to treat severe cases of hyperlipidemia. A common side effect is constipation, and these drugs interfere with the absorption of many other drugs (e.g., warfarin, digitalis, ß-blocker, and thyroxine). Laboratory studies or drug levels should be monitored when sequestrants are used together with those drugs.

12. How do nicotinic acids work?

Because of side effects (i.e., GI distress, elevated liver enzymes, hypotension, arrhythmia, hyperglycemia, and flushing), nicotinic acids are tolerated best when started at a low dosage and then increased slowly. A low-dose aspirin taken before nicotinic acid may alleviate the flushing. Glycemic control in diabetic patients may require adjustment if nicotinic acids are used, because nicotinic acid can cause hyperglycemia. The incidence of heart attacks has proved to be reduced in secondary prevention trials. Nicotinic acids decrease triglyceride, LDL-C, and VLDL-C levels and may increase HDL-C.

13. HMG-CoA reductase inhibitors?

HMG-CoA reductase inhibitors (e.g., lovastatin, pravastatin, and simvastatin) interfere with cholesterol synthesis and result in lowering LDL-C and VLDL-C. Because they have a stronger effect in reducing LDL-C (reduction of 25–40%), HMG CoA reductase inhibitors seem to be good drugs for CAD prevention. Side effects include diarrhea, elevated liver enzymes, myopathy, and rhabdomyolysis. Combination therapy of HMG CoA reductase inhibitors with fibric acids or nicotinic acids should be avoided because of the possibilities of hepatotoxicity, myopathy, and rhabdomyolysis.

14. What are the other hypolipidemics?

Fibric acids (e.g., gemfibrozil, fenofibrate, and clofibrate) lower triglyceride and increase HDL-C. Their mechanisms may be related to inhibiting peripheral lipolysis and reducing hepatic uptake of free fatty acids. Since they only have a mild effect on lowering LDL-C, they are not considered as a main drug for CAD prevention. Side effects include GI discomforts, elevated liver enzymes, abdominal pains, potential cancer risks, and myopathy. Fibric acids or nicotinic acids are good for treating hypertriglyceridemia.

The effect of CAD prevention has not been established by using **probucol** yet. The mechanism of action may be associated with the absorption and elimination of cholesterol. Probucol reduces LDL-C and also HDL-C. The reduction of HDL-C could be a concern with its use.

BIBLIOGRAPHY

1. Abrams WB, Berkow R: The Merck Manual of Geriatrics. Rahway, NJ, Merck & Co., 1990.
2. Cassel CK, Walsh JR: Geriatric Medicine. New York, Springer-Verlag,1984.
3. Denke MA, et al: Hypercholesterolemia in elderly persons: Resolving the treatment dilemma. Ann Intern Med 112:780–792, 1990.
4. Ettinger WH, et al: Lipoprotein lipids in older people. Results from the cardiovascular health study. Circulation 86:858–869, 1992.

5. Hazzard WR, et al (eds): Principles of Geriatric Medicine and Gerontology, 3rd ed. New York, McGraw-Hill, 1994.
6. HDL cholesterol predicts coronary heart disease mortality in older persons. JAMA 274:538–544, 1995.
7. Krumholz HM, et al: Lack of association between cholesterol and coronary heart disease mortality and morbidity and all-cause mortality in persons older than 70 years. JAMA 272:1335–1340, 1994.
8. Reikel W: Care of the Elderly: Clinical Aspects of Aging, 4th ed. Baltimore, Williams & Wilkins, 1995.
9. Summary of the second report of the National Cholesterol Education Program (NCEP) expert panel on detection, evaluation, and treatment of high blood cholesterol in adults (Adult Treatment Panel II). JAMA 269:3015–3023, 1993.

30. THYROID DISORDERS IN THE ELDERLY

Mary Ann Forciea, M.D.

1. Why is the thyroid gland important to aging?

The spectrum of thyroid dysfunction in the elderly is broad. Illnesses due to thyroid dysfunction are common enough to be seen regularly in any primary care practice with significant numbers of elderly patients. Alterations in thyroid hormone have even been proposed as the cause of aging itself.

2. What does the thyroid gland actually do?

The thyroid gland secretes thyroid hormone and parathyroid hormone. Parathyroid hormone is important in calcium regulation. The primary role of thyroid hormone is the regulation of metabolism. In humans, the thyroid gland incorporates dietary iodide molecules into the storage compound, thyroglobulin. When affected by the pituitary hormone thyroid-stimulating hormone (TSH), glandular epithelium releases L-thyroxine (T4), which contains four iodide molecules, and modest amounts of triiodothyronine (T3), which contains three iodides. T4 circulates largely bound to serum proteins and is converted in peripheral tissues to T3. T3 is the active form of the hormone at the cellular level in most tissues. Pituitary TSH production and release are triggered by hypothalamic thyrotropin-releasing hormone (TRH).

3. Is thyroid function different in older patients?

Healthy aging produces very little change in thyroid hormone homeostasis. No clinically significant alterations in circulating levels of T4, T3, or TSH are seen. Circulating levels of T4 are preserved despite alterations in both thyroidal production and peripheral degradation of T4. Pituitary response to exogenous TRH administration is also preserved. Age-related alterations in the ability of the thyroid to concentrate dietary iodine (as measured by the radioactive iodine uptake) does decrease with age; one study has shown that the absolute iodine uptake in 80–90-year-olds is 60% of that seen in subjects aged 20–39 years. End-organ responsiveness to T4 also varies in reports: in humans, the basal metabolic rate (BMR) is unchanged, but in animals, liver enzyme induction decreases.

4. How is thyroid function evaluated in older patients?

The evaluation of thyroid function is safe, reliable, and relatively inexpensive. Serum levels of circulating T4 and TSH are widely available. T4 is usually measured as **total T4**, i.e., T4 bound to serum proteins and the small amount of T4 circulating free. Because T4-binding proteins can fluctuate in various situations (e.g., exogenous estrogen use), most laboratories also report a measurement of binding protein availability, the **T3 resin uptake** (T3RU). This measurement has nothing to do with the patient's T3; the T3 in the name refers to *exogenous* radioactive T3(*T3) added in the laboratory to the patient's serum. A known amount of resin that will adsorb the "leftover" *T3 is also added. If large numbers of binding protein sites are unoccupied in the patient sample (as in hypothyroidism), most of the *T3 will stick to the protein and little will be available on the resin—thus, the T3RU will be low. In hyperthyroidism, binding sites will be full of the patient's T4, little *T3 will stick to the patient's proteins, and large amounts of *T3 will adhere to the resin—thus, the T3RU will be high. In patients on estrogen, total T4 will be high because of increased binding proteins; many sites will be available so that the resin contains little *T3, and the T3RU is low. The T3RU is reported as the percentage of added *T which appears in the resin, usually 35–45%. In many laboratories, the T3RU result is normalized to the value seen in control serum in that assay. The T3RU is then reported as a number (0.85–1.15, with the control sera as 1).

Correcting the total T4 by the T3RU generates an estimate of active hormone. This product is often called the **free thyroxine** index (FTI). Actual measurements of **free T4** and **total T3** can be obtained and are useful in special situations. **Thyroid autoantibodies** can be measured in most clinical laboratories. **Iodine uptake** is measured in the nuclear medicine laboratory; images generated are used as the thyroid scan.

5. What types of hypothyroidism are usually seen in the elderly?

Hypothyroidism is seen frequently in older patients. The prevalence of overt hypothyroidism is approximately 5%, with more women affected than men. Subclinical hypothyroidism (also called the "failing gland" syndrome) may precede overt hypothyroidism and can be seen in up to 15% of patients in some series. These patients are clinically euthyroid, serum T4 levels are normal, but TSH levels are elevated.

A group of patients at special risk for late hypothyroidism are those with laryngeal cancer who undergo extensive neck surgery and radiation, or who have undergone prior thyroid surgery and neglected follow-up. Myxedema coma is a severe form of hypothyroidism with altered consciousness and is an emergency.

Autoimmune thyroiditis is the most common cause of hypothyroidism in the elderly, with prior thyroid surgery or ablation the next most common cause. Pituitary insufficiency can produce thyroid hypofunction, a state referred to as secondary hypothyroidism.

6. How do you recognize hypothyroidism?

Patients with hypothyroidism are often unaware that anything is wrong. The onset of symptoms, such as lethargy, depression, confusion, dry skin, constipation, myalgia, and cold intolerance, are often mistaken by the patient and family as part of "old age." On physical exam, hypothyroid patients often appear pale and sallow (due to carotenoid pigments that can accumulate in the skin). The voice may sound low and hoarse. Classically, the outer third of the eyebrows is thinned or absent, but this finding is not specific for hypothyroidism in the elderly. The skin feels dry; the hair is also dry and brittle. The thyroid gland itself may be small. The examiner may occasionally find a surgical scar across the lower neck in a patient who underwent thyroid surgery and subsequently neglected follow-up or thyroid medication. Carpal tunnel syndrome may develop due to myxoid infiltration of the tendon sheath. The hallmark physical finding in hypothyroidism is a change in the patient's reflexes, with a relatively normal upstroke but a delay in the relaxation phase. This change is sometimes best appreciated by palpating the muscle belly while percussing the tendon.

Because of the occult nature of many of the signs and symptoms in older patients, hypothyroidism is often diagnosed with laboratory screening tests. All older patients should have a TSH determination as part of their health evaluation. Experts disagree as to the periodic need for repeat testing in a healthy older patient with a normal TSH, but most suggest a minimum of testing every 3 years. Patients with pituitary disease or in special situations should be screened with T4 and T3RU.

7. Is the treatment of hypothyroidism different in the elderly?

Thyroid hormone replacement is simple and relatively inexpensive. Patients should understand that they are almost certain to require thyroid replacement for life. Older patients may require lower doses of exogenous T4 to achieve full replacement. Replacement therapy is done with T4 (L-thyroxine), which can be given once daily. Therapy should be begun gradually because of the cardiac stimulation that can be associated with T4.

In the elderly, therapy is often begun with L-thyroxine, 0.0125 mg daily. In 2 weeks, if no cardiac problems have developed, the dose can be increased to 0.025 mg daily. Thereafter, the dose can be increased by 0.025 mg every 3–4 weeks, to a total dose of 0.075 mg. Each patient's final replacement dose must be individually assessed. After 3 months at 0.075 mg of L-thyroxine, a TSH level is checked. If the TSH remains higher than normal, the dose can be increased by 0.025 mg, and the process repeated until the TSH level remains in the normal range. If the TSH is suppressed (below normal), the dose of L-thyroxine can be reduced by 0.025 mg and the process repeated.

Patients with pituitary insufficiency present special difficulties in treatment because the correction of thyroid homeostasis may precipitate adrenal insufficiency and adrenal crisis. An endocrinologist should guide treatment in such patients.

8. What is the failing gland syndrome?

Early in the development of hypothyroidism, patients will develop elevations in TSH levels as their production of T4 begins to fall. The laboratory pattern will be that of a modest elevation in TSH with still normal T4. In former years, these patients were followed with repeat blood tests at 4–6 month intervals, and when a progressive pattern of TSH elevation was seen, L-thyroxine replacement was begun. Recent studies have shown that the presence of antithyroid antibodies in serum assays closely predicts which patients will progress to hypothyroidism. These antibody-positive patients can be begun on replacement therapy immediately.

9. When do you suspect hyperthyroidism in an older patient?

In most adults and many elderly patients, hyperthyroidism causes symptoms and signs related to "adrenergic" excess: agitation, tremor, sweating, palpitations, prominent stare, and weight loss. Patients may report heat intolerance, hyperdefecation (multiple formed stools each day), and hair and skin changes, but these are rarely the presenting complaint.

Apathetic hyperthyroidism is an unusual presentation of thyroid overactivity seen almost exclusively in older patients. Such patients appear depressed instead of agitated and display few of the adrenergic symptoms of hyperthyroidism. They are most often discovered in diagnostic evaluations of weight loss, depression, or atrial fibrillation. Diagnostic strategy and therapy of the apathetic variant are identical to classical hyperthyroidism. Research into the physiologic basis of the apathetic variant has focused on possible alterations in the adrenergic receptor family during aging.

10. Describe the physical findings in a hyperthyroid patient.

Physical examination in patients with classic hyperthyroidism reveals a nervous, agitated patient. He or she is likely to be dressed in lightweight clothing and may display a fine tremor with a rapid frequency. The skin is soft and smooth and may be slightly sweaty. Examination of the eyes reveals a bulging appearance of the globes (proptosis), a low rate of blinking, and sometimes show a rim of white sclera circling the iris (exophthalmos). Extraocular movement may be impaired, especially on lateral gaze, due to myxoid infiltration of the abducens muscles. While asking the patient to track an object from upward gaze to downward, the examiner may note a delay in the lid following the iris (lid lag).

The thyroid gland is usually enlarged; auscultation may reveal a bruit over the thyroid due to increased blood flow. Older patients may have developed fibrosis in the thyroid gland which restricts enlargement, and so older patients may be hyperthyroid even with a small thyroid gland. The cardiac rhythm may be rapid but sinus (sinus tachycardia) or may be rapid and irregular (atrial fibrillation). The fingertips may be red and painful (thyroid acropaxia); the nailbeds may separate from the fingers leaving dystrophic finger and toenails. Examination of the shins may disclose large thickened areas due to myxoid infiltration of the muscles, lesions which are called pretibial myxedema. Bone mineral density is reduced.

The ocular involvement in hyperthyroidism due to Graves' disease may precede other organ involvement or may occur alone (euthyroid Graves' ophthalmopathy). CT scans of the orbit reveal the characteristic muscle infiltration.

11. Are the causes of hyperthyroidism different in older patients?

Graves' disease, which is produced by autoimmune stimulation of the thyroid gland by antibodies resembling TSH, is the most common cause of hyperthyroidism in the elderly. Overproduction of thyroid hormones by isolated areas of thyroid glandular epitheliun which has escaped control and has become autonomous is the next most common cause; it is seen much more commonly in the elderly than in young patients. This autonomous area may be confined to a **solitary nodule** or, more often, to one nodule in a **multinodular goiter**. When the overproduction reaches levels that produce hyperthyroidism, the state is called toxic multinodular goiter, or Plummer's disease.

12. What diagnostic tests are indicated in hyperthyroidism?

The clinical suspicion of hyperthyroidism is confirmed initially with serum assays of T4, T3RU, and TSH. The TSH level is low due to suppression of the pituitary by elevated levels of circulating T4. Rarely, elderly or iodine-deficient hyperthyroid patients may secrete more T3 than T4, revealing an elevated T3 with a normal T4 (T3 toxicosis). A total T3 level should be requested in these patients. In early hyperthyroidism, the only abnormality may be a reduced response of pituitary TSH secretion in response to exogenous TRH. The etiology of the hyperthyroidism can be sought with nuclear medicine studies of thyroidal uptake of I-123. In Graves' disease, which is caused by autoimmune stimulation of the thyroid gland by an antibody similar to TSH, uptake is high and diffuse. In thyroiditis, the gland itself is undergoing inflammatory destruction; uptake is low. In toxic multinodular goiter, uptake is high in the autonomous nodule but suppressed in the rest of the gland. A characteristic image will be seen on a thyroid scan. Factitious hyperthyroidism, due to intentional or accidental overdose of exogenous thyroid hormone, can be suspected when I-123 uptake is low and screens for thyroid autoantibodies are negative.

Laboratory Results in Commonly Encountered Clinical Thyroid Syndromes

	TOTAL T4	T3RU	TSH	SPECIAL STUDIES
Hypothyroidism	Low	Low	High	—
Hypopituitarism	Low	Low	Low	—
Hyperthyroidism	High	High	Low	I-123 uptake scan for etiology TRH suppression for diagnosis in borderline cases
T3 toxicosis	Normal	High-normal	Low	T3 level should be measured in old or iodine-deficient patients
Factitious hyperthyroidism	High	High	Low	I-123 uptake is low Thyroid autoantibodies negative
Exogenous estrogen	High	Low	Normal	—
Malnutrition	Low	High	Normal	—
Failing gland	Low-normal	Low-normal	Slightly high	—
Euthyroid sick	Low	Low	Normal	—

13. What are the options in the treatment of older hyperthyroid patients?

Therapy for hyperthyroidism is aimed at relief of symptoms and cure. Historically, thyroidal overactivity was treated with surgical removal of most of the thyroid gland (subtotal thyroidectomy), but suppressive therapy with medications and organ-specific radioisotopes has largely replaced surgery. Beta-blockers, such as propranolol (Inderal), are very effective in curtailing the adrenergic symptoms such as agitation and tremor and may reduce heart rate. Thyroidal production of T4 and T3 can be reduced by antithyroid medications such as propylthiouracil (PTU) and methimazole. These drugs must be taken daily and have a high rate of serious side effects, such as granulocytopenia.

Thyroid tissue can be ablated by oral doses of I-131, which has a longer half-life than I-123. After treatment with I-131, overall production of thyroid hormones is reduced. In the elderly, I-131 is generally the safest treatment regimen: no long-term medications are required, the fall of

T4 is gradual, and theoretical risks of late malignancies are less concerning. Some endocrinologists recommend 2–4 weeks of pretreatment with antithyroid drugs before I-131 to reduce the amount of preformed T4 released during thyroid destruction.

After any form of treatment, patients must be monitored at regular intervals for late hypothyroidism due to either the primary disease process or therapy.

14. Define thyroid storm.

Patients with hyperthyroidism who undergo physiologic stress, such as infection, illness, or surgery, may develop a complication known as thyroid storm. They exhibit high fever (even to 106° F) and severe cardic dysfunction. Treatment is an emergency and should be directed by an endocrinologist.

15. What is factitious hyperthyroidism?

Factitious hyperthyroidism is caused by overdoses of thyroid replacement medication, either intentional or accidental. Patients may misunderstand instructions or may intentionally overdose in the hopes of losing weight. Errors in prescription may occur by physicians or pharmacists. The risk of error is greatest with L-thyroxine at the low dose of 0.025 mg being mistaken for the suppressive dose of 0.250 mg. The doses of L-thyroxine are universally color-coded, and patients should be instructed to report any unexpected change in the color of their tablets. Thyroidal uptake of I-123 will be low in these patients.

16. What causes a goiter?

Goiters are enlarged thyroid glands caused by long-term overproduction of colloid within the gland. This overproduction is caused in most elderly patients by congenital partial defects in the enzymes involved in incorporation of iodide into colloid. T4 production is slightly reduced, TSH is slightly elevated, and the gland slowly enlarges. The enlargement can be stopped by providing exogenous T4 (L-thyroxine) in replacement doses large enough to suppress TSH production. Very large goiters can compress the trachea and may need partial surgical resection. In areas of the world where dietary iodide is unavailable (generally areas far from the sea), iodide deficiency is the most common cause of goiter. In the United States, dietary goiter is now mainly seen in recent immigrants.

17. What is toxic multinodular goiter?

Also known as Plummer's disease, toxic multinodular goiter is a hyperthyroid state produced when one nodule in a goiter becomes autonomous and is no longer subject to pituitary regulation. This condition is seen almost exclusively in the elderly. Patients appear hyperthyroid and have the classic thyroid I-123 scan. Therapy with I-131 is ideal: the active nodular tissue is destroyed, and the normal tissue that was suppressed escapes damage and returns to normal function. Patients with small amounts of autonomous tissue may rapidly develop hyperthyroidism when exposed to large amounts of exogenous iodide, as in radiographic contrast dye or iodinated drugs such as amiodarone.

18. How are "cold" thyroid nodules detected?

In palpating the thyroid gland, the examiner may note an asymmetry which on further exam is felt to be a nodule. In the elderly, this nodule often represents the most superfical nodule of a goiter, may be an isolated colloid cyst, or may represent a focus of thyroid cancer. In former years, the next diagnostic step would be a thyroid I-123 scan; nodules that concentrated the I-123 ("hot" nodules) were believed to be composed of functioning tissue and were likely benign. Nodules that failed to concentrate I-123 ("cold" nodules) could not be assessed. Surgery to remove these cold nodules was usually recommended, but many specimens revealed normal tissue. In the last 15 years, the initial diagnostic step has become a fine-needle aspiration of the nodule. The cytopathologist can help differentiate benign nodules from malignant ones. Patients with benign nodules are often begun on thyroid replacement therapy to inhibit TSH-directed enlargement, and the nodules are monitored by sequential measurement in the office. An increase in size on replacement therapy is usually an indication for repeated aspiration.

19. Is thyroid cancer seen in older patients?

Primary cancer of the thyroid is uncommon but not rare. Cancers present most often as thyroid nodules. Unfortunately, since thyroid cancers cause so few symptoms, many cancers are not found until metastases have developed. The most common cancer diagnosed in nodules is well-differentiated and likely to be completely resected. Follicular carcinoma is less common but more aggressive. Anaplastic thyroid carcinoma is a very aggressive malignancy often diagnosed because of metastatic lesions before a primary nodule is appreciated.

20. What is the sick euthyroid syndrome?

Patients who are ill are often catabolic: they must breakdown their own protein stores to supply their metabolic needs. The body responds to this stress by suppressing TSH production and allowing T4 levels to fall slightly to spare further protein degradation. This physiologic state can be confirmed by documenting elevated levels of reverse T3, produced by an alternative pathway of T4 degradation. Studies have shown that replacement with exogenous T4 makes these patients sicker. Ill patients with low-normal T4 and T3RU levels and low TSH levels should not be started on L-thyroxine. Their thyroid function should be monitored as they recover.

BIBLIOGRAPHY

1. Francis T, Wartofsky L: Common thyroid disorders in the elderly. Postgrad Med 92(3):225–233, 1992.
2. Griffin JE: Hypothyroidism in the elderly. Am J Med Sci 299:334–345, 1990.
3. Hansen JM, Skousted L, Siersboek-Nielson K: Age dependent changes in iodine metabolism and thyroid function. Acta Endocrinol 79:60–65, 1975.
4. Hershman JM, Pekary AE, Berg L, et al: Serum thyrotropin and thyroid hormone levels in elderly and middle aged euthyroid persons. J Am Geriatr Soc 41:823–828, 1993.
5. Isley WL: Thyroid dysfunction in the severely ill and elderly. Postgrad Med 94(3):111–128, 1993.
6. Mokshagundaom, S, Barzel US: Thyroid disease in the elderly. J Am Geriatr Soc 41:1361–1369, 1993.
7. Rae P, Farrar J, Beckett G, Toft A: Assessment of thyroid status in elderly people. BMJ 307:177–180, 1993.

31. URINARY TRACT INFECTIONS

Dorothy A. Slavin, M.D., and Elias Abrutyn, M.D.

1. How are urinary infections defined and diagnosed?

Traditionally, urinary tract infection (UTI) has been defined clinically as symptoms of frequency, urgency, dysuria, and/or suprapubic discomfort in the presence of significant bacteriuria. The presence of $> 10^5$ colony-forming units (CFU)/ml of an organism in a midstream urine sample has been considered significant bacteriuria. However, this definition misses some symptomatic patients with $< 10^5$ CFU bacteria/ml. A recent article suggests more sensitive criteria for defining significant bacteriuria:

$> 10^2$ CFU coliform/ml or $> 10^5$ CFU noncoliform/ml in a symptomatic female
$> 10^3$ CFU bacteria/ml in a symptomatic male
$> 10^5$ CFU bacteria/ml in two cultures taken 1 week apart in asymptomatic female or male

Pyuria, defined as pus in the urine, is determined by the presence of > 10 leukocytes/mm^3 in an unspun urine sample using a hemocytometer or by a positive leukocyte esterase test on a urine dipstick. The dipstick method has a sensitivity of 75–96% and a specificity of 94–98% but should not be used alone to diagnose UTI in the elderly because pyuria may be present without bacteriuria.

2. How do the signs and symptoms of UTI differ in older and younger patients?

Younger patients often present with the typical symptoms and signs of UTI, such as frequency, urgency, dysuria, abdominal or flank pain, fever, and chills. Elderly patients may exhibit these typical signs and symptoms, remain asymptomatic, or present with nonspecific signs and symptoms, including a change in functional capacity, fatigue, anorexia, nausea, vomiting, mental status changes, or hypothermia.

3. What are the risk factors for the development of UTI?

For women:

Sexual intercourse
Use of a pessary, diaphragm, or spermicide
Conditions that prevent complete bladder emptying
Alterations in the vaginal flora due to a lack of estrogens (particularly in postmenopausal women)

For men:

Prostate enlargement leading to bladder outlet obstruction
Anal intercourse
Lack of circumcision
Sexual partner with vaginal colonization by uropathogens

For both men and women:

Genitourinary instrumentation, such as catheterization or cystoscopy
Conditions that result in soiling of the perineum, such as immobility, dementia, or cerebrovascular accident
Conditions associated with incomplete bladder emptying, such as neuropathy from spinal cord injuries or diabetes mellitus

For persons with indwelling urinary catheters:

Female sex, due to colonization of the periurethral area with fecal flora and tracking of these bacteria along the urethra into the bladder
Duration of catheterization, with a 5%/day incidence of bacteriuria in persons with indwelling catheters with closed drainage systems

Absence of systemic antibiotic use, which allows for bacterial colonization soon after the catheter is placed

Violations in sterile catheter care

4. Does an initial episode of UTI in an elderly man warrant further evaluation of the genitourinary tract?

The incidence of UTI in men increases with age, in part due to bladder outlet obstruction with prostatic enlargement. Evaluation of an elderly man presenting with an initial UTI should include:

- Urinalysis
- Urine culture
- Serum test for blood urea nitrogen (BUN) and creatinine levels
- Prostate examination
- Postvoid residual measurement

Based on these results and the patient's response to treatment, further evaluation may include ultrasound or intravenous pyelogram.

5. What is the difference between reinfection and relapse? What is the significance to elderly patients?

Reinfection is recurrence of infection with a bacteria different from the organism originally isolated. Relapse is recurrence with the same organism, indicating the presence of a persistent focus of infection.

Whenever possible, it is important to distinguish between the two. Reinfection may be treated with a short course (3 days) of therapy, whereas relapse requires a longer course of therapy and may indicate the need for further evaluation of the genitourinary tract. Relapse may be due to a persistent focus of infection, such as perinephric abscess, nephrolithiasis, or prostatitis. In the elderly, relapse may result from incomplete bladder emptying due to diabetes mellitus, uterine prolapse, or prostate enlargement.

It may be difficult to distinguish relapse from reinfection in a particular patient; in such circumstances, recurrence may be the more appropriate term.

6. What is the definition of a complicated UTI?

Although no definition of complicated UTI is universally accepted, most definitions include patients with functional or anatomic abnormalities of the urinary tract and patients with underlying diseases, such as diabetes mellitus. Examples include:

- Patients with upper tract obstruction (calculi, strictures, masses), bladder outlet obstruction (prostate enlargement, urethral strictures), incomplete bladder emptying (neurogenic bladder, bladder diverticula, uterine prolapse)
- Patients with a persistent focus of infection, such as prostatitis, renal abscess, renal calculi, chronic indwelling urinary catheter, ureteral stents, or nephrostomy tubes
- Infections in immunocompromised hosts and infections due to resistant organisms.

It is generally recommended that complicated UTIs be treated with at least 14 days of therapy, although this recommendation has never been adequately tested in randomized, controlled clinical trials.

7. What is the appropriate duration of therapy for uncomplicated UTIs?

Uncomplicated UTIs in females of any age may be successfully treated with a 3-day course of antibiotic therapy. Appropriate agents include trimethoprim-sulfamethoxazole and fluoroquinolones. Short courses of therapy should not be used in males or in patients with pyelonephritis, complicated UTI, or relapsed UTI.

8. Do elderly patients with pyelonephritis need to be hospitalized for two weeks of intravenous antibiotics?

Because of the potential for gram-negative sepsis, elderly patients with moderate-to-severe symptoms of pyelonephritis should be admitted to the hospital. Blood and urine cultures should be done before starting antibiotic therapy. Empiric intravenous antibiotic therapy should be based on the results of a Gram stain of the urine. Once a clinical response is obtained with resolution of symptoms, fever, and leukocytosis, elderly patients with pyelonephritis may complete a 14-day course of oral antibiotics. Mild cases of pyelonephritis may be considered for outpatient therapy.

9. Do urinary pathogens differ in elderly and younger patients?

Yes, although *Escherichia coli* is the most commonly isolated organism in both groups. Approximately 80–90% of community-acquired UTIs in young women are due to *E. coli*; 10% are due to *Staphylococcus saprophyticus*, and the remaining 5–10% due to gram-negative organisms other than *E. coli*. In elderly women, 60–70% of community-acquired UTIs are due to *E. coli*; the remaining 30–40% are due to other gram-negative organisms, such as *Klebsiella, Proteus*, or *Pseudomonas* species, or gram-positive organisms, such as *Staphylococcus* or *Enterococcus* species. In elderly men, gram-positive organisms account for a greater proportion of isolated organisms (as many as 30–40%).

10. Should asymptomatic bacteriuria be treated in patients without indwelling urinary catheters?

Asymptomatic bacteriuria is defined as > 10^5 CFU/ml of an organism in a urine sample on two occasions within 1–2 weeks. Asymptomatic bacteriuria is frequently found in elderly people, with prevalence rates of 20% in elderly women and 10% in elderly men. The corresponding rates in younger women and men are 5% and 0.1%, respectively. Despite its prevalence in elderly populations, routine screening for asymptomatic bacteriuria is not indicated, and treatment should not be undertaken. Arguments for not treating asymptomatic bacteriuria include the following:

- Asymptomatic bacteriuria is usually transient.
- There is no way to predict which patients with asymptomatic bacteriuria will develop symptomatic infection, but the incidence appears to be low.
- Asymptomatic bacteriuria and changes in the pattern of continence do not appear to be related. Treatment of asymptomatic bacteriuria is not likely to improve incontinence.
- A cause-and-effect relationship has not been established between bacteriuria and renal insufficiency (in the absence of urinary tract obstruction) in elderly people.
- Treatment of asymptomatic bacteriuria in elderly peoples has not resulted in decreased mortality.
- Even if treatment of a particular episode is successful, recurrence of bacteriuria is common.
- Treatment of asymptomatic bacteriuria may be associated with the emergence of resistant organisms.
- Antibiotic use, especially in the elderly, is often associated with adverse effects.
- The cost of treatment is considerable, and no major clinical benefit is apparent.

11. What is the significance of bacteriuria/pyuria in patients with chronic indwelling urinary catheters? Are urine cultures from catheters of any value in febrile, elderly patients?

After a short time, 100% of patients with an indwelling urinary catheter have bacteriuria, frequently polymicrobial. The incidence of bacteriuria increases with the duration of catheterization. Bacteria gain access to the bladder by carriage of organisms into the bladder during catheter insertion or by migration through the lumen or along the outside of the catheter. Growth of bacteria in biofilms on the inner surface of the catheter promotes encrustation, which may serve as a nidus for further bacterial growth and catheter obstruction. Therefore, cultures obtained from an indwelling catheter may not reflect organisms found in the bladder and upper tract.

12. What are the treatment recommendations for UTIs in elderly patients?

Some of the factors to be considered in choosing therapy for a UTI include:

Patient
Drug allergies
Concurrent medications
Renal function
Recent antibiotic use
Presence of indwelling urinary catheter
Result of urine Gram stain

Antibiotic
Cost
Route of administration
Spectrum of activity
Adverse effects

Treatment Options for UTIs Based on Presentation and Urine Gram Stain

	GRAM STAIN	TREATMENT	ALTERNATIVE
Uncomplicated	Gram-positive cocci	Amoxicillin/clavulanic acid	
	Gram-negative rods	Trimethoprim/sulfa-methoxazole	Fluoroquinolone
Pyelonephritis	Gram-positive cocci	Ampicillin/gentamicin	Vancomycin/gentamicin
	Gram-negative rods	Third-generation cephalosporin, fluoroquinolone	Extended spectrum penicillin, aztreonam

Oral ampicillin and amoxicillin are no longer recommended as first-line therapy for uncomplicated UTIs because of beta-lactamase production by gram-negative bacilli.

For pyelonephritis, particularly with sepsis, intravenous antibiotics should be administered once cultures of urine and blood are obtained. The regimen may be narrowed when final culture results are available.

Patients with mild symptoms of pyelonephritis who are able to tolerate oral medications may be considered for outpatient treatment.

13. Is there a role for prophylactic antibiotic therapy in UTIs?

Prophylactic antibiotic therapy is recommended to eradicate bacteriuria before genitourinary tract instrumentation. Prophylaxis aims to prevent gram-negative sepsis. It is also indicated for patients at increased risk for endocarditis. In general, prophylaxis begins the day before the scheduled procedure with a bactericidal agent.

14. What is the role of estrogens in the prevention or treatment of UTIs in postmenopausal women?

The use of estrogens results in replacement among the vaginal flora of gram-negative organisms with lactobacilli, which lower the vaginal pH and thus provide a hostile environment for pathogenic bacteria. In a well-designed study, the use of topical intravaginal estrogens was shown to decrease the frequency of UTIs in postmenopausal women with a history of recurrent UTIs.

15. Is there a role for cranberry juice in the prevention or treatment of UTIs?

The effects of cranberry juice are unclear. Possible benefits are obtained from increased fluid intake; acidification of the urine, which inhibits bacterial growth; or production of a metabolite, hippuric acid, which has antimicrobial activity.

A study of elderly women showed an odds ratio of 0.42 for bacteriuria with pyuria in women receiving 300 ml/day of cranberry juice compared with women receiving placebo. Bacteriuria with pyuria was found in 28.1% of urine samples from the placebo group compared with 15% from the treatment group. However, this study examined only women with asymptomatic bacteriuria, an entity that should not be treated. Therefore, the role of cranberry juice in the prevention or treatment of UTIs remains unknown.

BIBLIOGRAPHY

1. Abrutyn E, Mossey J, Berlin J, et al: Does asymptomatic bacteriuria predict mortality and does antimicrobial treatment reduce mortality in elderly ambulatory women? Ann Intern Med 120:827–833, 1994.
2. Avorn J, Monane M, Gurwitz JH, et al: Reduction of bacteriuria and pyuria after ingestion of cranberry juice. JAMA 271:751–754, 1994.
3. Baldessarre JS, Kaye D: Special problems of urinary tract infection in the elderly. Med Clin North Am 75:375–389, 1991.
4. Boscia JA, Abrutyn E, Kaye D: Asymptomatic bacteriuria in elderly persons: Treat or do not treat? Ann Intern Med 106:764–766, 1987.
5. Boscia JA, Abrutyn E, Levison ME, et al: Pyuria and asymptomatic bacteriuria in elderly ambulatory women. Ann Intern Med 110:404–405, 1989.
6. Johnson CC: Definitions, classification, and clinical presentation of urinary tract infections. Med Clin North Am 75:241–252, 1991.
7. Raz R, Stamm WE: A controlled trial of intravaginal estriol in postmenopausal women with recurrent urinary tract infections. N Engl J Med 329:753–756, 1993.
8. Sobel J: Urinary tract infections. In Mandell GL, Douglas RG Jr, Bennett JE (eds): Principles and Practice of Infectious Diseases, 4th ed. New York, Churchill Livingstone, 1995, pp 662–690.
9. Stamm WE: Catheter-associated urinary tract infections: Epidemiology, pathogenesis, and prevention. Am J Med, 91:65s–71s, 1991.

32. WOMEN'S HEALTH ISSUES

Michelle Battistini, M.D.

1. What are the most common complaints that cause an older woman to see a gynecologist?

Other than a routine exam, the most common reasons an aging woman visits a gynecologist are symptoms related to pelvic relaxation, vaginal discharge, vaginal bleeding, vulvar irritation or pruritus, and urinary incontinence. With increasing frequency, regardless of the primary reason for their visit, many women and their referring physicians have concerns and questions about hormone replacement therapy.

2. What is pelvic relaxation? How is it diagnosed?

Pelvic relaxation is the loss of normal and adequate supportive tissues along the vaginal canal, resulting in prolapse or herniation of pelvic structures into the vagina. The loss of support may occur universally or at specific sites along the length of the vagina.

The diagnosis of pelvic relaxation and the specific site of prolapse is made during physical examination with the patient in the dorsal lithotomy position or standing upright. If the examination is limited to the lithotomy position, a more accurate diagnosis is made by having the patient strain; this is accomplished by asking her to cough hard or to perform a Valsalva maneuver.

Pelvic Support Structures

STRUCTURE	NATURE	COMPONENTS	FUNCTION
Pelvic diaphragm	Muscular	Levator ani Pubococcygeus Puborectalis Iliococcygeus	Control of urination Maintenance of fecal continence Support of abdominal and pelvic viscera Integral role in birth process
Urogenital diaphragm	Muscular and fascial	Ischiocavernosus Bulbocavernosus Deep transverse Perineal	Supports external urethra Contains external urethral sphincter Maintains position of bladder neck Supports vaginal introitus Contains neurovascular supply to pudendum and clitoris
Endopelvic fascia	Thickened retroperitoneal fascia	Pubocervical fascia—anterior Mackenrodt's ligament, (cardinal ligament)—lateral and superior Uterosacral ligaments—posterior	Periurethral and vesical support Base of broad ligament Cul de sac support

3. How are disorders of pelvic relaxation classified?

The site of relaxation determines which organ will prolapse and the classification of the disorder.

Classification of Pelvic Relaxation Disorders

LOCATION OF ANATOMIC DEFECT	PROLAPSED ORGAN	DISORDER
Anterior vaginal segment	Urethra Bladder	Urethrocele Cystocele
Superior vaginal segment	Cervix/uterus/vaginal cuff Cul de sac	Cervical/uterine/vaginal vault prolapse Culdocele, enterocele
Posterior vaginal segment	Rectum Perineum	Rectocele Perineal laceration

4. What causes pelvic relaxation?

Usually multiple factors contribute to the weakening of pelvic support structures, including the following:

- Vaginal delivery
- Estrogen deficiency
- Sexual activity
- Chronic occupational stress
- Stress secondary to gravity
- Chronic cough
- Chronic constipation
- Surgical or acute trauma
- Neurologic disorders
- Congenital abnormalities

5. What symptoms are associated with pelvic relaxation?

Pelvic relaxation may be asymptomatic and detected only on physical examination. When women present with symptoms, the symptoms may be generalized or related to the specific organ that is prolapsed. Examples include:

- Vaginal fullness or pressure
- Pelvic pressure
- Backache
- Inability to empty bladder
- Difficulty with voiding
- Urinary incontinence
- Protrusion of organ outside vagina
- Difficulty with defecation
- Anal incontinence for flatus or stool
- Vaginal discharge or bleeding

Often women complain of feeling as though (1) they are "sitting on a ball"; (2) something is protruding from the vagina; or (3) they have a sensation of vaginal pressure, fullness, or fatigue. Urethroceles (see table in question 3) are frequently associated with urinary incontinence. Pure cystoceles may cause difficulty with bladder emptying; patients report having to reduce the cystocele manually or to assume various positions to void adequately. Incomplete bladder emptying may predispose to urinary tract infections and related symptoms. Rectoceles may be associated with incomplete defecation and a sensation of rectal fullness; patients may report the need to splint the vagina or perineum to defecate completely. Perineal defects may cause anal incontinence of flatus and feces. Complete prolapse of any of these structures may lead to surface irritation with resultant vaginal discharge or surface ulceration with vaginal bleeding. The severity of symptoms frequently, but not always, varies directly with the severity or degree of prolapse, which is determined at the time of physical examination.

6. Describe the system for grading the severity of pelvic relaxation disorders.

Pelvic Relaxation Disorders—Classification of Severity

EXTENT OF DESCENT	GRADE	SEVERITY	DEGREE
Normal position	Grade 0	Normal	Normal
Halfway to hymen	Grade 1	Mild	1st degree descensus
To hymen	Grade 2	Moderate	2nd degree descensus
Halfway past hymen	Grade 3	Moderately severe	Procidentia
Maximum descensus	Grade 4	Severe	Procidentia

7. What treatments are available for pelvic relaxation?

Pelvic relaxation can be treated with both surgical and nonsurgical therapeutic options. **Nonsurgical interventions** do not restore anatomic integrity to the pelvic structures; they are designed to relieve symptoms and prevent worsening of the condition. Nonoperative interventions strengthen muscular and fascial support structures, support herniated organs, and avoid exacerbating factors; they include the use of Kegel's exercises, estrogen therapy, vaginal pessaries, and stool softeners.

Surgical intervention includes procedures that are reparative or palliative. **Reparative surgical procedures** are designed to restore anatomic integrity to pelvic structures; they are site-specific and can be accomplished through an abdominal, vaginal, or combined approach. When a reparative option is chosen, a thorough preoperative evaluation of pelvic support structures is imperative. All sites of relaxation are repaired at the time of surgery to avoid recurrence. In addition, the preoperative and postoperative use of nonsurgical strategies to strengthen support tissues enhances the success of the repair and reduces the risk of recurrence. **Palliative procedures**, generally designed to obliterate the vaginal lumen, are performed less commonly today. They are usually reserved for the elderly patient who is no longer sexually active and has persistent or recurrent symptoms after other treatment options have been tried. The choice of treatment is based on several factors, including severity of symptoms, degree of prolapse, medical condition and preference of the patient, and success of prior conservative interventions. Age alone should not be considered a contraindication to surgical therapy.

Treatment of Pelvic Relaxation Disorders

Nonsurgical management	
Strategy	Intervention
Strengthen pelvic musculature	Kegel exercises
	Vaginal cones
	Biofeedback
	Electrostimulation
Strengthen non-muscular support	Estrogen therapy, topical or as replacement therapy
Mechanical support	Vaginal pessary use
Avoid exacerbating factors	Limit increases in intra-abdominal pressure (e.g., avoid heavy lifting)
	Stool softeners, high-fiber diets
	Review and adjust medications
Surgical management	
Reparative procedures—repair of all identifiable defects	
Defect location	Procedure
Anterior	Anterior colporrhaphy
	Periurethral suspension
Superior	Hysterectomy
	Vaginal vault suspension (abdominal or vaginal approach)
	Enterocele repair
Posterior	Posterior colporrhaphy
	Perineoplasty
Palliative procedures—obliteration of vaginal canal	
Defect location	Procedure
Anterior	Colpocleisis with or without incontinence repair procedure
	Hysterectomy
Superior	Colpocleisis, cervical amputation (Manchester-Fothergill procedure)
Posterior	Colpocleisis

8. What are vaginal pessaries? How are they used?

Vaginal supportive pessaries have been used for many years in the treatment of pelvic relaxation. The 17 different types of pessaries vary in shape and size, depending on their proposed purpose. They are composed of inert materials such as lucite and rubber; most modern pessaries are made of silicone. Pessaries can be used as a temporary treatment for symptomatic relief in women who are waiting for surgery or as permanent treatment in women who are poor surgical risks or choose a nonsurgical option. The most common pessaries used for treatment include:

• Ring, with and without support
• Gelhorn
• Donut
• Shaatz
• Gehrung

Pessaries require precision fitting by an individual experienced in their use. Poor sizing can cause obstruction of the urinary outflow tract and erosion of the vaginal epithelium with resultant ulceration. Patients should be instructed to report any difficulty with urination, foul vaginal discharge, or vaginal bleeding. Topical estrogen cream is often prescribed before pessary fitting to rejuvenate the vaginal walls. This treatment can be continued intermittently (1–2 nights/week) while the pessary is in place. Pessary hygiene includes periodic removal and cleansing of the pessary (every 8–12 weeks). Patients sometimes can be instructed in hygiene procedures, but most often they come to the office for pessary care.

9. What are Kegel exercises? How are they done?

Kegel exercises were introduced in the middle of the 20th century by Dr. Kegel as a treatment primarily for urinary stress incontinence. They are designed to strengthen the pubococcygeus muscle (PCM). Because the PCM plays a major role in pelvic support, Kegel exercises also may be used in the treatment of pelvic relaxation. Patients are instructed to contract the PCM, hold for three seconds and then relax for three seconds. They do so for 20 minutes, 3 times/day, repeating the exercise from 100–300 times. To assist the patient in identifying the correct muscle, different techniques are used. Patients can be told to tighten the muscle that holds gas in the rectum or to stop their urine in midstream and feel the muscle used to do so. Often it is useful to teach Kegel exercises during the pelvic exam. Slight pressure is applied to the muscle through the vaginal wall; the patient is then instructed to squeeze the fingers. Perineometers, vaginal cones, and biofeedback devices are used to facilitate the proper exercise technique.

10. What is menopause?

Many women need to define their position along the spectrum of declining ovarian function. Frequently they ask questions such as "Am I through with menopause?," "Am I in the menopause?," or even "Just what is menopause?"

Menopause is permanent cessation of menstruation, which marks the loss of ovarian endocrine activity seen during the reproductive years. The median age of menopause in North America is 51.5 years, with a normal range of 48–55 years. The hallmark of menopause is loss of ovarian production of estradiol, the potent estrogen of the reproductive years. Ovarian production of androstenedione is also reduced. Production of testosterone is the same or slightly increased because of stromal stimulation by elevated levels of the gonadotropins, follicle-stimulating hormone (FSH) and luteinizing hormone (LH). However, serum testosterone levels fall due to the reduced level of androstenedione precursor. Although there is essentially no ovarian production of estrogen after menopause, circulating levels of estrogen are variable and can be significant, primarily in the form of estrone, a less potent form. Estrone and, to a lesser extent, estradiol are formed from the peripheral conversion of androstenedione and testosterone, primarily in adipose tissue.

The years of waning ovarian function prior to menopause are often referred to as the **transition**. This period of fluctuating ovarian function is manifested by cycle irregularities and various symptoms related to fluctuations in hormone levels. **Perimenopause** refers to the few years immediately before and after cessation of menses. The term **climacteric** is often used to describe the years from the transition through menopause and into the postmenopausal period. How a woman experiences menopause and the years thereafter is as varied as life itself and depends on the complex interplay of hormonal, physical, and psychosocial factors.

Hormone	Serum Levels Postmenopause	Serum Levels Premenopause
Estradiol	5–40 pg/ml	20–600 pg/ml
Estrone	5–40 pg/ml	15–200 pg/ml
Androstenedione	20–50 ng/dl	100–150 ng/dl
Testosterone	10–40 ng/dl	20–80 ng/dl

11. What are the symptoms of menopause?

The most common acute symptom of menopause, the hot flush or flash, is related to vasomotor instability secondary to reduced estrogen levels in the thermoregulatory centers in the brain. Hot flushes are experienced by 85% of menopausal women and are the most common reason for seeking treatment of menopause. Flushes tend to occur more commonly at night and may cause significant sleep disturbance. Hot flushes can be precipitated by environmental factors such as stress, alcohol, hot foods, and warm weather. They frequently worsen with tamoxifen therapy. For most women, the frequency and severity of flushes tend to decrease and subside within the first 3–5 years after menopause; in up to one-third of women, however, they may persist longer. Vaginal changes secondary to reduced estrogen levels include decreased lubrication and loss of elasticity, frequently leading to symptoms of dryness, dyspareunia, pruritus, and atrophic vaginitis. Urinary symptoms of urgency, frequency, and worsening of incontinence reflect the estrogen receptivity of the bladder and urethra.

12. What is the role of estrogen replacement therapy (ERT) after menopause?

Estrogen receptors are found in virtually every organ system throughout the body. Symptoms and medical consequences represent the end-organ response to reduced estrogen levels characteristic of menopause. ERT is indicated for treatment of symptoms and prevention of the long-term medical consequences of reduced estrogen levels. The consequences of the hormonal events of menopause occur in a woman who is also aging. It is important, yet sometimes difficult, to differentiate for women and their families which changes are related to aging, which to the hormonal effects of menopause, and which to a combination of both. Other effects of ERT include maintenance of skin turgor, decreased joint pain, and increased sense of well-being.

13. What are the indications for ERT?

Indications for Hormone Replacement Therapy

SYMPTOM CONTROL	MEDICAL BENEFITS
Vasomotor instability—hot flushes	Prevention of osteoporosis
Sleep disturbances	Reduction of cardiovascular risk
Dyspareunia, vaginal dryness, atrophic vaginitis	? Amelioration of Alzheimer's dementia
Urinary urgency, frequency	? Reduction of colon cancer risk
Urinary stress incontinence	

The two major, well-documented medical benefits of ERT are osteoporosis prevention and reduction of cardiovascular risk. ERT initiated shortly after the menopause prevents the accelerated bone loss that occurs during the first 5–7 postmenopausal years. Long-term use is associated with a 50% reduction in fracture risk. ERT in the elderly, even when initiated long after menopause, has been shown to reduce the risk of hip fracture. Addition of progestin enhances this effect. Estrogen is currently the drug of choice for osteoporosis prevention and is used with other therapies in the treatment of osteoporosis.

Perhaps the most significant effect of ERT from an individual and public health perspective is its effect on the reduction of cardiovascular morbidity and mortality. The incidence of fatal and nonfatal myocardial infarction is reduced by 50% with ERT. The incidence of significant stenosis documented at catheterization is lower in women who use estrogen compared with nonusers. Long-term survival is significantly better (98% vs. 69%) in users than in non-users. The impact progestin has on the beneficial effects has yet to be determined. Preliminary data suggest that ERT may play a role in the prevention and progression of Alzheimer's dementia. Definitive documentation of this effect, however, awaits further research. ERT may reduce the risk of development of colon cancer, but this also awaits further documentation.

14. Describe the mechanisms by which estrogen achieves its beneficial effects.

Reduction of bone loss	Antiresorptive action on osteoclasts in bone
	Increased efficiency of calcium absorption in GI tract
	Decreased renal calcium excretion
Reduction of cardiovascular risk	Improved lipid profile
	Decreased total cholesterol
	Increased high-density lipoprotein (HDL) cholesterol
	Decreased low-density lipoprotein (LDL) cholesterol
	Increase in coronary blood flow
	Antioxidant–antiatherogenic effect

15. Does ERT cause cancer?

One of the most common reasons for avoidance of ERT after menopause is fear of cancer. It has been well documented that the use of unopposed estrogen in women with an intact uterus increases the risk for endometrial hyperplasia and endometrial cancer by a factor of 2–10. Risk increases with dose and duration of use. For this reason, it is standard to add a progestational agent, for at least 10 days a month, to the replacement regimen (PERT) in women who have not undergone hysterectomy. Some advocate 12–14 days of progestational exposure, especially when lower doses of progestational agents are used. Use of PERT according to this standard has actually been shown to lower the risk of endometrial cancer compared with women who use no hormones. The PERT regimen is also recommended in women without a uterus who have a history of endometriosis, because endometrial carcinoma originating in endometriotic implants has been reported.

Unfortunately, the effect of ERT and PERT on breast cancer risk is less clearly defined. Current reports continue to yield conflicting results. Short-term use ($\leq$ 5 years) of either ERT or PERT is not associated with an increased relative risk of breast cancer. Past use, regardless of duration, does not seem to increase risk. Still in question is the possibility of a small-to-moderate increase in risk among older women who are current users of long duration (> 10 years).

However, the current recommendation is that the benefits of ERT/PERT continue to outweigh the risks in light of the substantial benefits in terms of cardiovascular and osteoporotic disease. The lowest possible dose to accrue the greatest benefit should be used. No association has been proved between ovarian cancer and hormone replacement therapy (HRT).

16. Describe the standard regimens for HRT.

Standard Regimens for HRT

REGIMEN	ESTROGEN	PROGESTIN	ADVANTAGES	DISADVANTAGES
Unopposed	Day 1–25	None	Maximal established benefit	High incidence of endometrial hyperplasia
	Every day		No progestin side effects	Increased risk for endometrial cancer
				Requires annual biopsy if uterus present
Cyclic combined	Day 1–25	10–14 days Day 16–25 or day 13–25	Oldest standard regimen	Cyclic menstrual-like bleeding
			Adequate endometrial protection	Recurrence of symptoms on off days
				Premenstrual-like symptoms
Sequential	Every day	10–14 days/month (duration is dose dependent) Day 1–10 or 14 Last 10–14 days	Adequate endometrial protection	Progestin withdrawal bleeding
			No hormone-free days, less hormonal fluctuation, less symptom recurrence	Premenstrual-like symptoms
Continuous combined (most popular current regimen)	Every day	Every day	Eliminates cyclic bleeding	Irregular bleeding
			Reduces cyclic premenstrual side effects, including migraine headaches	Long-term endometrial protection yet to be established
			Easy regimen to use	
Periodic progestin	Every day	Weekdays (weekends off)	No cyclic and less irregular bleeding	Long-term endometrial protection yet to be established
			Less progestin exposure, reduced side effects	Complicated regimen to use
		Quarterly (14 days every 3 months)	Less progestin exposure, reduced side effects	Withdrawal bleeding heavier than monthly episodes
				Long-term endometrial protection yet to be established

17. What are the standard doses of estrogen? Of progestins?

Standard Doses of Estrogen

ESTROGEN	BRAND NAME	DOSE
Conjugated equine estrogens	Premarin	0.625 mg
Estropipate	Ogen	0.625–1.25 mg
Micronized estradiol	Estrace	1.0 mg
Transdermal 17-estradiol	Estraderm, Climara	0.05 mg
Estropipate	Ortho-est	0.625–1.25 mg
Esterified estrogen with methyltestosterone	Estratest Estratest H.S.	1.25/2.5 0.625/1.25
Esterified estrogen	Estratab	0.625–1.25 mg

Standard Doses of Progestins

PROGESTIN	BRAND NAME	DOSE
Medroxyprogesterone acetate	Provera Cycrin Amen	Cyclic/sequential—5–10 mg Continuous—2.5, 5.0 mg Periodic—10 mg × 14 days
Micronized progesterone	Progesterol	Cyclic/sequential—200 mg
Norethindrone	Micronor Norlutin NorQD	Cyclic/sequential—2.5–5.0 Continuous—0.35–2.1
Norethindrone acetate	Aygestin Norlutate	Cyclic/sequential—5–10 mg Continuous—1 mg
D/L-norgestrel	Overette	Cyclic/sequential—0.075 mg

18. Does HRT cause hypertension or strokes?

No. This common misperception is based on the association of early high-dose oral contraceptives with an increased risk of hypertension and cardiovascular disease. The estrogens and progestins used in HRT are different from formulations in the various oral contraceptives, and the dosages are one-fifth to one-seventh of the dosages in oral contraceptives. ERT and PERT are not associated with an increased risk of hypertension. Furthermore, well-controlled hypertension is not a contraindication to HRT. Because a small number of women may develop an idiosyncratic elevation of blood pressure, routine blood pressure monitoring is advocated. An increased risk of cerebrovascular events with the use of HRT has not been identified. In fact, long-term use appears to be associated with an overall reduction in mortality attributable to cardiovascular disease. The use of HRT in women with established cardiovascular disease is supported by reports from various sources of overall improved survival and decreased mortality.

19. Can a woman with a history of thromboembolic disease use HRT?

The standard regimens used in HRT do not adversely affect coagulation factors and are not associated with an increased risk of thromboembolic events. HRT is not contraindicated in women with a remote history of thrombosis associated with trauma. In women with a history of hormonally related thrombosis, the use of HRT should be based on individual risk/benefit analysis and counseling. In women with symptoms of or at increased risk of cardiovascular disease or osteoporosis, it is appropriate to offer HRT after adequate counseling. Acute thromboembolic disease is a contraindication to HRT.

20. When is HRT contraindicated?

Absolute contraindications	Relative contraindications
Unexplained vaginal bleeding	Seizure disorders
Acute liver disease	High triglyceride levels
Impaired liver function, acute or chronic	Migraine headaches
Recent vascular thrombosis	(with exceptions)
Carcinoma of breast (except in certain circumstances)	Atraumatic thrombophlebitis
Carcinoma of the endometrium (with some exceptions)	Current gallbladder disease

After appropriate diagnosis and management of vaginal bleeding, HRT can be considered according to standard indications and contraindications. Liver dysfunction, whether acute or chronic, may result in unacceptably high levels of estrogen due to altered liver metabolism. HRT is generally contraindicated in patients with a history of an estrogen-sensitive neoplasm, most commonly breast or endometrial cancer. In certain circumstances, however, such patients may use HRT after extensive counseling about risk and benefit. These decisions need to be made individually. HRT has been used in patients with a history of stage I, low-grade adenocarcinoma of the uterus with no demonstrable increase in risk of recurrence. Limited case series involving survivors of breast cancer have reported no negative impact on recurrence or survival, but such reports cannot serve as a basis for generalized use of HRT in this population. In conditions listed as relative contraindications, risk may or may not outweigh the benefits of HRT, and decisions need to be made individually. In addition, adjustments of dose or route of administration may limit risk (e.g., transdermal as opposed to oral route in patients with cholelithiasis).

21. What are the most common side effects of HRT?

The most common complaints are usually related to the addition of a progestational agent. Many of these side effects can be managed with improved patient education or by changing the progestational agent, dosage, or route of administration. **Resumption of menstrual-like bleeding** with the use of cyclic PERT is one of the most common reasons for discontinuance. Bleeding normally occurs near or at completion of the course of progestin administration. Use of a continuous course of progestin usually eliminates these cycles. Although 50% of patients may experience irregular bleeding on initiation of a continuous regimen, 60–70% achieve amenorrhea within 1 year.

Women may complain of **premenstrual-like symptoms**—such as depression, irritability, breast tenderness, and bloating—with cyclic administration of a progestational agent. Options include a lower dose for a longer duration, substitution of a continuous regimen, or changing the progestational agent. Recently, the use of medroxyprogesterone acetate, 10 mg for 14 days every 3 months, has been suggested as an alternative. This regimen appears to provide adequate endometrial protection, although the periodic bleeding episodes are somewhat heavier than with monthly administration. European authors report success with use of a progestin-releasing IUD, which offers endometrial protection while limiting side effects. Unopposed ERT can be considered when all other measures fail to relieve progestational side effects, but such patients must undergo annual endometrial biopsy for detection and treatment of endometrial hyperplasia.

Breast symptoms, such as fullness, tenderness, or increase in size, are commonly noted with initiation of HRT. Patient education and reassurance often alleviate the anxiety associated with these changes. Breast symptoms typically subside with continued use.

Exacerbation of migraine headaches may occur with cyclic regimens but frequently subsides with initiation of a continuous regimen. Often, changing the estrogen or route of administration may resolve these and other less common complaints.

Although women on HRT often complain of **weight gain**, significant changes in weight have not been consistently noted; patients should be counseled about exercise and nutrition.

22. What are the indications for endometrial biopsy other than unopposed ERT?

Routine endometrial biopsy before initiation of HRT is no longer indicated. The risk of endometrial hyperplasia and carcinoma is reduced with combined regimens but is never absolutely zero. Therefore, sampling of the endometrium is indicated in women with an abnormal bleeding pattern. Bleeding earlier than 2 days before completion of the progestational agent in a cyclic regimen is typically considered abnormal. The more difficult determination is the definition of abnormal bleeding with a continuous regimen. Persistent prolonged bleeding or heavy bleeding is usually considered an indication for biopsy.

23. Should all women take HRT?

The debate continues as to whether menopause is an endocrinopathy warranting treatment in all appropriate women or a normal life stage warranting treatment only for specific indications. Statistics show that most postmenopausal women choose not to take HRT. HRT should be encouraged for women with unwanted symptoms or at increased risk for osteoporosis or cardiovascular disease. Women without contraindications who choose HRT should be supported in their decision. All women should receive counseling about proper nutrition, adequate calcium intake, regular exercise, and routine preventive health care.

24. Is vaginal bleeding after menopause a sign of serious disease?

In women not receiving HRT, all postmenopausal bleeding, regardless of amount, should be considered secondary to cancer until proved otherwise. However, only up to 30% of cases of postmenopausal bleeding are due to a malignant or premalignant condition; the remainder result from various benign causes. Although cancer of the endometrial lining is the most common malignant cause of postmenopausal bleeding, other gynecologic malignancies may present with vaginal bleeding and should be considered in the diagnostic work-up. Nongenital sites, such as the urinary and gastrointestinal tracts, also should be examined. Consider the possibility of trauma. Resumption of intercourse may result in lacerations of an atrophic lower genital tract and hemorrhagic bleeding. The emotional nature of this situation should be appreciated.

Causes of Postmenopausal Bleeding

Gynecologic sources—upper genital tract	Gynecologic sources—lower genital tract	Nongynecologic sources
Endometrial polyp	Trauma, vulvar or vaginal lacerations	Urethral caruncle
Atrophic endometrial lining	Vaginitis, infection with or without atrophy	Urethral lesions, benign or malignant
Endometrial hyperplasia, simple or complex	Vulvar intraepithelial neoplasia (VIN)	Hemorrhoids
Endometrial hyperplasia, complex with atypia	Vaginal intraepithelial neoplasia (VAIN)	Rectal polyps or other lesions
Endometrial carcinoma	Cervical epithelial neoplasia (CIN)	
Uterine malignancy of another nature (sarcoma)	Vulvar carcinoma	
Carcinoma of the fallopian tube	Vaginal carcinoma	
Ovarian neoplasm	Cervical carcinoma	

25. Describe the evaluation of postmenopausal bleeding.

Evaluation includes a thorough history and physical examination to determine the site of origin of the bleeding, a Papanicolaou smear, and an in-office endometrial sampling. Diagnostic hysteroscopy and dilatation and curettage (D&C) are performed if in-office sampling is impossible or insufficient because of cervical stenosis or if results are not conclusive. Ultrasonic evaluation of the endometrial stripe thickness is also used in the work-up of postmenopausal bleeding. A measurement of 4 mm or less in a postmenopausal woman not taking HRT is reassuring but does not preclude the need for histologic evaluation of the endometrial lining. Additional diagnostic studies, such as pelvic ultrasound and evaluation of the urinary tract or GI tract, may be indicated by the preliminary work-up.

Evaluation of Postmenopausal Bleeding

Baseline	Additional (as directed by above)
History	Pelvic Ultrasound
Physical examination with pelvic and rectal exam	Hysteroscopy and dilatation and curettage
	Urinalysis
Pap smear, HemOccult stool test	Evaluation of urinary tract
Endometrial sampling (in office)	Evaluation of gastrointestinal tract

26. Define postmenopausal osteoporosis. What is the scope of the problem?

Osteoporosis is a systemic skeletal disease characterized by a reduction in bone mass and microarchitectural deterioration. It results in an increased susceptibility to fracture. Osteoporosis is a significant public health problem in the United States, affecting 20 million people and accounting for > 275,000 hip fractures annually. In addition, osteoporosis is a significant burden in terms of health care costs, carrying an annual price tag of 8 billion dollars.

27. What are the classifications of osteoporosis?

Osteoporosis may be a primary disease or a condition secondary to various other disease states or medications. **Primary** osteoporosis affects mainly the aging population and is referred to as involutional osteoporosis. **Juvenile** osteoporosis is a rare form of primary osteoporosis that affects children and young adults. **Involutional** osteoporosis describes gradual and progressive bone loss that occurs in postmenopausal women (type I) or in aging men and women (type II).

28. Describe the major characteristics of involutional osteoporosis.

Characteristics of Involutional Osteoporosis

	TYPE I—POSTMENOPAUSAL	TYPE II—SENILE
Age	50–65 yr	75 yr and older
Gender	Women	Men and women
Bone type	Trabecular	Cortical and trabecular
Fracture site	Spine, wrist	Hip, proximal humerus, tibia, pelvis
Cause	Estrogen deficiency	Age-related factors: Decreased adrenal function Decreased calcium absorption Secondary hyperparathyroidism

Osteoporosis, like other chronic disease states, remains asymptomatic until late in its course when it presents with fractures that may occur spontaneously (e.g., in the spine) or as the result of trauma (e.g., in the hip or wrist). Frequently, the precipitating trauma is minimal. Osteoporotic fractures of the spine, known as **compression fractures**, cause loss of height and postural deformities (e.g., kyphosis of the thoracic spine or "dowager's hump," loss of lumbar lordosis) and are a significant source of pain and functional impairment. Osteoporotic **hip fractures** are associated with significant morbidity and mortality. There is a 15–20% excessive mortality rate after hip fracture; less than one-third of patients return to their previous level of function after 1 year.

29. How is osteoporosis diagnosed?
Osteoporosis is often diagnosed late in its course, when a characteristic fracture occurs. Early in its course, it can be diagnosed by measurement of bone mass. Bone mass measurement has been shown to predict fracture risk accurately, much as cholesterol screening predicts heart disease. The risk of fracture is inversely related to bone density. With each standard deviation of decline, the risk doubles. Risk also depends on factors such as age and risk of falling.

Techniques for Measuring Bone Density

MODALITY	SITE MEASURED	RADIATION EXPOSURE	SCAN TIME	COST	COMMENTS
Single photon absorptiometry (SPA)	Radius	10 mrem	15 min	$75	Radionuclide source; requires bath water
Dual photon absorptiometry (DPA)	Spine, hip	5 mrem	20–40 min	$100–150	Radionuclide source; expensive isotope
Dual energy x-ray absorptiometry (DEXA)	Spine, hip	1–3 mrem	5–15 min	$75–150	Precise, lower radiation exposure
Quantitative computed tomography (QCT)	Spine	100–1000 mrem	10–20 min	$100–200	Higher costs and radiation exposure

30. What are the current indications for bone density measurement?
- Estrogen deficiency—when information will be used to make decisions about estrogen replacement
- Osteopenia or vertebral abnormalities on x-ray—to confirm diagnosis of osteoporosis and assist in management decisions
- Chronic glucocorticoid therapy—assessment of bone loss to assist decisions about medication adjustment
- Primary hyperparathyroidism—to identify candidates for surgical intervention based on extent of skeletal disease
- Osteoporosis—to assess response to therapy

31. Describe the management of osteoporosis.

Prevention is the preferred approach in osteoporosis management. Strategies include adequate calcium intake, a program of weight-bearing exercise, estrogen replacement after menopause, and avoidance of associated risk factors, such as alcohol, tobacco, and diets high in sodium, caffeine, and protein. Treatment of osteoporosis includes measures to decrease the risk of fracture and related morbidity, such as pharmacologic agents that maintain or increase bone density and relieve pain; exercise to increase muscle strength and improve fitness; adequate calcium intake; and fall prevention strategies.

32. Which pharmacologic agents are used in the treatment of osteoporosis?

Antiresorptive agents	Stimulators of bone formation
Estrogen*	Fluorides
Progestins	Anabolic steroids
Calcitonins*	Parathyroid hormone and peptides
Bisphosphonates	
Etidronate	
Clodronate	
Pamidronate	
Tiludronate	
Alendronate *	
Calcium	
Vitamin D derivatives	
Calciferol and cholecalciferol	
Calcitriol	

* Recommended and approved for use in postmenopausal osteoporosis.

BIBLIOGRAPHY

1. American College of Obstetricians and Gynecologists: Guidelines for Women's Health Care. Washington, D.C., American College of Obstetricians and Gynecologists, 1996.
2. Baden WF, Walker T (eds): Surgical Repair of Vaginal Defects. Philadelphia, J.B. Lippincott, 1992.
3. Favus MJ: Primer on the Metabolic Bone Diseases and Disorders of Mineral Metabolism, 2nd ed. New York, Raven Press, 1993.
4. Kase NG, Wiengold AB, Gershenson DM: Principles and Practice of Clinical Gynecology. New York, Churchill & Livingstone, 1990.
5. Office of Technology Assessment: The Menopause, Hormone Therapy, and Women's Health. Washington DC, U.S. Government Printing Office, 1992.
6. Scott JR, DiSaia PJ, Hammond CB, et al (eds): Danforth's Obstetrics and Gynecology, 7th ed. Philadelphia, J.B. Lippincott, 1994.
7. Sobel NB: Primary care of the mature woman. Obstet Gynecol Clin North Am 21:299–314, 1994
8. Speroff L, Glass RH, Kase NG (eds): Clinical Gynecologic Endocrinology and Infertility, 5th ed. Baltimore, Williams & Wilkins, 1994.

33. ANEMIA IN THE ELDERLY

Janet Abrahm, M.D.

1. Are all patients with a low hemoglobin and hematocrit anemic?

No. Patients with a normal red cell mass may appear to be anemic if they have an increased plasma volume. Patients with congestive heart failure, hypothyroidism, or hyperviscosity syndrome may therefore appear to be anemic when they are not. All three of these conditions are seen more commonly in older adults than middle-aged and young individuals.

2. What are the common types of anemia in the elderly?

Common microcytic anemias include iron deficiency, lead poisoning, and congenital disorders not previously diagnosed (hemoglobinopathies or hereditary spherocytosis). The anemia of chronic disease and infiltrative marrow processes are usually normocytic. Macrocytic anemias are usually due to B_{12} or folate deficiency, but a significant portion reflect myelodysplasia. Patients can also have congenital or acquired hemolytic anemias.

3. How are iron deficiency and lead poisoning diagnosed?

In otherwise healthy patients, an iron saturation (Fe/total iron-binding capacity [TIBC]) of < 15% indicates **iron deficiency**. However, in patients with inflammatory, infectious, or hepatocellular disease, the iron saturation may appear to be >15% despite an iron-deficient status. In these patients, a ferritin level ≤ 100 µg/l indicates iron deficiency.

The anemia of **lead poisoning** can mimic that caused by iron deficiency. Lead poisoning may arise from an untreated occupational exposure (welders, metal workers) or from ingestion of lead leached into fluids from earthenware or lead-glazed pottery. In both iron deficiency and lead poisoning, the cells are microcytic, but in lead poisoning, the red cells have a characteristic basophilic stippling. Abdominal complaints, neuropathy, and hypertension may also be present. Chelation therapy is required.

4. How should patients with iron deficiency be treated?

Iron is poorly absorbed in the elderly. Patients should ingest foods that contain heme iron, such as red meats or liver, or foods containing non-heme iron along with foods rich in vitamin C, such as citrus fruits or dark-green leafy vegetables. (Vitamin C enhances the absorption of non-heme iron). Iron supplements are usually poorly tolerated in elderly patients because they exacerbate constipation and cause gastric irritation. Enteric-coated iron supplements, however, should not be used; their iron is released distal to its site of intestinal absorption. Parenteral iron replacement with Imferon should be considered for patients with ongoing iron losses (e.g., from inflammatory bowel disease or vascular malformations).

5. What are the common microcytic congenital disorders? How are they diagnosed?

The alpha- and beta-thalassemias and hemoglobin E disease. Alpha-thalassemias occur in people of African origin, beta-thalassemia in persons of Iranian or Mediterranean origin, and hemoglobin E disease in those of Southeast Asian descent.

In the thalassemias, cells are microcytic, but the red cell count is elevated. Patients with beta-thalassemia also have target cells, fragments, and basophilic stippling. Hemoglobin electrophoresis will be diagnostic in both iron-replete patients with beta-thalassemia and in hemoglobin E disease. The alternate hemoglobins (E, F, and rarer variants) and increased levels of A_2 appear. Electrophoresis is normal in alpha-thalassemia, and genetic studies are required for its diagnosis.

6. What is the "anemia of chronic disease"?

This is a normocytic, normochromic anemia that occurs in most patients with an inflammatory chronic disease, such as rheumatoid arthritis or active infection, that has persisted for 1–2 months. While the exact mechanism is unknown, contributing factors likely include the many cytokines released, including interleukin-1, tumor necrosis factor, and interferons alpha and gamma. Re-utilization of iron is impaired, and serum iron and TIBC levels are decreased despite normal or increased amounts of marrow iron.

7. How can the anemia of chronic disease be distinguished from that of other causes?

The figure illustrates one way to diagnose an anemic patient whose red cell indices are reported to be normal. The first step is to review the peripheral blood smear, as that can often make the diagnosis.

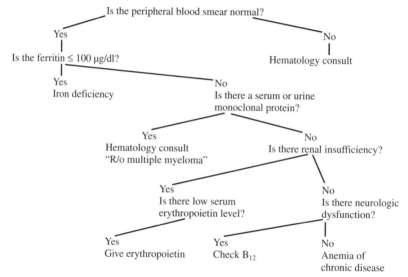

Evaluation of Patients with Normocytic, Normochromic Anemia

1. If the marrow is infiltrated by cancer, many of the red cells will have abnormal shapes (e.g., teardrops), platelets often are large, and both red and white cell precursors are seen. This blood smear is termed *myelophthistic* or *leuko-erythroblastic*. A bone marrow aspirate and biopsy are necessary to confirm this diagnosis.

2. If there is a primary marrow process, such as acute or chronic leukemia or the myelodysplastic syndromes, abnormalities of the white cells and platelets will also be present. Review of the peripheral smear is often diagnostic. In most cases, however, bone marrow aspirate or biopsy is required to make this diagnosis, as well.

If the laboratory reports or you see these types of abnormalities, then a hematology consultation is required.

3. If, however, the smear is normal, a serum ferritin level will distinguish iron deficiency from the anemia of chronic disease. For example, a patient with rheumatoid arthritis who takes nonsteroidal agents and whose ferritin is ≤ 100 µg/dl is iron-deficient, whereas a patient with a level > 100 µg/dl has the anemia of chronic disease.

4. In patients who are not iron-deficient, multiple myeloma must be excluded by serum and urine protein electrophoreses. Myeloma occurs most commonly in the fifth and sixth decades but can occur in older patients as well. If a monoclonal protein is present, it can be caused by one of a number of plasma cell disorders, including multiple myeloma. A hematology consultation is therefore required here, as well.

5. In patients without iron deficiency or myeloma who have renal insufficiency, low serum erythropoietin levels confirm that the anemia is due to renal failure. Treatment with erythropoietin reverses this anemia.

6. In those without renal insufficiency, it is important to exclude B_{12} deficiency. While this disorder usually produces a macrocytic anemia (see Question 10), about 15% of patients with neurologic dysfunction from B_{12} deficiency (loss of position sense, loss of sensation, or dementia) have normal red cell size. Therefore, in the elderly population with any of these neurologic findings, evidence for B_{12} deficiency must be sought.

8. Do all patients with macrocytic anemias have megaloblastic anemias?

No. Macrocytic anemia in the elderly may be due to a megaloblastic process, myelodysplasia, or, rarely, hypothyroidism or severe liver dysfunction.

9. How should an elderly patient with macrocytic anemia be evaluated initially?

Thyroid function tests should be obtained, and the peripheral blood smear should be reviewed to distinguish macrocytosis from megaloblastosis and from myelodysplastic syndromes (MDS). Patients with hypothyroidism will have macrocytosis alone; those with liver failure will have target cells and acanthocytes. The white cells will appear normal and the platelets will be normal (in hypothyroidism) or reduced (in liver failure).

In megaloblastic disorders, macro-ovalocytes appear and granulocytes are hypersegmented. In patients with MDS, the neutrophils may be hypogranulated or hyposegmented. Pseudo-Pelger-Huët cells (with nuclei resembling a pair of glasses) are seen in about 20–30%.

10. What are the common causes of megaloblastic anemias in the elderly? How should they be treated?

Megaloblastic anemias arise from tissue deficiencies of B_{12} or folic acid due to inadequate intake or impaired utilization. As many as one-third of elderly patients with a history of gastric surgery may be B_{12}-deficient. Even in those without gastric surgery, atrophic gastritis or agents that inhibit acid production (e.g., cimetidine or omeprazole) can cause B_{12} deficiency. While intrinsic factor production is usually normal in these patients, the lack of acid and pepsin renders them unable to liberate B_{12} from the food protein which binds it. Diet is otherwise not implicated in B_{12} deficiency, as B_{12} is found in all animal products. However, strict vegetarians can become deficient in 5–6 years. B_{12}-deficient patients need 5 days of parenteral B_{12} (1000 µg/day) followed by weekly shots for 1 month and then monthly shots for life. Those with neurologic manifestations require more intensive replacement.

Folate deficiency usually occurs from lack of dietary intake, increased excretion (in alcoholics), or impaired absorption due to achlorhydria. Rarely, folate deficiency occurs in patients with a marked increase in folate requirement from a severe exfoliative skin disease (such as psoriasis) or aggressive hemolytic anemia. Dark-green leafy vegetables, the best source of folate, are not usually a major part of the diet of the elderly. Oral folic acid (1 mg/day) is adequate replacement.

A number of medications cause folate deficiency. The folate deficiency induced by methotrexate (used in dermatologic and rheumatologic diseases), phenytoin, or trimethoprim-sulfamethoxazole can be reversed by concomitant administration of folic acid, without interfering with the therapeutic effect of the drugs. That induced in AIDS patients receiving trimethoprim-sulfamethoxazole, however, cannot be reversed, even by folinic acid. Patients receiving zidovudine or antineoplastic chemotherapy will also have megaloblastic anemias that do not respond to supplemental B_{12} or folate.

11. When is a bone marrow aspiration/biopsy indicated in an elderly patient with a macrocytic anemia?

If macrocytic and megaloblastic processes are eliminated, a bone marrow should be considered to diagnose myelodysplastic syndromes (MDS) and obtain prognostic information. MDS includes a number of related stem cell disorders: refractory anemia, refractory anemia with ringed sideroblasts, refractory anemia with excess blasts, refractory anemia with excess blasts in transformation, and chronic myelomonocytic leukemia. Patients with MDS have deficiencies in one or more cell lines (red or white cells, or platelets) and may develop a form of acute leukemia that is unresponsive to conventional anti-leukemic chemotherapy. The cause of MDS is often unknown, but in many patients it is caused by chemotherapy-induced marrow injury. Patients who received adjuvant chemotherapy for ovarian or breast cancer or chemotherapy for myeloma or lymphoma are at increased risk of developing MDS.

The most important prognostic information is obtained from the karyotype abnormalities of the malignant clone. Patients with multiple chromosomal abnormalities or who have deletion of the long arm of chromosome 7 (7q–) have a median survival of only 1 year. Those with no detectable abnormalities or deletion of the long arm of chromosome 5 (5q–), on the other hand, have an excellent prognosis. Marrows are usually obtained, therefore, both to make the diagnosis and to obtain this prognostic information.

12. How is MDS treated in elderly patients?

Unfortunately, patients over age 60 are not candidates for the only curative therapy, bone marrow transplantation. They experience much more toxicity than younger patients from this procedure, and the consequent risks outweigh the benefits. Besides supportive care, there are few tolerable, effective treatments for the associated cytopenias or leukemias. Some advocate a trial of pyridoxine, though this is rarely effective. Combinations of growth factors can sometimes reverse the cytopenias, though transfusion support is often needed. Occasionally, removal of a massively enlarged spleen that is sequestering red cells is effective. Patients die either from complications resulting from the cytopenias or leukemic transformation.

13. When should hemolysis be considered as the cause of anemia in an elderly patient?

Acute hemolysis in the elderly presents in the same way as it does in younger patients, with jaundice, dark urine, and weakness, though cardiovascular complaints may also occur. Chronic hemolysis, however, may be asymptomatic except for gallstones, early satiety from splenomegaly, or shoulder pain from splenic infarct. Patients may not even appear jaundiced, though most have splenomegaly. They will, however, have a low haptoglobin level and an elevated reticulocyte count, bilirubin, and lactate dehydrogenase.

14. What are the common causes of congenital hemolytic anemias?

Hereditary hemolytic anemias are usually due to hereditary spherocytosis, enzymopathies, or hemoglobinopathies. Hereditary spherocytosis may first present in the seventh decade. Gallstones may become clinically apparent, or splenomegaly may be noted for the first time during a physical exam for a life insurance policy. Glucose-6-phosphate dehydrogenase (G6PD) deficiency may manifest when the patient is first exposed to a medication causing an oxidant stress. Phenazopyridine, primaquine, and the sulfa drugs sulfamethoxazole (found in Septra and Bactrim), sulfacetamide, sulfanilamide and sulfapyridine all must be avoided in patients with G6PD deficiency.

Mild hemoglobinopathies (e.g., sickle trait, alpha-thalassemia, or mild variants of beta-thalassemia) similarly may have gone undiagnosed. Hematuria in an elderly patient might be the first presentation of sickle cell trait. However, sickle trait and the other hemoglobinopathies mentioned do not affect the patient's lifespan, except in unusual circumstances. A parvovirus infection, for example, may cause a severe, symptomatic anemia. In these patients the red cell survival is shorter than normal. A parvovirus infection will transiently stop red cell production, causing the anemia to worsen significantly and become symptomatic, possibly for the first time. In addition, some thalassemic patients may have incorrectly been thought to suffer from iron deficiency, as their cells are also small. If they received iron for prolonged periods, they may develop iron overload, which can present as heart or liver failure or as arthritis.

15. How are the hereditary hemolytic anemias diagnosed?

In hereditary spherocytosis, spherocytes appear on the smear, and the direct and indirect Coombs' tests (see Question 19) are negative. The diagnosis can be confirmed by performing an osmotic fragility test, along with a 48-hour autohemolysis test.

G6PD levels are assayed in the red cells after the reticulocytosis following the hemolysis resolves. Testing the red cells for G6PD during the period of reticulocytosis can give a falsely normal value because reticulocytes have higher levels of G6PD than older cells. Except for alpha-thalassemia, hemoglobinopathies are detected by hemoglobin electrophoresis, as noted earlier.

16. What are the common types of acquired hemolytic anemias in the elderly?

Acquired hemolytic anemias are caused by microangiopathic or immune processes. The antibodies causing the immune hemolytic anemias may be autoantibodies (idiopathic, disease-related, or drug-induced) or alloantibodies (from a transfusion).

17. How are microangiopathic hemolytic anemias diagnosed and treated?

Elderly patients develop microangiopathic hemolytic anemia from uncontrolled hypertension, aortic dissections, leaking artificial valves (especially aortic), widespread metastatic cancer, or certain chemotherapeutic agents. Very rarely, they develop idiopathic thrombotic thrombocytopenic purpura (TTP).

Red cells fragments and early red cell precursors are present on the blood smear; in TTP, there will also be very few platelets. Medication for the blood pressure, surgery to correct the vascular or valvular disease, or plasmapheresis for those with idiopathic TTP is usually effective. There is usually no effective therapy for patients with TTP from widespread cancer or chemotherapy.

18. What are the causes of immune hemolysis in the elderly?

The usual causes are autoimmune hemolytic disorders. These are either idiopathic or associated with underlying lymphoproliferative disorders (e.g., chronic lymphocytic leukemia, lymphoma). The antibodies are of the IgG or IgM class. The former are active at usual body temperatures and so are considered "warm" antibodies; the latter are most active in the cold and so are called "cold" antibodies. The cold antibodies cause **cold agglutinin disease**, a very difficult form of hemolytic anemia to treat.

Drugs can also produce antibody-mediated hemolytic anemia. Ten percent of patients on methyldopa or L-dopa develop antibodies, but rarely (in 10% of those with antibodies) does the patient develop hemolysis. Penicillin-induced hemolysis is mediated through a hapten mechanism, while sulfa drugs and quinidine induce an immune complex-mediated hemolysis.

A less common antibody-mediated process is the **delayed hemolytic transfusion reaction**. These reactions are caused by alloantibodies raised in response to a non-ABO red cell antigen that was absent on the patient's red cells but present on red cells in the transfusion. Seven to 10 days after the transfusion, the newly formed antibodies cause lysis of transfused red cells that have the foreign antigen. The patient suddenly develops dark-colored urine, jaundice, and, if a large number of units were transfused, symptoms of anemia.

19. How are the autoimmune hemolytic anemias diagnosed and treated?

Immune hemolytic anemias are diagnosed by performing a direct and an indirect Coombs' test, which detects the presence of IgG, IgM, or complement on the patient's red cells (direct Coombs) or IgG or IgM in the patient's serum (indirect Coombs). In the direct Coombs' test, the patient's red cells are incubated with reagents that cause red cells coated with antibodies to agglutinate. The test is positive in patients with immune hemolytic anemias, as the cause of the anemia is the coating of the patient's cells with antibody. The indirect Coombs' test detects antibodies in the serum. The patient's serum is reacted with red cells from a variety of donors, and the cells are examined for agglutination. Usually, this test is also positive, because patients with immune hemolytic anemias usually make more antibody than can bind to the red cells. The excess antibody appears in the serum.

Steroids are the initial therapy for idiopathic **warm antibody-mediated hemolysis,** but splenectomy is also often required to remove the major site of antibody recognition and red cell destruction. However, in addition, specific chemotherapy for the underlying cancer is required to reverse the immune hemolysis associated with lymphoma or chronic lymphocytic leukemia.

For patients with **cold agglutinin disease** associated with mycoplasma or Epstein-Barr virus infection, no therapy is usually required. For the idiopathic forms, the patient is usually advised to stay in a warm climate. Steroids are not routinely effective and immunosuppresive chemotherapeutic agents have mixed success.

20. How are the drug-induced immune anemias diagnosed and treated?

Drug-induced antibodies are also detected by the Coombs' tests. They are positive for IgG in the case of penicillin and methyldopa/L-dopa-induced hemolysis, but the direct Coombs will be positive only for complement in hemolysis induced by quinidine and sulfa drugs. If patients on methyldopa or L-dopa have antibodies but no evidence of hemolysis, the drugs can be continued. If hemolysis has occurred, however, the drugs must be stopped.

21. And the delayed hemolytic transfusion reaction?

A delayed hemolytic transfusion reaction is confirmed by an indirect Coombs' test, which, in this case, detects the specific serum antibody responsible for the hemolysis. The direct Coombs' test will usually be negative, because the red cells which bound the antibody (and would have made the direct Coombs positive) have been hemolyzed.

As the process is self-limited, no specific therapy is usually required. Patients subsequently receive transfusions only with red cells lacking the antigen to which the antibody was directed.

BIBLIOGRAPHY

1. Atony AC: Megaloblastic anemias. In Benz EJ, et al (eds): Hematology: Basic Principles and Practice, 2nd ed. New York, Churchill Livingstone, 1994, pp 4552–4586.
2. Brittenham GM: Disorders of iron metabolism: iron deficiency and overload. In Benz EJ, et al (eds): Hematology: Basic Principles and Practice, 2nd ed. New York, Churchill Livingstone, 1994, pp 492–523.
3. Greenberg PL: Myelodysplastic syndrome. In Benz EJ, et al (eds): Hematology: Basic Principles and Practice, 2nd ed. New York, Churchill Livingstone, 1994, pp 1098–1121.
4. Guyatt GH, Oxman AD, Ali M, et al: Laboratory diagnosis of iron deficiency anemia: An overview. J Gen Intern Med 7:145–153, 1992.
5. Schilling RF: Anemia of chronic disease: A misnomer. Ann Intern Med 115:572–573, 1991.
6. Schwartz E, Benz EJ Jr, Forget BG: Thalassemia syndromes. In Benz EJ, et al (eds): Hematology: Basic Principles and Practice, 2nd ed. New York, Churchill Livingstone, 1994, pp 586–610.
7. Schwartz RS, Silberstein LE, Berkman EM. Autoimmune hemolytic anemias. In Benz EJ, et al (eds): Hematology: Basic Principles and Practice, 2nd ed. New York, Churchill Livingstone, 1994, pp 710–729.

34. PAIN MANAGEMENT

Janet Abrahm, M.D.

1. What are the major types of pain? How do they present?

There are three main types of pain: somatic, visceral, and neuropathic. **Somatic pain**, such as postoperative pain or pain from bony metastases, arises from cutaneous or deep tissues. The pain is usually very well-localized and is dull or aching in character.

Visceral pain, arising from organ infiltration, compression, or stretching, is poorly localized, deep, squeezing and pressure-like. It may be referred to cutaneous sites, such as the diaphragmatic pain that is felt in the shoulder region. When it is acute, there is often associated nausea, vomiting, or sweating. Patients with an acute myocardial infarction, cholecystitis, bowel obstruction, or liver enlargement due to tumor infiltration present with visceral pain.

Neuropathic pain arises from traumatic or ischemic injury to the peripheral or central nervous systems or from nerve infiltration, compression, or other damage. The pain is usually severe, burning, or vise-like, but it is occasionally shooting, like an electric shock. Patients with diabetic or alcoholic neuropathy or herpes zoster have neuropathic pain, as do patients with spinal cord compression.

Pain complaints may also arise in people who have no anatomical lesions. The pain complaint may be the only manner in which the patient is able to express nonspecific feelings of distress caused by anxiety, financial problems, anger, loneliness, depression, or grief over poor health or lost relatives. Since these concerns may exacerbate any concomitant painful sensations, alleviating them can treat the cause of the distress and thereby significantly decrease the need for pain medications.

2. What are the components of an adequate pain assessment?

Effective pain management requires repeated, comprehensive assessment of the patient's pain(s). While the elderly experience pain to the same degree as younger patients, they often under-report their pain, ascribing it to normal changes expected with aging. Scales that quantify patient reports of pain are valid, reliable, and reproducible. They should be used, much as a blood sugar determination is used in diabetes, to monitor the efficacy of therapy.

If, for example, you are using a scale of 0 (no pain) to 10 (the worst pain imaginable), the change in the rating 1 hour after pain medication is given will indicate how to adjust the medication. The physician must determine both the intensity of the pain and the functional distress caused by the pain (e.g., is it interfering with the patient's ability to eat, sleep, interact with others, move, walk, or talk, or with emotions or concentration). The goal is to lower the pain to a level acceptable to the patient.

3. How does chronic pain differ in its manifestations from acute pain?

Patients in chronic pain do not present the common autonomic manifestations of acute pain (i.e., tachycardia, elevated blood pressure, sweating, or facial grimacing). Such patients will often be quiet and withdrawn, manifesting little spontaneous movement; they can be depressed or irritable and will complain of discomfort if moved. When their pain is relieved, however, they often become mobile and engaged and involved with other people.

4. What common nonpharmacologic methods are effective for pain control?

Hypnosis: Simple hypnotic techniques to minimize patient anxiety and pain include rehearsing the planned test or procedure, distraction techniques (e.g., listening to music) and dissociation (e.g., daydreaming or imagining to be somewhere else). Even without formal hypnotic induction, the words used by the practitioner to describe procedures are very important. Using the phrase "You will feel something; everyone feels this a little differently" in place of "This is going to hurt a lot!" gives the patient permission to alter the sensation and may also diminish the experience of pain.

Hyperstimulation analgesia: Ice massage, using a paper cup filled with ice, is a form of hyperstimulation analgesia that is particularly well-accepted by elderly patients with cancer pain. **Acupuncture** can be helpful for patients with osteoarthritis or neuropathic pain. It is the intensity, not the precise site, of the mechanical stimulation that induces the anesthesia. This anesthesia is not simply due to placebo effect. **Transcutaneous electrical nerve stimulation** (TENS) devices using electrical hyperstimulation are indicated for patients with dermatomal pain, such as post-herpetic neuralgia or radiculopathy from spinal cord compression. For optimal effect, a physiatrist or physical therapist familiar with the device should train the patient in its use.

Other: For arthritis pain, **dry heat** or **hydrotherapy** is often used, as is **physical therapy**, which maximizes function and minimizes disability. **Orthotic devices** or prostheses to reduce joint loading and minimize abnormal stresses can limit pain as well as progression of joint damage. Removing fluid from the joint can also provide relief. In certain patients with extensive deformities, synovectomy, joint replacement, or **other surgeries** are indicated for pain relief. **Trigger point injection** can provide relief for many patients with myofascial or certain neuropathic pain syndromes (e.g., post-thoracotomy pain).

5. How are the nonpharmacologic and pharmacologic therapies used for different types of pain?

Pain Regimens for Geriatric Patients

SEVERITY	FREQUENCY	TYPE	AGENTS
Mild	Intermittent	Somatic, visceral	Acetaminophen Nonacetylated salicylates (aspirin, NSAIDs)* Trigger point injection Nonpharmacologic means (hypnosis, ice massage, wet or dry heat) Orthotic devices
Moderate	Intermittent	Somatic, visceral	Combination agent (ASA, acetaminophen with codeine, oxycodone) Acupuncture Hypnosis
	Intermittent or continuous	Neuropathic	Combination agent Tricyclic antidepressant or anticonvulsant Steroids, capsaicin TENS, hypnosis Peripheral nerve, ganglion block, lysis
Severe	Intermittent	Somatic, visceral, neuropathic	Strong short-acting opiates† Tricyclic antidepressants Nonacetylated salicylates or acetaminophen
	Continuous	Somatic, visceral, neuropathic	Substitute a sustained-release or long-acting opiate for the short-acting opiate† in the regimen for severe, intermittent Steroids Peripheral, central nerve ablation

* Significant toxicities at therapeutic doses in geriatric patients. ASA = acetylsalicylic acid; NSAIDs = nonsteroidal anti-inflammatory drugs.
† Short-acting: oxycodone (alone), Dilaudid (hydromorphone), Levodromeran (levorphanol), immediate-release morphine.

6. Which patients would benefit from non-narcotic analgesics?

Non-narcotic analgesics (aspirin, acetaminophen, NSAIDs) should be given to patients with **mild pain,** especially of somatic or visceral type. Nonacetylated salicylates which do not impair prostaglandin synthesis, such as salicylic acid and choline magnesium salicylate, cause less toxicity and therefore should be the first-line agents for elderly patients. It is important to prescribe an adequate dose of the drug at regular intervals, switching to another non-narcotic analgesic only when maximal doses of the first are ineffective. The limited metabolism of salicylates can, however, lead to salicylate toxicity if the patient takes the pills more often than recommended. The non-narcotic analgesics should be continued in patients with moderate pain when narcotic analgesics are added, as they will potentiate the pain-relieving effect of the narcotic.

7. What drugs are particularly helpful for patients with bone pain?

The non-narcotic analgesics are especially useful in patients with bone pain, as they decrease local prostaglandin release and may thereby reduce the sensitization of pain receptors. Effective new agents for patients with bone pain caused by cancer include the bisphosphonates (e.g., pamidronate) and strontium-89. The treatment of low back pain of nonmalignant origin requires a combination of pharmacologic, nonpharmacologic, rehabilitative, psychologic, and occasionally surgical and anesthetic strategies.

8. What problems may occur in elderly patients using NSAIDs?

Renal insufficiency, peptic ulcer disease, and bleeding diatheses. Renal function should be assessed 1 or 2 weeks after initiation of the NSAID.

9. What agents are helpful for patients with neuropathic pain?

Tricyclic antidepressants (amitriptyline, nortriptyline), anticonvulsants (phenytoin, carbamazepine), capsaicin, and steroids are non-narcotic analgesics with particular efficacy in relieving moderate or severe neuropathic pain.

Post-herpetic neuralgia, which occurs in 1–2% of geriatric patients each year, is not very responsive to narcotic medications. It is very effectively treated, however, with amitriptyline, beginning at 10–25 mg hourly during sleep and increasing as tolerated to 100–150 mg. Nortriptyline (Pamelor) may be tolerated, as it has fewer anticholinergic side effects. Dosing begins at 50 mg at bedtime. Serum levels comparable to those required for antidepressant effect are usually required. Topical capsaicin (0.075%), TENS devices, and nerve block or lysis are also useful.

Trigeminal neuralgia, which occurs mostly in geriatric patients, responds to the anticonvulsant carbamazepine (Tegretol). It is started at 100 mg twice daily, with careful monitoring for decreases in the white blood cell count. Doses need to be increased very slowly, as tolerated, to maximize efficacy.

10. How can compliance with a narcotic prescription be ensured?

Narcotic analgesics are the mainstay of therapy for patients with moderate to severe pain of any type, whether of malignant or nonmalignant origin. Education of the patient and family is often required to dispel the misconceptions about narcotic therapy. The fear of addiction is a common cause of inadequate dispensing of narcotics and a barrier to their acceptance by patients. The physician can increase compliance by providing a full explanation of the differences between addiction and physical dependence, along with reassurance that patients with malignancies who take narcotics do not become addicts. Patients may also fear that if they take narcotic medications for moderate pain, these agents will no longer be effective if more severe pain occurs. A functional goal of therapy, such as returning to a favorite hobby or reinstituting normal activities of everyday life, may enable the patient and family to accept the narcotic.

11. Which narcotic medications should be used in elderly patients?

A wide variety of medications are available for use by the oral, rectal, transdermal, or parenteral route. These include the short-acting agents codeine, oxycodone, hydromorphone, and morphine and the longer-acting agents levorphanol, transdermal fentanyl, and morphine in sustained-release preparations. Oxycodone (5 mg/pill) is the opiate in the combination agents Percodan (with aspirin) and Percocet and Tylox (with acetaminophen).

The choice of agent should be dictated by the frequency and type of the pain being treated. **Intermittent, moderate to severe pain** lasting hours to several days is amenable to oral short-acting (3–4 hr) analgesics with appropriate potency. **Severe pain** of relatively constant intensity should be treated with oral long-acting morphine preparations (given every 8–12 hrs) or fentanyl, absorbed through a transdermal patch (renewed every 72 hours). Meperidine is the least useful narcotic for patients with long-lasting moderate to severe pain. It provides pain relief for only about 1–2 hours, and its metabolite can cause seizures.

Combinations of a non-narcotic analgesic along with an opiate (e.g., Percodan) are very useful, even for patients with moderate somatic or visceral pain of nonmalignant origin. Patients with pain of bony origin, such as severe osteoarthritis or rheumatoid arthritis, are ideal candidates for these agents.

Fewer than 1% of people who use narcotics for pain become addicted to them. They may continue to need them to keep their pain at a tolerable level and may even develop a physiologic dependence, but they will not start stealing TV sets. They will not begin to crave the drugs or seek them to "get high."

12. What other routes are available for patients who cannot take narcotics orally?

Narcotics: Analgesic Equivalents

	PARENTERAL (MG)	ORAL (MG)
Morphine	10	30
Oxycodone	—	30
Hydromorphone	1.5	7.5
Levorphanol	2	4
Meperidine*	75	300

* Chronic use may cause seizures.

Narcotics can be given rectally, transdermally, or via subcutaneous, intravenous, or spinal infusions. For patients with severe pain, intravenous drug delivery using a **patient-controlled analgesia system** is recommended.

Rectal opiates in short-acting formulations (morphine, oxymorphone, and hydromorphone) have about the same potency and half-life as orally administered agents and therefore have to be given frequently. Sustained-release morphine preparations have the same potency and half-life when administered rectally as they do orally, but they are not approved for rectal use. Patients switched from oral or rectal to parenteral routes of the same medication, or who are given another opiate because they have unacceptable side effects from the first, must have the dose altered accordingly to avoid overdose or undertreatment.

A **transdermal fentanyl system** continuously delivers fentanyl from its reservoir into the skin, achieving a relatively constant plasma fentanyl concentration at 14–20 hours after the initial patch is placed. New patches are placed every 72 hours. Rescue medication (10% of the total 24 hour dose) must be provided during the first 48 hours of use of the patch. This patch is not recommended for patients who need immediate pain relief. Elderly patients or those with respiratory insufficiency may require lower doses. Because drug remains in the skin reservoir after the patch is removed, in overdose, naloxone infusion may be required until the drug is eliminated from the skin depot.

13. How is a patient converted from oral or parenteral morphine to a transdermal fentanyl patch?

The table provides information on converting dosages. For example, a patient who has been receiving 90 mg of sustained-relief morphine every 12 hours should be given a 50-µg fentanyl patch ($90 \times 2 = 180$ mg morphine daily—135–224 mg oral morphine on the table—corresponding to a 50–µg fentanyl patch). A patient on a morphine drip of 2 mg/hr should be started on 75 µg of fentanyl (2 mg/hr $\times$ 24 hrs = 48 mg parenteral morphine daily—38–52 mg parenteral morphine—corresponding to 75 µg of fentanyl).

Dosage Conversions

FENTANYL (µg/hr)	MORPHINE (mg/day)	
	PARENTERAL	ORAL
25	8–22	45–134
50	23–37	135–224
75	38–52	225–314
100	53–67	315–404
125	68–82	405–494
150	83–97	495–584

14. Which medications can add to the pain-relieving effect of the opiates and so minimize the dose needed?

Low doses of tricyclic antidepressants (TCAs, such as nortryptiline, 50 mg given at bedtime) are well-tolerated and are effective within 2–3 days. Though nortryptiline has the fewest anticholinergic side effects of the TCA class, it should not be given to patients with known glaucoma, urinary retention, or first-degree heart block. Side effects (usually associated with amitriptyline) may include autonomic effects, which can be mild (dry mouth, constipation) or more severe (postural hypotension, glaucoma, or urinary retention).

15. How should the constipation and sedation associated with narcotics be managed?

Laxatives must be given routinely, not on an as-needed basis, to patients treated with any narcotics. Bowel irritants such as Senokot or resins such as lactulose are the most effective agents. Docusate is not effective, and fiber only exacerbates the problem.

Benzodiazepines, barbiturates, and chloral hydrate are not recommended as sleep medications for patients receiving narcotics, as they produce excessive daytime sedation. The TCA nortriptyline is preferred as a sleep medication, as low doses (e.g., 50 mg) potentiate pain relief, have few anticholinergic side effects, and produce moderate sedation. When possible, medications that produce sedation as a side effect (e.g., cimetidine or diphenhydramine) should be discontinued.

Dextroamphetamine (2.5–7.5 mg orally) or methylphenidate (Ritalin, 10 mg orally with breakfast) permit lowering of the narcotic dose by one-third to one-half while maintaining equivalent analgesia and less sedation. Doses can be slowly escalated as needed. The effect of the amphetamine is short-lived (2–3 weeks) but can be important in helping patients be as alert and pain-free as possible for an important event, such as a child's wedding or an important anniversary. Methylphenidate is contraindicated in patients with cardiac disease, as serious arrhythmias may occur. Patients may also become overstimulated or anxious and develop insomnia, paranoia, or confusion. Paradoxically, however, many elderly patients with depression respond well to similar doses of methylphenidate, with increased appetite and a better sense of well-being.

Naloxone reverses narcotic-induced respiratory and CNS depression, but caution should be exercised before administering naloxone to a patient chronically receiving narcotics: severe withdrawal may be precipitated. In such patients, rather than administering the usual 0.4-mg/ml dose, dilute the 0.4 mg of naloxone into 10 ml of saline, and give only enough to reverse respiratory depression, not enough to awaken the patient.

16. Discuss the special problems presented by narcotics and adjuvants in the elderly.

Pharmacokinetics both of narcotics and psychotropic adjuvant medications are altered in the elderly. Elderly patients (age 70–89) have decreased narcotic clearance, which leads to a prolonged duration of effect. Effective doses are one-half to one-quarter of those needed in younger patients. Long-acting agents such as methadone, sustained-release morphine, or fentanyl patches should be used with caution in the frail elderly, as the drug may accumulate and cause excessive toxicity. Drugs with short half-lives are preferred, and initial doses should be half those used with younger patients. The acute urinary retention due to opiates (especially in patients with prostatic hypertrophy) and hypotension and tachycardia caused by TCAs can be more frequent and of more clinical severity in this population.

17. What are the special problems of pain control in patients with dementia?
Little is known about the problem of giving pain medications to elderly patients with dementia. However, patients with AIDS dementia have been found to be much more sensitive to the adverse side effects of opiates. Sedation and confusion have been especially troublesome but have responded to psychostimulants such as methylphenidate or to antipsychotics such as haloperidol without diminution of the pain relief. It might be reasonable, therefore, to add psychostimulants or antipsychotic agents in appropriate elderly demented patients who develop these side effects from the opiates used to control their pain. Whenever possible, nonpharmacologic therapies, such as relaxation, hypnosis, or other cognitive therapies, should be employed.

BIBLIOGRAPHY

1. Donovan MI: Clinical assessment of cancer pain. In McGuire DB, Yarbro CH (eds): Cancer Pain Management. Philadelphia, W.B. Saunders, 1987, p 105.
2. Ferrel BA: Pain management in elderly people. J Am Geriatr Soc 39:64–73, 1991.
3. Foley KM: Management of cancer pain. In DeVita VT, Hellman S, Rosenberg SA (eds): Cancer: Principles and Practice of Oncology, 4th ed. Philadelphia, J.B. Lippincott, 1993, p 2417.
4. Kaiko RF, Wallenstein SL, Rogers AG, et al: Narcotics in the elderly. Med Clin North Am 66:1079, 1982.
5. Portenoy RK: Pain management in the older cancer patient. Oncology 6:86–98, 1992.
6. Portenoy RK, Farkash A: Practical management of non-malignant pain in the elderly. Geriatrics 43:29–47, 1988.
7. Wall PD, Melzack R (eds): Textbook of Pain, 3rd ed. Edinburgh, Churchill Livingstone, 1994.

35. URINARY INCONTINENCE

Grace A. Cordts, M.D.

1. What is urinary incontinence?

Urinary incontinence (UI) is a significant cause of disability and dependency, especially among the elderly. It is estimated that 15–30% of community-dwelling older people and 50% of institutionalized older people suffer from UI. UI is defined as the involuntary loss of urine, severe enough to cause social or hygienic problems. Potential adverse effects include social isolation, depression, stress, skin breakdown, recurrent urinary tract infections, falls, and high economic costs.

2. How do you identify patients with UI?

At least one-half of older patients with incontinence can improve without extensive evaluations and interventions. The problem arises in identifying people with UI. Because of the long-held belief that UI is a normal part of aging, many patients do not seek help from their primary care provider. Even if patients complain of UI, many health care professionals are reluctant to discuss the problem or to offer adequate evaluation and treatment. The importance of identifying and treating UI is reflected in the fact that UI was one of the first clinical guidelines to be tackled by the Agency for Health Care Policy and Research (AHCPR).

Questions about UI should become a part of the health care provider's initial and ongoing evaluation. Health care providers should ask elderly patients and, if appropriate, their family and caregivers about UI. Questions such as "Do you have trouble holding your urine?" are effective ways to open discussion of UI. They can be followed with specific questions, such as, "Do you ever lose urine when you don't want to?," "Do you ever have difficulty getting to the bathroom?," and "Do you ever wear a pad to collect your urine?" If the answer to any of these questions is yes, further evaluation should be undertaken.

3. How is UI classified?

The initial clinical classification consists of two categories: acute reversible forms and persistent incontinence. Acute reversible UI has a sudden onset and is usually associated with an acute medical illness or an iatrogenic cause. Persistent UI occurs over time and is unrelated to acute events. Acute reversible factors may contribute to and worsen persistent UI.

4. What can cause acute reversible UI?

D	**D**elirium
R	**R**estricted mobility, retention
I	**I**nfection, inflammation, impaction
P	**P**olyuria, pharmaceutics

Patients with delirium may become unaware of the urge to void or be unable to get themselves to a toilet. When the delirium resolves, urinary continence returns.

Any condition that acutely restricts mobility can precipitate functional incontinence or worsen persistent incontinence. Such conditions include fractured hip, stroke, Parkinson's disease, use of restraints, or exacerbation of arthritis.

Urinary retention due to medication or anatomic obstructions can cause overflow incontinence.

Acute urinary tract infections can cause new onset of UI. Inflammatory conditions such as atrophic vaginitis and urethritis may precipitate incontinence. Fecal impaction is a common cause of acute UI.

Any condition that causes polyuria can precipitate UI. Glucosuria and calciuria are common metabolic problems. Congestive heart failure and venous insufficiency cause edema and nocturia, precipitating nocturnal urinary incontinence. The list of medications that precipitate incontinence is long. Examples include alcohol, calcium channel blockers, beta-adrenergic agonists, alpha-adrenergic agonists, alpha-adrenergic blockers, narcotic analgesics, psychotropics, anticholinergics, and diuretics.

5. How is persistent UI classified?

Persistent UI can be classified in several ways, including anatomic, pathophysiologic, and clinical. The clinical classification is most useful for practicing physicians because it helps direct clinical evaluation and intervention. The clinical categories include the following:

1. **Stress incontinence**—involuntary loss of urine when intra-abdominal pressure increases, as during coughing, sneezing, or exercising. A common cause is relaxation of pelvic floor musculature. It is the most common cause of UI in people under the age of 75 years. It is more common in women but may occur in men if the anatomic sphincters are damaged after transurethral surgery or radiation therapy. Patients complain of losing urine when laughing, coughing, or standing. The amount of urine lost varies from a small amount that requires no intervention to large amounts that require intervention.

2. **Urge incontinence**—involuntary loss of urine associated with the sensation of the desire to void. Urge incontinence is usually, but not always, associated with involuntary detrusor contractions (detrusor overactivity). Neurologic problems are often associated with this type of incontinence, including stroke, dementia, Parkinson's disease and spinal cord injury. If a neurologic disorder is present, it is called detrusor hyperreflexia; if no neurologic disorder is present, it is called detrusor instability. Patients complain that they do not have enough time to get to the bathroom after they have the urge to void. It is the most common cause of incontinence in people over 75. One variation of urge incontinence is detrusor hyperactivity with impaired contractility. Patients have involuntary contractions but do not empty the bladder completely. They have symptoms of urge incontinence and high postvoid residuals. They may also have symptoms of obstruction, stress incontinence, and overflow incontinence. It is important to identify this condition because it can mimic other types of incontinence and may be treated inappropriately.

3. **Overflow incontinence**—involuntary loss of urine associated with overdistention of the bladder. It is caused by an anatomic obstruction, such as prostate enlargement; neurogenic factors, such as diabetes or multiple sclerosis, that result in an underactive or acontractile bladder; or medications. Patients usually complain of small amounts of urine leakage without the sensation of bladder fullness.

4. **Functional incontinence**—involuntary loss of urine secondary to factors outside the lower urinary tract. Common causes are severe dementia, severe musculoskeletal problems, environmental factors that make access to a bathroom difficult, and psychological factors. This is a diagnosis of exclusion; even frail elderly patients with significant dementia and physical impairments can have treatable causes of UI.

Frequently, UI in elderly patients presents with a variety of symptoms and a urodynamic picture of more than one type of UI. Correct treatment requires identification of all components.

6. Discuss the neurophysiology and anatomy of continence.

To be continent, a person must be able to recognize that his or her bladder is full and to get to a bathroom. Although this sounds easy, it is a complex physiologic process involving autonomic reflexes and volitional control. It involves the bladder, urethra, and pelvic floor musculature as well as their neural pathways.

Anatomically, the lower urinary tract consists of the bladder, urethra, internal sphincter, and external sphincter. The bladder is made up of a smooth muscle, called the detrusor muscle, that can contract in all directions. The urethra is 4 cm in women and 20 cm in men. The urethral mucosa in women is maintained by estrogen. The mucosa atrophies in estrogen-deficient states. There is a 90° angle between the bladder and urethra. Normal pelvic geometry allows intra-abdominal pressure to be distributed equally to the urethra and bladder. Therefore, when intra-abdominal pressure increases from coughing or laughing, urinary leakage is prevented. The internal sphincter is located at the base of the bladder and consists of smooth muscle. The external sphincter, which is made up of smooth muscle and striated muscle, allows voluntary interruption of voiding.

The lower urinary tract is innervated by parasympathetic, sympathetic, and somatic nerves. Parasympathetic cholinergic nerves from the sacral micturition center innervate the bladder. Stimulation causes the bladder to contract. The bladder base, neck, and internal sphincter are supplied by alpha-adrenergic sympathetic nerves from the hypogastric plexus. Stimulation of these nerves causes contraction of the bladder neck and urethra. Beta-adrenergic fibers from the hypogastric plexus connect to the detrusor muscle. Stimulation causes bladder relaxation. In addition, sympathetic nerve fibers inhibit parasympathetic tone. Stimulation of the pudendal nerve, which innervates the pelvic floor musculature, results in increased tone of the pelvic floor muscles. (See figure below.)

Thus, urine storage can be considered primarily a sympathetic process. Stimulation of the sympathetic fibers causes relaxation of the bladder and contraction of the bladder neck and urethra. Urination can be viewed as primarily a parasympathetic process with stimulation of the nerves causing contraction of the bladder.

Higher centers in the brainstem, cerebral cortex, and cerebellum can influence the lower urinary tract and thus affect voiding. As the bladder fills, sensory impulses are sent to the detrusor motor nucleus in the pons. This nucleus fires, causing the detrusor to contract and the sphincter to relax, allowing urination. Neurons in the frontal lobe can inhibit the pontine nucleus and thus stop urination. Disorders of the cerebral cortex, such as stroke, Parkinson's disease, or dementia, and disorders of the brainstem can cause incontinence. Knowledge of the anatomy and physiology helps to elucidate the cause of incontinence and possible treatment modalities. (See figure, next page.)

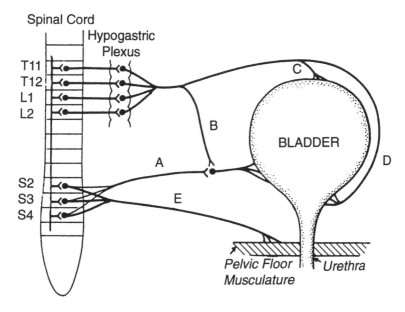

	TYPE OF NERVE	FUNCTION
A	PARASYMPATHETIC CHOLINERGIC (Nervi Erigentes)	Bladder contraction
B	SYMPATHETIC	Bladder relaxation (by inhibition of parasympathetic tone)
C	SYMPATHETIC	Bladder relaxation (β adrenergic)
D	SYMPATHETIC	Bladder neck and urethral contraction (α adrenergic)
E	SOMATIC (Pudendal nerve)	Contraction of pelvic floor musculature

Parasympathetic, sympathetic, and somatic innervation of the bladder. (From Ouslander JG: Geriatric Urinary Incontinence. Disease-a-Month 38:67–149, 1992, with permission.)

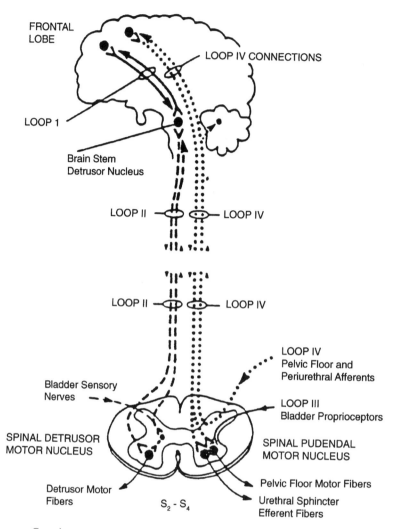

Central nervous system connections to the bladder and periurethral musculature.

7. What normal changes in the urinary tract are associated with aging?

As with all systems of the body, age-related changes affect the lower urinary tract. Such changes predispose an elderly person to incontinence but do not cause incontinence per se. Thus, incontinence is not a normal part of aging. Aging involves decreases in estrogen, bladder capacity, urethral pressure, and urinary flow rate and increases in uninhibited detrusor contractions, postvoid residuals, nocturnal urine production, and prostate size. Despite these predisposing factors, usually an added insult precipitates incontinence. Such insults are typically reversible causes outside the lower urinary tract. Treating the added insult often cures the incontinence.

8. What is the goal of the basic evaluation of UI?

The goal of the initial evaluation is to confirm UI and to identify transient causes, patients who need further evaluation, and patients who can begin treatment without extensive testing. This goal can be accomplished with a careful history, a complete physical exam, simple bedside testing, and a few laboratory tests.

9. What is the focus of the history in a UI evaluation?

A thorough history begins the work-up, as in any other medical evaluation. The history should focus on details of the symptoms, looking for clues to determine the type, pathophysiology, and precipitating factors:

- Duration and characteristics of UI
- Timing and amount of both continent and incontinent urination
- Fluid intake; type and amount—caffeine, alcohol
- Other symptoms, such as nocturia, dysuria, frequency, hematuria, pain
- Associated events—cough, surgery, new diabetes, new medications
- Alterations in bowel or bladder function
- Use of absorbent pads or other protective devices
- Previous treatment of UI and its effects

The medical history should focus on problems such as diabetes, congestive heart failure, venous insufficiency, cancer, neurologic problems, stroke, and Parkinson's disease. The genitourinary history should include any abdominal or pelvic surgery, childbirth, or urinary tract infections. A review of medications, both prescribed and over-the-counter, is important. Many classes of drugs are particularly associated with UI, including sedative-hypnotics, diuretics, anticholinergic agents, adrenergic agents, and calcium channel blockers. There is usually a time connection between the use of these medications and onset of incontinence or worsening of chronic incontinence.

10. What should the physical exam include?

The goals of the physical exam are to identify causes precipitating incontinence and to help establish pathophysiology. In addition to a complete general physical exam, the physician should concentrate on the abdomen, genitalia, rectum, neurologic function, and, in women, the pelvis. The **abdominal exam** should focus on identifying bladder fullness, tenderness, masses, or evidence of surgery. The condition of the skin and anatomic abnormalities should be identified during the **genital exam**. The **rectal exam** is primarily for identifying stool impaction and evaluating sphincter tone, perineal sensation, and the bulbocavernous reflex. Prostate nodules can be identified during the rectal exam, but the rectal exam is not accurate in determining prostate size. The **pelvic exam** evaluates for mucosal atrophy, atrophic vaginitis, masses, muscle tone, pelvic prolapse, and either cystocele or rectocele. The **neurologic evaluation** is partially accomplished during the rectal exam, when perineal sensation, anal tone, and the bulbocavernous reflex are tested. The neurologic exam also should evaluate for treatable diseases, such as Parkinson's disease or spinal cord compression. The physical exam should also include an assessment of **functional and cognitive status**, focusing on the patient's ability to recognize the urge to void and to use the toilet.

11. Which simple bedside evaluation should be done?

Simple urodynamic testing can be done at the bedside without the use of expensive technical equipment. Postvoid residual (PVR) should be estimated by physical exam. A specific measurement can be made with ultrasound or urinary catheterization. Stress-induced leakage can also be evaluated at the bedside with direct visualization. This evaluation should be done when the patient has a full bladder with the urge to void. The patient is asked to cough while in the lithotomy and standing positions. Leakage can easily be seen. Bladder filling can be evaluated by a simple technique outlined by Ouslander,[3] although interpretation of the data involves potential errors. Information can be obtained on first urge to void, presence or absence of involuntary bladder contractions, and bladder capacity.

12. Which laboratory studies should be done?

Urinalysis should be done for all patients to evaluate hematuria, pyuria, bacteriuria, glycosuria, and proteinuria. Serum electrolytes, blood urea nitrogen, creatinine, glucose, and calcium are assessed to determine baseline renal function and conditions causing polyuria.

13. Are voiding records useful?

Voiding records track voiding patterns. They are used to record the timing and amount of continent and incontinent voids and symptoms associated with UI. They can clarify symptoms or identify factors contributing to UI. They can be used in an ambulatory or institutional setting. They are kept for 1–3 days. The records can also be used to monitor therapeutic response. Keeping the records can be a therapeutic intervention because it makes patients aware of precipitating factors associated with incontinent episodes.

14. Who should be referred?

Most geriatric patients with UI can be helped by health care professionals without invasive testing. Patients should be referred to specialists for more invasive evaluation and testing in the following settings:

- Hematuria without infection
- UI with recurrent symptomatic urinary tract infections
- PVR > 200 ml
- Prostate nodule
- Diagnosis is unclear and a rational plan cannot be developed from bedside evaluation
- Failure to respond to adequate therapeutic trial
- Symptomatic pelvic prolapse
- Other symptoms that indicate a more serious underlying problem
- Recent history of lower urinary tract surgery, pelvic surgery, or radiation treatment

15. What are the mainstays of treatment?

Treatment of UI consists of behavioral, pharmacologic, and surgical interventions. The rule of thumb in choosing a therapeutic option is that the least invasive and least dangerous should be used first. A combination of surgical, behavioral, and pharmacologic treatment may help. The optimal treatment strategy depends on the patient, type of UI, and risk-benefit ratio of each intervention. The success of each modality depends on the accurate identification of the cause of UI.

16. Describe the behavioral techniques.

Behavioral techniques present little risk to the patient and may provide a decrease in UI frequency. General strategies include education of the patient or caregiver and positive reinforcement when progress is made. Specific techniques include bladder training, habit training, prompted voiding, and pelvic muscle exercises. High-tech techniques that can supplement and enhance behavioral methods include biofeedback, electrical stimulation, and vaginal cone retention.

Bladder retraining involves progressive increases in the intervals between mandatory voiding with distraction or relaxation techniques. It requires that the patient resist or inhibit the sensation to void. It has been shown to be helpful in urge and stress incontinence.

Habit training requires scheduled toileting. It is most successful when the timed toileting is matched with patient's natural voiding pattern. It is best used with functional incontinence and requires staff or caregiver involvement.

Prompted voiding attempts to teach patients to recognize their continence status and to request toileting. It has been used successfully in patients with cognitive impairment in nursing homes.

Pelvic muscle or Kegel exercises involve repetitive contraction of the pelvic floor muscles. By strengthening the pelvic floor, these exercises help to increase closing pressure on the urethra and support of the pelvic structures. They are helpful for stress and urge incontinence.

An adjunct to behavioral techniques is evaluation of the **physical and social environment**, including toilet access, clothing that makes disrobing easier, chairs that are easy to rise from, and accessible call system.

17. Which medications are helpful in treating UI?

Several drugs can be helpful in UI; they are used to increase bladder storage and to facilitate bladder emptying. The initial dose of any of these drugs should be low. The patient must be monitored closely for side effects and urinary retention. The drug is titrated slowly to maximize benefit and minimize side effects.

Drugs beneficial in **urge incontinence** have anticholinergic and smooth muscle-relaxant properties. Examples include propantheline, oxybutin, imipramine, calcium channel blockers, and flanoxate. Low-dose oxybutin seems to be the most useful for elderly patients. The starting dose of oxybutin should be 2.5 mg in the evening.

Drugs effective for **stress incontinence** have alpha-adrenergic agonist properties because of the high number of alpha-adrenergic receptors in the bladder neck and base and proximal urethra. Estrogen is also beneficial because of its direct effect on urethral mucosa. The drugs most often used are phenylpropanolamine and estrogen. Both are more helpful in patients with mild-to-moderate stress incontinence and no major anatomic abnormalities.

Drugs for **overflow incontinence** stimulate bladder contractions or relax the sphincter. These agents include cholinergic agents, such as bethanechol, and alpha-adrenergic blockers, such as prazosin. Prazosin has been used in men with prostate enlargement because of the number of alpha-adrenergic receptors in the capsule of the prostate.

18. When is surgical intervention appropriate?

Surgical intervention for UI should be considered in patients with stress or overflow incontinence and in patients with pathology in the lower urinary tract that contributes to UI. Successful surgical intervention requires careful assessment of the cause of UI and careful correlation of anatomic and physiologic findings with the surgical procedure. Age alone should not be a deterrent to indicated surgery, but estimation of surgical risk is extremely important. Patients with mixed causes of UI need to be assessed carefully to determine how much the surgical procedure will affect the outcome. For instance, patients with stress and urge incontinence may not benefit from surgery for stress incontinence if detrusor instability is present. There are various types of surgical procedures for restoring continence. Of interest, recently available procedures include injection of collagen or Polytef paste into periurethral tissue to provide increased resistance to urine outflow in patients with sphincter weakness. The long-term efficacy is not yet known.

19. What other measures or devices can be used for the management of UI?

Absorbent pads and garments are available in wide variety. They should be used only after evaluation of UI and trial of proper treatment. Early use of absorbent pads can lead to difficulty in achieving continence. When used improperly, they also contribute to skin breakdown.

Penile clamps can be useful in stress incontinence in elderly men. If they are not properly used, complications such as penile erosion and edema can occur.

Pessaries are useful in incontinence associated with pelvic prolapse. Patients require frequent monitoring. The pessaries must be changed every 3 months. Complications include fistula formation and ulcerations of the vagina (see figure, following page).

External catheters are preferable to indwelling catheters, but they are associated with urinary tract infections. Again, they must be properly used to avoid mechanical irritation, contact dermatitis, and penile obstruction.

Intermittent catheterization involves insertion of a catheter into the bladder every 4–6 hours for drainage. This option is preferable to indwelling catheters because of its lower incidence of symptomatic UTIs and stone formation. Frail elderly patients and caregivers are able to use this technique.

Indwelling catheters should not be used in the routine management of UI. Complications include sepsis, stone formation, epididymitis, abscess formation, and leakage. Indwelling catheters should be used only when persistent urinary retention causes symptomatic infections or renal compromise that cannot be treated surgically or medically and intermittent catheterization is not feasible. Indwelling catheters may be appropriate in patients with a terminal illness when frequent clothing and bed changes are painful; in patients with significant skin problems that are made worse by UI; and in patients who have not responded to specific treatments and prefer a Foley catheter.

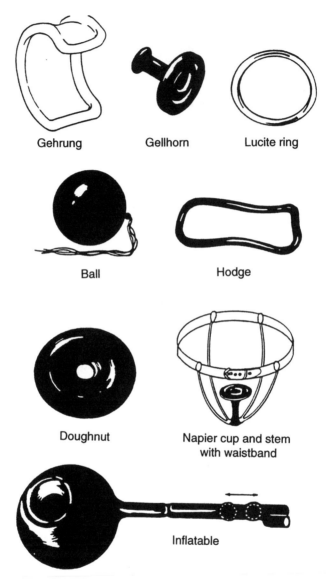

Gehrung   Gellhorn   Lucite ring

Ball   Hodge

Doughnut   Napier cup and stem
with waistband

Inflatable

Types of pessaries.

20. What community resources are available to the patient and primary care practitioner for UI?

The increase in awareness of UI and its consequences has led to an abundance of information for both practitioner and patient. The Clinical Practice Guidelines on Urinary Incontinence in Adults can be obtained by calling the AHCPR Clearinghouse at 1-800-358-9295. The guidelines are also available in a format suitable for patients and their families. Continence clinics using nonsurgical techniques for UI are becoming more common. Contacting medical centers or aging clearinghouses can identify these clinics. The following national organizations also can help people with incontinence:

Help for Incontinent People   Simon Foundation for Continence
P.O. Box 544   P.O. Box 835
Union, SC 29379   Wilmette, IL
(864) 579-7900   (800) 23-SIMON

BIBLIOGRAPHY

1. Baum N, Suarey G, Appel RA: Urinary incontinence: Not a "normal" part of aging. Postgrad Med 90:99–109, 1991.
2. Du Beau CE, Resnick NM: Evaluation of the causes and severity of geriatric incontinence: A critical appraisal. Urol Clin North Am 18:243–256, 1991.
3. Ouslander JG: Geriatric urinary incontinence. Disease-a-Month 38:67–149, 1992.
4. Pannell FC: Urinary incontinence for the primary care physician. Ct Med 57:299–308, 1993.
5. Resnick NM, Yalla SV: Management of urinary incontinence in the elderly. N Engl J Med 313:800–805, 1985.
6. Urinary Incontinence Guideline Panel: Urinary Incontinence in Adults: Clinical Practice Guidelines. AHCPR Pub. No. 92-0038. Rockville, MD, Agency for Health Care Policy and Research, Public Health Service, U.S. Department of Health and Human Services, 1992.
7. Vernon MS: Urinary incontinence in the elderly. Primary Care 16:515–528, 1989.

36. STROKE

Steven E. Arnold, M.D.

1. What is a stroke?

Stroke is an injury to the brain caused by occlusion or rupture of a cerebral artery. It is the third most common cause of death in the United States and, perhaps even more grim, the leading cause of adult disability. The challenges of stroke prevention and care are particularly compelling for geriatricians, given the burgeoning elderly population and the fact that the most significant risk factor for stroke is age.

2. What are the major categories of stroke? Are they important to recognize?

The stroke syndrome is characterized by rapid onset and a pattern of focal signs and symptoms that reflect injury in a specific vascular territory. The two broad categories of stroke are (1) ischemic stroke, resulting from thrombosis or embolism, and (2) hemorrhagic stroke due to primary intracerebral or subarachnoid hemorrhage. Thrombotic strokes are the most common and account for approximately 65% of all strokes, whereas embolic stroke accounts for 20–25%, intracerebral hemorrhage for 5%, and subarachnoid hemorrhage for 5%.

Diagnosing the type and location of stroke is critical for appropriate management and prevention of recurrence. For instance, hemorrhagic stroke has a mortality rate 3–5 times greater than that of ischemic stroke and requires more critical and specialized care. Although information about the early temporal profile may be difficult to obtain, a stroke's mode of onset can yield clues about whether the lesion is thrombotic, embolic, or hemorrhagic in origin. The symptom profiles for stroke vary according to type and vascular territory.

3. Describe the mode of onset for different types of strokes.

Thrombotic strokes

Variable onset of neurologic symptoms

Frequently preceded by transient ischemic attacks (TIAs) that herald permanent deficits

Neurologic deficits are often rapid in onset but may be fluctuating, stepwise, or stuttering ("stroke in evolution")

Embolic strokes

Sudden onset with maximal neurologic deficit present from the start

Intracerebral hemorrhage

Sudden onset

Often occurs in setting of elevated blood pressure and during activity

Subarachnoid hemorrhage

Sudden onset

Tends to occur during activity and may be associated with elevated blood pressure

Invariably accompanied by a crashing headache (which is a rare or minor symptom in other types of stroke)

Often proceeds to coma, from which the patient may emerge in a confusional state

4. Describe the major clinical syndromes of stroke.

Middle cerebral artery

Contralateral hemiplegia

Contralateral hemisensory loss

Contralateral homonymous hemianopia

Ipsilateral gaze preference

Aphasia (dominant hemisphere)

Affective disturbance (especially in nondominant hemisphere)
Neglect (especially in nondominant hemisphere)
Anterior cerebral artery
Contralateral leg/foot paralysis   Ideomotor apraxia
Gait disturbance   Perseveration
Abulia   Urinary incontinence
Posterior cerebral artery
Contralateral homonymous hemianopia
Dyslexia
Memory impairment
Contralateral hemiparesis (mild)
Contralateral hemisensory loss
Variable brainstem signs (e.g., ipsilateral third nerve palsy contralateral involuntary movements, hemiplegia, ataxia)
Internal carotid artery
Transient monocular blindness
"Watershed" signs
  Homonymous hemianopia
  Aphasia (dominant hemisphere)
  Neglect (nondominant hemisphere)
  Variable sensorimotor deficit
Signs of middle, anterior, and posterior cerebral artery infarction (as above)
Vertebral artery
Ipsilateral cerebellar ataxia   Ipsilateral vocal cord paralysis
Ipsilateral face dysesthesia   Dysphagia
Contralateral trunk and limb dysesthesia Nausea and vomiting
Vertigo   Ipsilateral Horner syndrome
Nystagmus
Basilar artery
Wide spectrum of clinical symptoms   Nystagmus
Contralateral hemiplegia or quadriplegia Nausea, vomiting
Contralateral hemisensory loss   Deafness, tinnitus
Horizontal gaze palsies   Coma
Ipsilateral facial paralysis   "Locked-in" syndrome
Internuclear ophthalmoplegia
Lacunar syndromes
Pure motor hemiparesis   Hemichorea/hemiballismus
Pure sensory stroke   Homolateral ataxia and crural paresis
Dysarthria/clumsy hand syndrome

5. What causes stroke?

Primary thrombotic occlusion typically occurs in a blood vessel already partially occluded by atherosclerosis. The earliest lesion is a "fatty streak" that evolves into a fibrous plaque. The rate of progression from atheromatous stenosis to virtual occlusion is highly variable but may be as short as weeks. The source of most **cerebral embolisms** is the heart; much less commonly, embolic material may be released from ulcerated atherosclerotic plaques in the aortic arch and origin of the great vessels. The sites of embolic occlusion within the brain are more variable than in athrothrombotic disease, although there is some predilection for right hemisphere lesions, based on tendencies of blood flow. **Lacunar infarcts** are a particular type of ischemic stroke involving the deep perforator arterial and arteriolar branches of the major cerebral blood vessels. Pathologically, they are due to lipohyalinosis or microatheroma.

Intracerebral hemorrhage is usually due to either rupture of the small penetrating arteries of the brain in the setting of hypertension or amyloid angiopathy. **Subarachnoid hemorrhage**

is most commonly due to rupture of a congenital saccular aneurysm, which typically occurs at sites of arterial bifurcation or branching. Most aneurysms are asymptomatic until they rupture. Subarachnoid hemorrhage can also be caused by arteriovenous malformation or tumors.

Thrombotic
- Atherosclerotic plaque—may be due to stenotic ischemia or "local" ulcerated plaque embolization

Common carotid bifurcation	Proximal basilar artery
Proximal vertebral artery	Middle cerebral artery stem
Internal carotid siphon	

- Rare causes

Antiphospholipid antibodies	Cerebral vein thrombosis
Clotting inhibitory factor deficiencies	Polycythemia vera
Arteritides	

Embolic
- Cardiac source

Mural thrombus	Bacterial endocarditis
Atrial fibrillation	Marantic endocarditis
Myocardial infarction	Libman-Sacks endocarditis
Valvular disease	Atrial myxoma
Patent foramen ovale	

- Atherosclerotic plaques in aortic arch or origin of great vessels

Lacunar
- Strongly associated with age, diabetes mellitus, and hypertension

Intracerebral hemorrhage
- Rupture of small penetrating vessels in setting of hypertension
  - Putamen
  - Thalamus
  - Pons
  - Cerebellum
- Amyloid angiopathy—tends to be lobar
- Hemorrhagic conversion of an ischemic infarct

Subarachnoid hemorrhage
- Cerebral aneurysm
  - Anterior communicating artery
  - Internal carotid artery at origin of posterior communicating artery
  - Middle cerebral artery bifurcation
- Arteriovenous malformation
- Tumor

6. What other conditions can mimic TIAs or stroke?

A number of other neurologic processes that cause transient as well as nontransient deficits can be misdiagnosed as TIA or stroke. In fact, it has been estimated that 10–15% of initial diagnoses of stroke are incorrect. Seizures (especially simple and complex partial seizures), confusional states, and cardiogenic syncope lead the list of alternative diagnoses confused with stroke. Other conditions that can simulate stroke or TIA include migraine and migraine equivalents, subdural hematoma, brain tumor, hypoglycemia, demyelinating disease, brain abscess, encephalitis, and panic attack. Obviously, management of these various conditions differs greatly.

7. What are the major modifiable risk factors for stroke?

Much of the steady decline in stroke mortality over the last 50 years may be attributed to the identification and treatment of risk factors, particularly hypertension. This decline has been most prominent among the elderly, but it appears to be slowing or even reversing in recent years. Stroke remains the third leading cause of death. Some risk factors, such as age, male gender,

African-American heritage, and heredity are nonmodifiable, whereas other medical and lifestyle factors may be modified. To decrease the still high incidence of stroke, there needs to be yet greater emphasis on education and management of the modifiable risk factors.

Individuals with **hypertension** (> 160/95) are at a 3–4-fold greater risk for stroke than those without; given the prevalence of hypertension, it is the most important modifiable risk factor. Both diastolic and systolic components are important, and even borderline hypertension carries an increased risk. The incidence of stroke increases with the level of systolic blood pressure and not merely the presence of hypertension. Although the relative risk of hypertension for stroke may diminish somewhat with advancing age, it remains highly significant. Indeed, in a study of efficacy of treatment of hypertension, the largest reduction in prevalence of hypertension and incidence of stroke occurred in patients 75 years and older, emphasizing that control of hypertension in the elderly prevents stroke.

Cardiac disease is the next most important risk factor for stroke. Coronary artery disease, congestive heart failure, and left ventricular hypertrophy (as determined by EKG) increase the risk 2–4-fold, independently of hypertension. Atrial fibrillation, either nonvalvular or associated with rheumatic heart disease and mitral stenosis, increases the relative risk of stroke by 5–17-fold, depending on the presence of associated valvular disease. In the Framingham Study, 15% of strokes were associated with atrial fibrillation; this association steadily increases with age (36% of strokes in octogenarians are associated with atrial fibrillation). The risk associated with chronic atrial fibrillation is especially high in elderly patients with concurrent hypertension or congestive heart failure.

Diabetes mellitus increases the risk of stroke by 2–4-fold and is also associated with greater mortality and morbidity due to stroke.

The contribution of **hyperlipidemia** to stroke remains more controversial than previously noted risk factors. Although blood lipids have clearly been related to the incidence of coronary artery disease, the Framingham Study did not show a clear relationship between cholesterol level and stroke. Other clinical trials of cholesterol-lowering therapies also failed to show an associated risk reduction for stroke. Increased low-density lipoprotein and decreased high-density lipoprotein have been associated with the presence and severity of carotid atherosclerotic disease in some but not all studies. Low serum cholesterol levels increase the risk of death from intracranial hemorrhages in men. Despite the controversy regarding stroke and the paucity of evidence that therapy for hyperlipidemia benefits the elderly, it appears prudent to monitor and make an effort to lower elevated blood lipids, particularly as coronary artery disease is the main cause of death among stroke patients.

Cigarette smoking is another important modifiable risk factor for stroke, with several large scale studies estimating a relative risk of 1.5–2.9. The incidence of stroke among quitters falls substantially within 2 years. In 5 years the risk is the same as that of nonsmokers.

There is somewhat less consensus about the risk of **alcohol consumption**. Light or moderate alcohol consumption may be protective for ischemic stroke, similar to its effect on coronary artery disease, whereas chronic, heavy drinking increases the risk of stroke up to 4-fold. Heavy use is a risk factor for lobar intracerebral hemorrhage in young and middle-aged individuals.

Other potential risk factors that have recently been recognized include atrial septal aneurysm, patent foramen ovale, aortic arch atheroma, anticardiolipin antibodies, and free protein S deficiency. These factors may be especially important in younger populations with cryptogenic stroke; their significance in the geriatric population is undetermined.

Major Risk Factors for Stroke

NONMODIFIABLE	MODIFIABLE MEDICAL FACTORS	LIFESTYLE FACTORS
Age	Systolic and diastolic hypertension	Cigarette smoking
Male gender	Cardiac disease (especially atrial	Excessive alcohol
African-American heritage	fibrillation)	Sedentary
Family history	Diabetes mellitus	
	?Hyperlipidemia	
	Hypercoagulable state	

8. What are the options for primary stroke prevention?

Stroke prevention strategies target the modifiable risk factors. In general, although the risk factors for stroke are not exactly the same as those for coronary artery disease, the main cause of death in patients with cerebrovascular disease is cardiac disease. Therefore, the same recommendations are made for stroke as for coronary artery disease. Hypertension, diabetes mellitus, hyperlipidemia, tobacco abuse, alcoholism, and obesity should be managed with a combination of dietary and lifestyle changes and, when necessary, medication.

9. When should anticoagulation be considered for primary stroke prevention in patients with cardiac disease?

For primary prevention of stroke in patients with a well-established cardiac source for embolic stroke (chronic atrial fibrillation, dilated cardiomyopathy, valvular heart disease, prosthetic valves), anticoagulation with warfarin is clearly effective, and the risk of bleeding complications is generally acceptable. Patients over the age of 75 share in this decreased risk, although they experience a significantly higher risk of major hemorrhage; thus, the decision to anticoagulate is made on a case-by-case basis. Antiplatelet therapy with aspirin, 325 mg, has fewer bleeding complications and has been shown to reduce the risk of stroke in patients with atrial fibrillation, albeit with significantly less efficacy (about half) than warfarin. Initial results from recent trials combining low-dose warfarin and aspirin have not been encouraging.

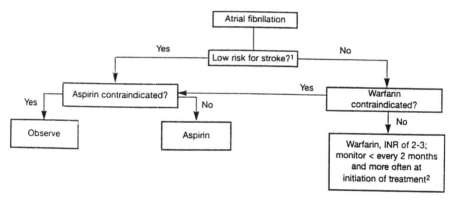

[1] Low stroke risk: age < 60 years with none of the following: previous transient ischemic attack/stroke, hypertension, diabetes mellitus, congestive heart failure, echocardiogram with left atrial enlargement or global left ventricular dysfunction.

[2] INR: International Normalized Ratio is a measure of prothrombin time that adjusts for differences in thromboplastin reagents used by different laboratories. INRs between 2 and 3 are currently considered optimal for atrial fibrillation patients.

Atrial fibrillation.

10. What is the initial management for a patient with acute stroke?

For all patients with acute stroke, rapid clinical evaluation and initiation of treatment are critical. Treating stroke as anything less than an emergency is substandard care. Beyond the history and physical examination, the initial emergency room evaluation should include an EKG, chest x-ray, complete blood count, platelet count, prothrombin and partial thromboplastin times, chemistry profile, erythrocyte sedimentation rate, syphilis serology, and arterial blood gas. It is imperative to distinguish hemorrhage from infarction as soon as possible because further acute management decisions depend on this distinction. Therefore, a noncontrast CT scan of the head should be performed urgently; this technique easily differentiates hemorrhage from infarction in almost all cases.

In patients with ischemic infarction, high blood pressure should not be lowered rapidly unless it is > 220 systolic or 120 diastolic or unless other indications, such as heart failure or aortic dissection, are present. In contrast, for patients with hemorrhage, elevated blood pressure should be lowered and maintained within the normal range. Other general management should include treatment of hypoglycemia or hyperglycemia (> 170 mg/dl), monitoring of cardiac status, oxygen for hypoxemia, and monitoring for cerebral edema and seizures. Accumulating evidence indicates that specialized stroke units can save lives and improve outcome and should be used if available. In addition, many medical centers have ongoing treatment trials for ischemic stroke (e.g., thrombolytic or neuroprotective agents), and referral to these centers should be considered.

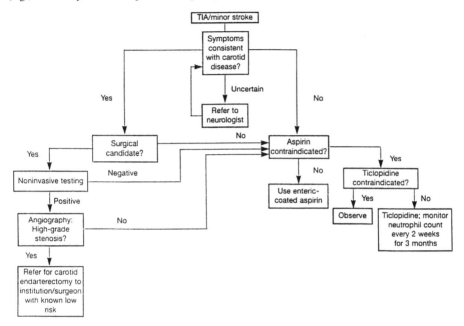

Transient ischemic attack (TIA)/minor stroke. (This algorithm is not intended to be a comprehensive management strategy for patients with TIA or minor stroke.)

11. Does a TIA require immediate diagnosis and management?

TIAs should be evaluated and treated according to the same principles as stroke. TIAs are warning signs of stroke, and their aggressive management can prevent permanent disability and death. The rate of a completed stroke after TIA may be as high as 57% within 2 years, and most occur within the first year. The risk of stroke in the first few days after a TIA is unclear; however, it is considered to be highest during this time. Therefore, all patients with a recent TIA (within 10 days) should be evaluated urgently.

12. Describe the diagnostic work-up of a new stroke or TIA.

At present, there is no uniformly accepted algorithm for diagnosis of stroke. Which tests to perform and how aggressively they should be used is based on individualized decision making that considers multiple factors, such as age, clinical presentation, risk factors, other health considerations, and intent to treat. At a minimum, evaluation should include the admission tests listed in question 10, CT scan of the head, and noninvasive carotid artery evaluation to identify atherosclerotic disease. Duplex scanning is the most revealing noninvasive method because it combines ultrasound real-time imaging with a Doppler probe and is quite accurate in detecting significant disease up to the carotid bifurcation. Ultrasound techniques are of little use for vertebrobasilar disease. Additional diagnostic tests and procedures for selected patients include transthoracic echocardiography (and transesophageal echocardiography if a cardioembolic source is highly suspected); transcranial Doppler; magnetic resonance imaging (MRI); MR angiography to assess suspected intracranial arterial stenoses; cerebral angiography to identify any cerebrovascular disease; and tests for coagulopathies (e.g., protein C and S, antiphospholipid antibodies, antithrombin III deficiencies, especially in younger patients with no other obvious cause). For cases of suspected subarachnoid hemorrhage, lumbar puncture is indicated if clinical suspicion is high and CT is nondiagnostic. Early angiography is also indicated for subarachnoid hemorrhage, especially in more robust, less impaired patients, for whom early aneurysm repair is the treatment of choice. Positron emission tomography (PET) and single-photon emission computed tomography SPECT, although not widely available, may be useful in assessing TIAs in patients with no anatomic lesion or early stroke prior to tissue infarction.

13. What is the role of anticoagulation in acute stroke?

Anticoagulation is clearly effective in preventing recurrent cardioembolic stroke. Patients with cardioembolic stroke due to atrial fibrillation, recent myocardial infarction, valvular disease, or patent foramen ovale should be anticoagulated if there are no contraindications. Heparin should be administered on admission for at least 48 hours before being replaced by warfarin if there are no systemic contraindications, if no hemorrhage is seen on imaging studies, if the infarct is not large (hemorrhagic conversion is a greater risk in large than in smaller strokes), and if there is no evidence of bacterial endocarditis. For patients with atrial fibrillation who are not candidates for long-term anticoagulation, low-dose heparin may be considered. Aspirin alone also reduces the risk of further embolization in atrial fibrillation, although not nearly as much as warfarin. The role of anticoagulation is more controversial for patients with atherothrombotic ischemic stroke. Many physicians feel compelled to anticoagulate patients with atherothrombotic stroke in evolution, but the value of this strategy has not been demonstrated. Anticoagulation is of no benefit in completed stroke.

14. What is the role of thrombolytic agents or neuroprotective agents in acute stroke?

Several protocols have been established to study the efficacy of intravenous and intra-arterial thrombolytic agents (e.g., recombinant tissue plasminogen activator, urokinase, prourokinase) in "hyperacute" stroke, i.e., in the first 6 hours after the event. Initial results have shown some promise in improving neurologic status, especially for strokes in the vertebrobasilar territory. However, this therapy remains experimental, the time window excludes most patients, and the results of more extensive studies are pending. The potential role of various neuroprotective agents in interrupting the cascade of molecular events that lead to neuron death after ischemic injury are at even earlier stages of investigation.

15. What are the major complications of acute stroke?

The most common and significant medical complications after stroke include deep vein thrombosis and pulmonary embolism, aspiration pneumonia, urinary tract infections, and decubitus ulcers. Cardiac arrhythmias are also common after stroke, and EKG monitoring is indicated in the first few days. Three major neurologic complications, particularly with large strokes, are cerebral edema, seizures, and hemorrhagic transformation of ischemic infarcts. Cerebral edema is especially important in cerebellar infarctions because it may cause brainstem herniation. Hyperventilation, osmotic therapy, or even surgery may be needed for cerebral edema. Corticosteroids have not been shown to be effective in cerebral infarction or hemorrhage with or without edema. Seizures should be treated with anticonvulsants. If anticoagulation is being considered for stroke in evolution or other circumstances, a repeat CT scan before initiation of heparin should be performed to check for hemorrhagic conversion.

16. When should carotid endarterectomy be recommended?

Three major controlled studies have clearly demonstrated that carotid endarterectomy (CEA) reduces the risk of subsequent stroke in patients who have had TIAs or minor stroke and who have arteriographically confirmed high-grade stenosis (> 70%). It appears to be of no benefit in patients with less than 30% stenosis; patients in this group should be more vigorously evaluated for cardioembolic and other causes of stroke. As yet, results are inconclusive for patients with symptomatic, moderate carotid artery stenosis (30–69%), and evaluation of the efficacy and indications for CEA in this group is ongoing through the North American Symptomatic Carotid Endarterectomy Trial (NASCET). If ulcerated plaque is present in the setting of moderate stenosis, the risk of stroke increases and patients benefit from CEA. Surgical decisions in this setting should be made on an individual basis. Referrals to a NASCET center can be easily made through local neurologists, neurosurgeons, and vascular surgeons or by calling the NASCET hotline: 1-800-565-6331.

Recommendations for Carotid Endarterectomy

GRADE (%) OF STENOSIS	RECOMMENDATION
< 30 %	No. Search for cardioembolic or other sources
30–69%	Individualized decision: yes if ulcerated plaque
≥ 70%	Yes
Asymptomatic, ≥ 70%	Possibly

17. What are the major risks of CEA? Do they differ in the elderly?

The major risks of CEA include stroke and death as well as local complications such as hematoma, infection, or false aneurysm formation. Although successful CEA confers a relative risk reduction of 69% in the incidence of stroke over the ensuing 5 years, perioperative and arteriography-related risk for mortality and stroke must be taken into account. There is an approximately 3% aggregate risk of stroke or death in the perioperative period with an experienced team, including the risk of stroke associated with arteriography. As a bottom line, patients with CEA have a 4.8% risk of stroke within 5 years compared with 10.6% for patients without CEA.

The results of CEA for the elderly are controversial. Some studies indicate an increased risk of complications with advanced age, whereas one recent study of CEA in octogenarians found the procedure to be as safe and effective as for the general population. Patients with prohibitive surgical risk should be treated with antiplatelet agents and risk factor reduction.

18. What medical therapy can prevent recurrent stroke in patients with established atherothrombotic cerebrovascular disease?

Numerous controlled clinical trials have demonstrated the efficacy of antiplatelet agents for the secondary prevention of stroke in patients who have had TIAs or previous stroke. **Aspirin** has been the most extensively studied, and its use is associated with a 23% decrease in the risk of subsequent stroke or myocardial infarction. Controversy continues over the optimal dose, with recommendations ranging from 30–1300 mg. A recent survey found that most neurologists recommend 325 mg/day in deference to gastrointestinal symptoms; however, a retrospective study suggests that a dose > 500 mg/day is better for secondary stroke prevention.

Ticlopidine (Ticlid) is the other platelet antiaggregant with efficacy in secondary stroke prevention. It works by inhibiting ADP linkage of fibrinogen to platelets and has a greater global inhibitory effect than aspirin. In two large multicenter clinical studies, ticlopidine, 250 mg twice daily, was modestly more effective than aspirin in preventing strokes. However, adverse reactions, including diarrhea, rash, GI upset, and neutropenia, have limited its widespread use. Complete blood counts need to be obtained every 2 weeks for the first 3 months to monitor for neutropenia (which occurs in 2.4% of patients and is fully reversible on discontinuation).

The role of **warfarin** for prevention of carotid atherothrombotic stroke is unclear and awaits the results of a large multicenter center trial currently underway (Warfarin Aspirin Recurrent Stroke Study [WARSS]). Dipyridamole and sulfinpyrazone show no efficacy in secondary stroke prevention, either when used alone or in combination with aspirin.

19. How should asymptomatic carotid artery disease be managed?

Stenosis may be identified in asymptomatic patients on the basis of bruits heard during physical examination, vascular studies done for other reasons, or screening tests for unusual symptoms.

Asymptomatic carotid stenosis is an indicator of more extensive atherosclerosis and is associated with an increased risk of stroke. Recently, the Asymptomatic Carotid Atherosclerosis Study (ACAS) reported that for asymptomatic patients with high-grade stenoses, CEA in combination with aspirin and risk factor reduction lowers the relative risk for stroke compared with medical therapy alone. However, the relative risk reduction is not as great as for patients who have had TIAs or minor strokes. Consequently, consideration of other factors such as age, other medical illnesses, and risks of surgical and arteriographic complications become even more important in reaching a surgical decision. Whether or not surgery is recommended, risk factor modification and antiplatelet therapy should be initiated.

20. Who should be referred for rehabilitation after stroke?

Sensory, motor, cognitive, and language deficits are the presenting symptoms of stroke and, to varying degrees, the permanent residua. Mortality from stroke has declined with advances in technology and treatment; as a consequence, a greater proportion of patients survive with substantial neurologic impairment. The goal of rehabilitation is not cure, but rather adaptation to functional handicap—to maximize function in the service of enhancing quality of life. A host of factors must be considered in determining the appropriateness of referral for rehabilitation. Patients with mild deficits probably do not need specialized rehabilitative services, and patients who are stuporous, completely immobile, severely cognitively impaired, or severely ill medically will derive little benefit. Type and severity of neurologic deficit, presence and degree of cognitive impairment, physical endurance, patient and family goals, available social support, and psychological make-up contribute to the success of rehabilitative efforts and need to be carefully assessed. Age is not a factor; patients of all ages have shown substantial benefit in outcome from rehabilitation.

21. How common are depression and other psychiatric complications after stroke? How should they be managed?

Mood disturbances are common after stroke as a result of both organic and psychological factors. Depression may play a critical role in the success of a patient's recovery, rehabilitation, and adjustment to disability and should be assessed and treated aggressively. Depending on the diagnostic criteria, prevalence estimates for depression after stroke range from 23–63%. Because of frequent impairments in communication and cognition and the common bias that "anyone would be depressed after a stroke," clinical depression is underdiagnosed and undertreated. Yet its importance is underscored by studies indicating that depression in the postacute phase has an impact on physical recovery and subsequent function in the chronic phase. Treatment with antidepressant medication is as effective in poststroke depression as in generic depressive disorders and should be used. The newer selective serotonin reuptake inhibitors (SSRIs), such as sertraline, paroxetine, and fluoxetine, are especially well tolerated and effective. Other neuropsychiatric complications of stroke include delirium with agitation, paranoid reactions (especially in association with Wernicke's aphasia), impulse dyscontrol, and pseudobulbar affect (emotional incontinence). These complications can be distressing to patients, family, and caregivers alike and are often amenable to psychiatric management.

BIBLIOGRAPHY

1. Adams HP Jr., Brott TG, Crowell RM, et al: Guidelines for the management of patients with acute ischemic stroke. A statement for health care professionals from a special writing group of the Stroke Council, American Heart Association. Stroke 25:1901–1914, 1994.
2. Antiplatelet Trialists Collaboration: Collaborative overview of randomized trials of antiplatelet therapy. I: Prevention of death, myocardial infarction, and stroke by prolonged antiplatelet therapy in various categories of patients. BMJ 308:81–106, 1994.
3. Caplan LR: Stroke: A Clinical Approach. Boston, Butterworth-Heinemann, 1993.
4. Hass WK, Easton JD, Adams HP Jr, et al: A randomized trial comparing ticlopidine hydrochloride with aspirin for the prevention of stroke in high risk patients. Ticlopidine Aspirin Stroke Study. N Engl J Med 321:501–507, 1989.

5. Moore WS, Barnett HJM, Beebe HG, et al: Guidelines for carotid endarterectomy—A multidisciplinary consensus statement from the Ad-Hoc Committee, American Heart Association. Circulation 91:566–579, 1995.

6. Wolf PA, Abbott RD, Kannel WB: Atrial fibrillation: A major contributor to stroke in the elderly: The Framingham Study. Arch Intern Med 147:1561–1564, 1987.

7. Wolf PA, Cobb JL, D'Agostino RB: Epidemiology of stroke. In Barnett HJM, Mohr JP, Stein BM, et al (eds): Stroke: Pathophysiology, Diagnosis, and Management, 2nd ed. New York, Churchill Livingstone, 1992, pp 3–27.

37. PERIOPERATIVE MANAGEMENT IN THE ELDERLY

Jerry Johnson, M.D., and Harold Mignott, M.D.

1. Does chronologic age affect the risk for adverse postoperative events?

Although many studies show that older patients have a higher mortality rate than younger patients, chronologic age is not the major predictor of postoperative outcome when other factors are considered. The most important predictors of postoperative morbidity and mortality in the elderly are the urgency of the procedure and the presence of coexisting illness, particularly cardiac and pulmonary disease. Many studies of postop outcomes in the elderly combine patients undergoing elective and emergency surgeries and combine low-risk persons who have few coexisting diseases with higher-risk individuals who have multiple coexisting diseases. Chronologic age should not be viewed as an independent risk factor of postoperative complications based on these data, and surgery should not be denied solely on the basis of age.

2. Why is it important to understand preoperative assessment in the elderly?

Preoperative assessment in older patients is important because of the high probability that older patients will require surgery and because of the increased risk of morbidity and mortality in the elderly. Surgical rates are 55% higher in persons over age 65, and 40% of admissions of older patients to general hospitals are to surgical services.

Even though the trend in studies of perioperative outcomes in the elderly is toward a decreasing mortality rate, postoperative mortality is higher among the elderly than among younger adults. Surgical mortality of patients over age 65 undergoing cardiac revascularization procedures is about 5% compared to 1% in younger adults. Typical postoperative mortality rates of older patients undergoing major intra-abdominal surgery range from 3–5%, about twice that of persons under age 65. Generally, older patients account for 75% of all postop deaths compared to 25% for persons under age 65.

3. How does the type of surgical procedure affect postoperative outcomes?

Surgeries that involve the thoracic or abdominal cavities confer the greatest postoperative risk. Low-risk surgeries, with mortality rates substantially < 1%, include cataract surgery, hernia repair, and transurethral resection of the prostate. On the other hand, cardiac and peripheral vascular procedures such as abdominal aortic aneurysm repair confer the highest risk, ranging from 3–10% on average. Emergency surgery, surgery occurring within 24 hours of admission to the hospital, doubles to quadruples the risk of mortality for any given procedure.

4. What is the role of the general medical or geriatric medical consultant in evaluating a patient during the preoperative period?

The often-used concept of "clearing" the patient for surgery is misleading in that one cannot provide absolute assurance that no adverse events will occur in patients undergoing surgery in any age group. The goal of the preop assessment is to identify risk factors, quantify the magnitude of the risk factors (if possible), and offer recommendations to correct those factors that are correctable.

5. What chronic problems should be considered in the evaluation of the older patient?

In addition to acute medical problems (i.e., cardiac or pulmonary disorders and infections), the consultant also should screen for the presence of chronic problems:

Pre-existing dementia predisposes to delirium, which can then lead to a cycle of dehydration, malnutrition, deconditioning, and acute infections. However, studies have not evaluated dementia as an independent risk factor for death or morbitiy.

Depression predisposes to dehydration and deconditioning.

Malnutrition or undernutrition has been shown in several studies to be associated with significantly higher mortality (among patients with > 20% weight loss preoperatively). However, there is considerable controversy as to whether nutritional supplements in the preoperative phase improve surgical outcome. Most experts agree that delaying surgery to provide preoperative nutrition is not warranted except, possibly, for the severely malnourished.

Parkinsonism can lead to deconditioning, falls, and prolonged recovery.

Prostate disease can lead to urinary retention and subsequent infections.

All of these chronic disorders carry the risk of predisposing the patient to the development of pressure ulcers.

6. Does decreased mobility or exercise tolerance affect the postoperative outcome?

Decreased mobility or exercise tolerance is an important nonspecific predictor in the elderly, not only associated with cardiac adverse outcomes but also with mortality in general. Another study indicates that the inability to exercise sufficiently (attain a heart rate of 100 bpm) is predictive of postoperative cardiac ischemic events. In a study comparing active and inactive patients for surgical complications (active defined as able to leave home by one's own efforts at least twice weekly), all complications, including life-threatening complications, were more frequent in the inactive patients.

7. What information should be sought by the medical history?

The frequency of multiple comorbidities in the elderly necessitates a comprehensive history and physical examination. The **cardiac history** should attempt to identify the past evidence of coronary artery disease or congestive heart failure. A myocardial infarction in the previous 6 months, active congestive heart failure, and unstable angina confer substantial risk of postoperative cardiac complications. With the exception of extreme levels, chronic hypertension does not increase the risk of postoperative complications. However, evidence of recent fluctuations in blood pressure or new-onset hypertension may indicate instability during the procedure. The pulmonary history should attempt to identify the presence of COPD or asthma.

A past history of **thromboembolic events** involving the lower extremities or **pulmonary emboli** is a substantial risk factor for postoperative thromboembolic events. Some complications are seen most frequently in orthopedic surgery of the knee and hip and in pelvic or intraabdominal surgery for malignant conditions: 40–60% of patients undergoing hip fracture repair will sustain a deep venous thrombosis, and 20% will experience at least one pulmonary embolus.

8. What information can be obtained by the physical examination?

The **cardiac exam** should aim to detect the presence of active heart failure or a cardiac murmur, particularly aortic stenosis, the most common valvular disease in the elderly. The physician should listen carefully for an S_3 and examine the patient for an increased jugulovenous pulse. Bradycardia, tachycardia, and irregularities suggesting ectopic beats can be detected by physical examination. The pulses should be examined carefully, and any evidence of edema should be recorded. The physician should take note of decreased breath sounds, which may suggest COPD, or rales or bronchospasms, which may suggest pulmonary disease or heart failure.

The **neuropsychiatric exam** is aimed at detecting cognitive impairment, acute or chronic depression, evidence of Parkinson's disease, and focal weakness. The patient should be observed ambulating for evidence of potential deconditioning and gait instability, which may be exacerbated during the postoperative period.

9. Which preop indexes are useful in predicting postop complications?

Anesthesiologists have long used the **Dripps' Physical Status Scale**, which classifies patients in five groups from Class I, healthy persons, to Class V, patients who are moribund and not expected to survive 24 hours with or without the operation. This scale, while useful in predicting the extreme classes, does less well as a predictor in classes II, III, and IV. More importantly, it gives no insight into correctable factors.

The **Cardiac Risk Index**, a predictor of postoperative cardiac outcomes in noncardiac surgery, is the best known predictive tool. Nine independent risk factors of adverse cardiac outcomes have been identified and assigned points as follows:

Third heart sound (S$_3$)	11 points
Elevated jugulovenous pressure	11
Myocardial infarction in past 6 months	10
EKG: premature atrial contractions or any rhythm other than sinus	7
EKG shows > 5 premature ventricular contractions per minute	7
Age > 70 yrs	5
Emergency procedure	4
Intrathoracic, intra-abdominal, or aortic surgery	3
Poor general status, metabolic or bedridden	3

These nine factors are then used to classify patients into 4 categories of risk as follows:

Class	Point Total	None or Minor Complication	Life-threatening Complication	Cardiac Death
Class I	0–5	99%	0.7%	0.2%
Class II	6–12	93	5	2
Class III	13–25	86	11	2
Class IV	≥ 26	22	22	56

Subsequent studies have indicated that Class I underestimates the risk of cardiac complications in patients undergoing peripheral vascular procedures. Rather than memorize the point system, bear in mind that individuals over age 70 who undergo an intra-abdominal, intrathoracic, or aortic procedure and who have any of the first five factors will total 13 points, sufficient to place them in one of the two highest risk categories by this scale.

10. Which routine preoperative tests should be obtained?

The purpose of preoperative testing is to uncover diseases and problems unrecognized by the history and physical examination or to confirm the diagnosis suspected by the history and examination. Routine tests that should be obtained in all elderly patients include the following:

Fasting glucose—screens for diabetes
CBC—may indicate the presence of infection or anemia
Electrolytes, BUN, and creatinine—reflects risk of arrhythmias
Chest x–ray—screens for occult pulmonary disease
EKG—detects ischemia or arrhythmia

11. When are noninvasive cardiac tests indicated?

Because of the concern about postoperative ischemic events, **thallium testing**, particularly with dipyridamole testing, has become almost a routine procedure before all surgery in the elderly in some medical centers. Such a routine approach is *not* indicated. The physician should obtain thallium testing in elderly patients with Q waves on the resting EKG, history of ventricular ectopy requiring treatment, diabetes, and known angina. Other preoperative studies, such as **Holter monitoring** or **exercise testing**, are not consistently useful in asymptomatic individuals.

An **echocardiogram** may be useful in persons in whom a systolic murmur is suspicious for aortic stenosis. Measures of left ventricular injection fraction are useful in quantifying risks in persons undergoing cardiac procedures. In noncardiac procedures, an echocardiogram is not indicated in the preoperative period in asymptomatic patients.

12. When is invasive monitoring required?

Right heart catheterization is indicated in patients undergoing major vascular procedures or in those with active heart failure, significant aortic stenosis, unstable angina, or recent MI.

Under other circumstances, right heart catheterization adds marginal information to that which can be obtained by a careful and thorough history and physical examination and other testing as described.

13. When are pulmonary function tests indicated?

All procedures do not confer an increased risk of pulmonary complications. Thus, age > 65 or 70 is not an absolute indication for pulmonary function testing (PFTs). Patients undergoing lung resection should always undergo PFTs first. Procedures that involve incisions of the upper abdomen or thorax should probably undergo PFTs, especially if the following factors are present: cough, known COPD, cigarette smoking, dyspnea, or other known pulmonary disease. On the other hand, orthopedic procedures and procedures of the lower abdomen confer minimal risk of pulmonary compromise and thus PFTs are not indicated in asymptomatic individuals.

Because body size and age affect PFTs, and because there is a paucity of data on normal PFTs in individuals over age 75, there is uncertainty as to the most appropriate cutoffs to apply in the elderly as predictors of respiratory complications. Furthermore, most studies of pulmonary risks have used individuals with known lung disease, particularly COPD. These data may not apply to the elderly in general. Nevertheless, the data suggest the following cutoffs as predictors of significant respiratory complications:

PCO_2 > 45 mmHg

FEV_1 < 2 liters (particularly < 1 liter)

Maximal ventilatory volume < 50% predicted

14. What specific preoperative recommendations are useful?

General: Cessation of smoking prior to surgery is helpful, but must be undertaken at least 2 weeks prior to surgery. Training in coughing and deep breathing should be undertaken prior to surgery. If COPD is present, aggressive use of bronchodilators should be implemented both pre- and postoperatively. Of course, any pulmonary infections must be treated prior to the operation.

Thromboembolism: Prophylaxis of thromboembolic events is based on the type of procedure and level of risk of the patient. For high-risk general surgery patients, i.e., patients undergoing surgery because of an intra-abdominal or pelvic malignancy, low-dose heparin begun on the day of surgery is effective. In the elderly, a dose of 5,000–7,500 units every 12 hours is usually adequate. Low-molecular-weight heparin with or without intermittent pneumatic compression is also effective. Among orthopedic surgery patients, such as those with hip fracture or undergoing elective hip or knee implantation, anticoagulation should be started on the day of surgery. Three successful approaches have been to give:

1. 10 mg warfarin the night before surgery, 5 mg the first postop day, and on subsequent days adjust the dose to prolong the prothrombin time by 3–4 seconds

2. 10 mg warfarin on the evening of surgery followed by daily warfarin to maintain an INR of 2.0–3.0

3. Low-molecular-weight heparin administered subcutaneously once a day

Minidose warfarin (1 mg) daily and aspirin are ineffective. Pneumatic compression stockings should be used in patients undergoing neurosurgery.

Cardiac medications: In patients at risk of postoperative ischemia, antianginal medications should be maximized. Heart failure should be corrected preoperatively. Antihypertensives should be continued at the preoperative dose.

Coronary artery revascularization: Prophylactic coronary artery bypass surgery (CABG) for the sole purpose of preventing a perioperative event is unwarranted. No randomized clinical trials have tested whether prophylactic CABG or angioplasty in the preoperative period is warranted, and the combined morbidity and mortality of both the coronary procedure and the intended operation must be considered. In general, the physician should perform a revascularization procedure preoperatively only if it would be performed in the absence of the surgical procedure.

15. What should be the focus of postoperative care?

In the postoperative period, a continuation of monitoring and treatment of those risk factors uncovered during the preoperative evaluation are most important. The critical factors at this point are ischemic heart disease, heart failure, arrhythmias, thromboemboli, respiratory complications, delirium, and general deconditioning. The patient should be monitored for the development of heart failure, angina or myocardial infarction, and arrhythmias. An EKG on days 1 and 2 will identify 96% of postoperative myocardial infarctions. Continued monitoring and prevention of deep venous thrombosis with anticoagulants are essential until the patient is mobile. Judicious use of narcotic medications is vital, but sometimes these agents must be discontinued because of delirium. Exercise is important for general reconditioning as well as prevention of thromboemboli. An individualized exercise program under the direction of a physical therapist is warranted in most patients.

BIBLIOGRAPHY

1. Ashton C, Petersen N, Wray N, et al: The incidence of perioperative myocardial infarction in men undergoing noncardiac surgery. Ann Intern Med 118:504–510, 1993.
2. Dalen JE, Hirsh J. Consensus conference on antithrombotic therapy: Prevention of venous thromboembolism. Chest 102(4 suppl): 391S–407S, 1992.
3. Eagle KA, Coley M, et al: Combining clinical and thallium data optimizes pre-operative assessment of cardiac risk before major vascular surgery. Ann Intern Med 110:859–886, 1989.
4. Goldman M, Caldera D, Southwick F, et al: Multifactorial index of cardiac risk in non–cardiac surgical procedures. N Engl J Med 297:845–850, 1977.
5. Jackson MC: Pre-operative pulmonary evaluation. Arch Intern Med 148:2120–2127, 1988.
6. Johnson J: Surgical assessment in the elderly. Geriatrics 43(suppl): 83–90, 1988.
7. Thomas DR, Ritchie CS: Preoperative assessment of older adults. J Am Geriatr Soc 43:811–821, 1995.

38. DERMATOLOGY

David Margolis, M.D., and Jeffrey Miller, M.D.

1. What happens to the skin as an individual ages?

Skin changes with aging include the formation of skin cancers and precancers, wrinkles and furrows, increased "dryness," easy bruising, and slower healing response. These changes are due to alterations in the architecture of the epidermis, dermis, and subcutaneous fat layer and in the interactions between these layers of the skin.

The keratinocyte is the major cell type found in the epidermis. These cells are prone to environmental insults which accumulate with age. The most important repetitive insult is from sunlight, and this is believed to be the chief risk factor for premature aging of the skin, such as the formation of wrinkles and all types of skin cancer. Aging and photodamage alter the way the epidermis and dermis interface, resulting in increased cutaneous fragility. Fibroblasts, which are the chief cellular component of the dermis and are responsible for the formation of much of the extracellular matrix of the dermis, enter a period of senescence with biologic aging of the body. Aged fibroblasts are unable to replicate and respond properly to growth factors, thereby leading to degenerative collagen and elastic components. The subcutaneous fat layer degenerates with age, contributing to the lax, inelastic feel of aged skin.

2. Why does the skin of older individuals flake?

The frequency of complaints related to dry skin increases with aging. This increased frequency is probably related to a decrease in the production of sebum and keratinocyte-produced fatty acids, an increase in water vapor permeability across the dermal-epidermal barrier, and harsher methods used to care for the skin. Clinically, these skin problems can be manifested as mild scaling to frank excoriation. Dry skin is often associated with pruritus.

Treatment includes the frequent use of emollients and moisturizers. Since the geriatric population is at increased risk of developing contact dermatitis, care must be exercised to ensure that any topical product used is not a sensitizing agent for that patient. These products may need to be applied as frequently as four times daily. Patients should also be instructed in gentle skin care, which includes the use of a moisturizing soap, infrequent bathing or showering using tepid water, and gentle drying of the skin by patting rather than rubbing.

3. How is pruritus approached in the elderly?

Many older persons present with the chief complaint of pruritus (itching). Pruritus may be due to a primary skin disease, systemic disease, or multifactorial or idiopathic causes. Xerosis, defined as rough, dry, scaling skin, is the most common cause of pruritus in the elderly. This type of pruritus is often called senile pruritus. Xerosis may be related to winter and its low humidity, excessive bathing, medications (e.g., opiates), and atopy (e.g., history of hay fever, eczema, asthma). Other causes of pruritus include psychogenic factors related to stress and depression and manifestations of systemic disease, such as renal, thyroid, hepatic, anemia, diabetes, and malignancy.

Therapy is directed at the underlying cause of the pruritus. Emollient cream and ointment (e.g., Dermasil), decreased bathing, application of nonmedicated soap (e.g., Dove) limited to the axilla and genital areas, moderate strength topical corticosteroids (e.g., fluocinolone or triamcinolone ointment), and systemic antihistamines are used for pruritus related to xerosis. If no skin disease is evident, an underlying systemic disorder needs to be investigated based on history and physical exam.

4. Why do the lower extremities become red and swollen?

Lower extremity swelling can be related to impaired venous or lymphatic flow. These abnormalities can be secondary to congenital disorders, such as lymphedema praecox, or acquired disorders, such as deep venous thromboembolism or congestive heart failure. Edematous limbs frequently become dermatitic and clinically may mimic cellulitis. In patients with venous disease, the chronicity of the edema may lead to sclerosis of the cutaneous structures and a skin finding called **lipodermatosclerosis**. Both dermatitis and lipodermatosclerosis are due to trauma to the cutaneous structures from the edema. In addition, a significant increased incidence of contact dermatitis is noted in edematous limbs.

It is important to understand the cause of the edema before treating it. For example, diuretics work well for edema related to congestive heart failure but poorly for venous-related edema, which responds to external compression. Treatment should include the use of topical emollients. Petrolatum is the least likely to cause a contact dermatitis. The use of topical steroids should be limited. They initially appear to be helpful but are treating only a symptom, dermatitis, and not the problem, limb edema.

5. What is shingles?

Shingles, or herpes zoster, is the reactivation of the latent herpes varicella-zoster virus usually in a dermatomal pattern. Reactivation tends to occur in the elderly population, as well as in patients who are immunosuppressed secondary to collagen vascular disease, malignancy, or medications. Patients often note a prodrome of burning in the involved dermatome. The disorder is then manifested by grouped vesicles or pustules within a dermatome. The most common sites of involvement are the trunk, face, and scalp. The disease may disseminate to involve more than one dermatome, a presentation which is more likely in immunocompromised hosts. The reactivation of varicella-zoster virus is usually self-limited with full resolution within 2 weeks. However, a sizable group of patients will develop chronic discomfort called post-herpetic neuralgia.

6. Define post-herpetic neuralgia.

No consensus exists for defining post-herpetic neuralgia. An acceptable definition is the persistence of skin discomfort in an area of recent varicella-zoster reactivation. However, the definition of persistence ranges from pain after all lesions are healed to pain that is present > 30–90 days after all lesions have been healed. Post-herpetic neuralgia most commonly occurs in the elderly with an increasing prevalence with increasing age. The discomfort can vary from burning to a sharp pain which can be debilitating.

Studies show that early treatment of the initial reactivation of varicella-zoster with oral antiviral agents can avoid the development of post-herpetic neuralgia. Early intervention with these agents is probably indicated for patients at highest risk to develop this sequela, the aged. Past reports examined the use of corticosteroids (prednisone, 60 mg, tapered over 3–4 weeks) and acyclovir (800 mg 5× per day for 10 days). Corticosteroids are probably helpful for pain management but do not ultimately alter the disease. Once post-herpetic neuralgia has occurred, treatments are relatively unsuccessful. The basis for these treatments is pain control and include electrical stimulation, acupuncture, tricyclic antidepressants (amitriptyline 25 mg every night), and narcotics.

7. Describe the different causes of leg ulcers.

Leg ulcers afflict approximately 1% of the population, with at least two thirds of those afflicted being over age 60 years. Causes of chronic leg ulcers include venous disease, arterial insufficiency, insensate ulcers, pressure ulcers, sickle cell ulcers, and vasculitis.

Insensate ulcers or neuropathic ulcers are usually related to diabetes mellitus but can be related to other diseases that cause a sensory neuropathy, such as leprosy, and are usually located on the plantar areas of the foot. The wound may be associated with a Charcot joint. Lower extremity wounds associated with **arterial insufficiency** are usually accompanied by claudication. Claudication is pain that occurs suddenly in the lower extremity after a metabolic challenge and is quickly relieved after resolution of this challenge. The most common chronic leg ulcer is related to **venous disease**. Venous disease occurs because of elevated ambulatory venous pressures. These pressures can be elevated because of obstruction of the deep venous system of the leg (e.g., clot), loss of valvular competence of the veins communicating between the deep and superficial venous system (e.g., varicose veins), or loss of the muscular tone of the calf. It is also not uncommon for an individual to suffer from more than one cause of leg ulcer (e.g., venous *and* arterial disease) concomitantly.

Treatment of chronic wounds depends on the correct diagnosis. Once the diagnosis is made, treatment should be based on removing the cause of the wound. For example, an individual with venous disease needs to have the ambulatory venous hypertension decreased by augmenting venous return with external compression, while an individual with arterial insufficiency needs improved arterial flow which may require surgical intervention. Good wound care should be provided for the ulcer. This includes the use of moist dressing, removal of necrotic tissue, and gentle cleansing.

8. What is the most common blistering disease in the elderly?

Bullous pemphigoid. Most cases appear in patients over age 60 years. Bullous pemphigoid is characterized by a chronic, nonscarring vesicular bullous eruption in which nongrouped bullae occur on normal or urticarial skin. Lesions are most common on flexural surfaces, with the oral mucosa affected in one-third of patients. Nikolsky's sign (induction of blister with lateral skin pressure) is negative. The blistering results from autoantibodies directed against a 230-kilodalton antigen which anchors the basal cells of the epidermis to the basement membrane. Biopsy of an early small blister reveals a subepidermal blister. Diagnosis is often confirmed through direct and indirect immunofluorescence which identify the patient's autoantibodies. The disease typically lasts a year with a variable number of flareups.

Bullous pemphigoid is to be distinguished from **pemphigus vulgaris**. Pemphigus vulgaris produces widespread erosions and flaccid bullae with a positive Nikolsky sign. Mucous membranes are commonly affected. Age of onset is frequently in the 4th to 5th decade. The blistering is caused by autoantibodies directed against adhesion molecules between keratinocytes in the epidermis. Direct and indirect immunofluorescence is diagnostic.

9. Do the elderly get acne?

Rosacea, a condition often confused with acne, commonly affects the middle-aged to elderly. Found in 10% of the general population, the disease is characterized by flushing, facial erythema and telangiectases, papules and pustules, and rhinophyma. Most patients present with facial erythema and telangiectases. The absence of comedomes and different age prevalence distinguish rosacea from acne. The differential diagnosis of rosacea includes carcinoid syndrome, seborrheic dermatitis, lupus erythematosus, contact dermatitis, and steroid-induced rosacea.

10. What is a reasonable approach to hair loss in the elderly?

At menopause in women and at age 20–40 years in men, thin hair and hair loss may become a severe problem. A good medical and drug history needs to be taken, and simple tests for thyroid function, free testosterone, and dihydroepiandosterone sulfate levels as well as complete blood count should be conducted in the appropriate setting. Correction of the medical problem may help, especially in nutritional and metabolic deficiency states. For example, replacement of iron in iron-deficiency anemia can restore hair growth. Spironolactone at a dose of 50–200 mg/day may be helpful if an androgen excess is uncovered. If there is no medical abnormality, other approaches include minoxidil 2% for androgenic alopecia and surgical approaches such as hair transplants and scalp reductions. Minoxidil must be applied twice daily and used for a minimum of 4 months before declaration of treatment failure. Shedding of hair occurs if the patient uses less than the recommended dose or stops treatment.

11. How common is melanoma?

The incidence of melanoma continues to rise throughout the world. In the United States, its incidence has nearly tripled in the past four decades, growing faster than that of any other cancer. By the year 2000, projections suggest that melanoma will develop in 1 in 75–90 white

Americans. African-Americans and Asians have decreased rates of melanoma because of greater degrees of pigmentation. It is important to note that the highest age-specific incidence rates occur in the elderly population. Recognizing risk factors for melanoma is important because prognosis is excellent with early detection and treatment of melanoma. Major risk factors for melanoma include:

Higher than average number of benign melanocytic nevi
Atypical nevi (> 6 mm size, irregular border, and variegated color)
Pigmentary characteristics of blue eyes, blond or red hair, and fair complexion
Personal history of melanoma
Family history of melanoma
Immunosuppression
Excessive sun exposure

12. What are the clinical signs of melanoma?

As a visible tumor, cutaneous melanoma can be recognized and detected early. An **ABCDE** rule has been established to help diagnose melanoma in any pigmented lesion.

A—**A**symmetry
B—**B**order irregularity
C—**C**olor variegation
D—**D**iameter > 0.6 cm (size of pencil eraser)
E—**E**levation

Melanoma should also be suspected if a patient reports any change in an existing mole or a new pigmented lesion. Also, itching and burning of a mole should raise suspicion for melanoma, but most patients with melanoma experience no symptoms. A definitive diagnosis requires an excisional biopsy for histologic examination.

13. Which nonmelanoma skin cancers are seen most commonly in the elderly?

Basal cell carcinomas and **squamous cell carcinomas** are common nonmelanoma skin cancers in the elderly. More than one-third of all cancers in the United States are nonmelanoma skin cancers. Basal cell carcinoma commonly presents as a translucent flesh-colored or pink pearly papule with prominent telangiectasias. Squamous cell carcinoma typically presents as a firm, erythematous nodules with elevated borders and occasional central ulceration. Both types of cancer commonly occur in sun-exposed areas, such as the head, neck, and arms. Basal cell carcinomas have a low risk of metastases (< 1/400 cases). Squamous cell carcinomas also have a low risk of metastases, except when they appear in the setting of immunosuppression or at sites of chronic inflammation, scar tissue, and radiation.

14. Are sunscreens important for the elderly?

Chronic exposure to the sun's ultraviolet rays, UVB and UVA, is thought to be the primary cause of skin cancer and skin aging. It is estimated that about 75% of the total lifetime dose of UV radiation is accumulated before age 20 years. Sunscreens are important in the battle against skin cancer and skin aging. Regular use of a sunscreen in the elderly population is important because this practice can minimize the risk of sun-induced skin cancer, slow the effect of photoaging, and prevent drug-induced photosensitivity.

15. How does sun protective factor (SPF) work?

The best chemical sunscreens provide UVA and UVB coverage. The effect of a sunscreen's SPF number depends on the patient's minimal erythemal dose (MED), defined as how long it takes the sunlight in a particular place, on a particular day, to turn skin barely pink. Whatever the patient's MED for a particular time and place, a sunscreen's SPF value can be used to estimate how long he or she can safely stay outdoors. Just multiply the MED by the SPF number.

Sensitivity to UVB radiation is determined by the melanin content of skin. This has led to the assignment of skin types I to VI based on sun sensitivity and pigment response. Sun exposure results in sunburn in a shorter period of time with skin type I compared to skin type IV. Therefore, a person's MED increases with higher skin types.

Skin Type	Complexion	MED UVB, (mJ/cm²)	Recommended SPF	Sunburn/Tanning History
I	Very fair	15–30	15–30	Always burns; never tans
II	Fair	25–35	15–30	Often burns; tans minimally
III	Light	30–50	15–30	Sometimes burns; tans gradually
IV	Medium	45–60	10–15	Rarely burns; tans easily
V	Dark	60–90	10–15	Never burns; tans easily
VI	Darkly pigmented	90–120	6–10	Never burns; deeply tans

16. Name the most common dermatologic conditions seen in the geriatric population.

Patients who presented to a geriatric clinic and noninstitutionalized volunteers who underwent a full skin examination were evaluated for skin conditions. Although this survey is limited by sample size and bias, the following skin conditions were commonly seen in this geriatric population (age > 65 years old):

Seborrheic keratoses (benign neoplasm of epidermal cells appearing as a pasted-on papule)
Actinic keratoses (precancerous neoplasm of the epidermis caused by sunlight)
Pruritus
Tinea pedis (fungal skin infection characterized by plantar scale)
Seborrheic dermatitis (chronic, superficial, inflammatory process especially affecting the scalp, eyebrows, and face)
Venous stasis dermatitis
Nonmelanoma skin cancers

BIBLIOGRAPHY

1. Bolognia JL: Aging skin. A J Med 98 (1A):99S–103S, 1995.
2. Koh HK: Cutaneous melanoma. N Engl J Med 325:171–182, 1991.
3. Kurban RS, Kurban AK: Common skin disorders of aging: diagnosis and treatment. Geriatrics 48(4):30–42, 1993.
4. O'Donoghue MN: Cosmetics for the elderly. Dermatol Clin 9:29–34, 1991.
5. West MD: The cellular and molecular biology of skin aging. Arch Dermatol 130:87–95, 1994.

39. PRESSURE ULCERS

Robert Goldman, M.D.

1. What are pressure ulcers? Where and how do they occur?

Pressure ulcers are areas of skin disruptions consisting of focal necrosis of epidermis, dermis, subdermis, fascia, muscle, or joint capsule. They are caused by excessive, prolonged pressure that produces ischemia to soft tissue over bony prominences (hot spots) such as the greater trochanter of the femur, sacrum, ischial tuberosity, or calcaneus. Injury may occur from prolonged sitting or lying without transient relief of pressure. Although commonly observed on patients that are bed-bound or bedfast, the term "pressure ulcer" is preferable to "bedsores" or "decubitus ulcers." Pressure ulcer better describes the cause, and because ulcers also occur on sitting patients, the other terms are not accurate descriptors.

2. What is the relationship of pressure to ulcer formation?

Unrelieved axial pressure of 4–6 times systolic blood pressure causes necrosis in as short as 1 hour, but pressure similar to systolic requires 12 hours to cause a similar lesion. Shear, defined as force tangential to the skin surface, causes ulceration at markedly lower axial pressure. Skin moisture aggravates both axial and shear forces and predisposes to breakdown; ischemic change occurs in response to compromised capillary perfusion. Periodic pressure relief increases resistance of tissue to breakdown. Therefore, sitting patients should be instructed to lift their buttocks from the seat at least 15 seconds every 30 minutes. Supine patients should be turned every 2 hours.

3. How are pressure ulcers assessed and classified?

The National Pressure Ulcer Advisory Panel (NPUAP) classification, which is partially based on the well-known Shea system, is recommended:

Stage I	Nonblanchable skin erythema (difficult to assess in patients with heavily pigmented skin)
Stage II	Breakdown into dermis, but not subcutaneous tissues (i.e., subdermis)
Stage III	Ulcer extends from subcutaneous depth to fascia
Stage IV	Ulcer extends from depth of the fascia to bone

Serial reassessments of area and depth, at no longer than weekly intervals, quantify healing and assess the success of current treatment strategies. The simplest method is to measure the length along major and minor axes. A more quantitative technique is to trace the ulcer margin onto an acetate sheet (i.e., for Xerox copy transparencies) with a laundry marker, placing polyethylene film (i.e., Saran Wrap) between the ulcer and the sheet. Photography assesses the ulcer's appearance and size. Depth should be documented with swabs.

4. What interventions relieve pressure and shear?

- Placing pillows or other cushioning between trochanteric prominences and bed for side-lying patients
- Keeping the bed as horizontal as possible
- Using heel protectors
- Using special beds and mattresses

There is a wide spectrum of choice, with maximal efficiency of pressure and shear relief correlated with maximal cost. For patients with stage IV ulcers or stage III ulcers with spinal cord injury, low air loss (e.g., SAR Low Air Loss Mattress System) or air fluidized systems (e.g., Clinitron) are suggested. Less effective for pressure reduction and much lower in price are foam mattresses (e.g., "egg crate" or "Sof-care" mattress). Seating systems for wheelchairs are issued to many patients who lack protective sensation or cannot shift weight. Examples are air-filled vinous (e.g., Roho), contoured foam with a gel insert (e.g., Jay), or contoured foam (e.g., polyurethane) with or without protective cover. A solid seat (rather than the usual sling seat) may be prescribed for stability. Doughnut-shaped air cushions are not recommended, because pressure at the margin of the cushion exceeds the safe limit.

5. Which patients are most likely to develop pressure ulcers?
The mnemonic **DECUBITUS** is suggested as a learning aid.

D   **D**elirium, **d**ementia, **d**ependence. Only a patient with a clear mind can act purposefully to relieve a noxious stimulus. Therefore, patients with altered mental status, such as coma or severe dementia, are at risk for skin breakdown. Patients at risk of pressure ulcers are partially or completely dependent on others. Patients who require one or two persons to assist them in getting into bed are at high risk for ulceration.

E   **E**lderly. Seventy percent of pressure ulcers occur in the elderly. Frailty, dependence, incontinence, chronic illness, and degenerative neurologic disease increase with age. Associated with aging are diminished pain perception and blunting of the inflammatory response. Histologic changes in skin include flattening of the dermal-epidermal junction and reduced elastin content, both of which increase susceptibility to shear and minor laceration. Ulcer closure is delayed because of reduced rates of both reepithelialization and contraction.

C   **C**ontractures. If severe, contractures prevent routine turning and positioning on most mattress types. Thus they contribute to delayed healing and increased incidence.

U   **U**rinary incontinence. Wet skin is easily macerated. If the urine is infected, the skin and any ulcers will be contaminated. (See chapter 35.)

B   **B**owel incontinence. Soiling may lead to bacterial colonization or local infection. The wet skin associated with diarrhea also contributes to ulcer formation.

I   **I**mmobility. Chronic bed rest leads to a decrease in lean muscle mass of 5% per week and contributes to osteoporosis and contractures through collagen remodeling within tendons and joint capsules. Immobility feeds a vicious cycle of wasting, contractures, pressure "hot spots," and worsening ulceration.

T   **T**ension O_2 low. Ischemia is related to ulcer formation. Anemia should be corrected (e.g., by iron supplementation). Edema impairs gas and nutrient exchange between healing tissue and the blood supply.

U   **U**ndernourishment. Inadequate caloric or protein intake may result in malnutrition and impaired ulcer healing. (See question 10.)

S   **S**pasticity, sensory loss, spinal cord injury. By several mechanisms, neurologic injury predisposes to pressure ulcer formation:
- Spasticity (increased muscle tone) predisposes to contracture formation and poor mobility.
- Lack of protective sensation, which leads to pressure ulcer formation, may be dermotomal with spinal cord injury or hemisensory with stroke.
- Spinal cord injury, especially above T6, is related to sympathetic nervous system dysfunction and impaired skin perfusion at sites of pressure.

6. What are occlusive or semiocclusive dressings? How are they used in pressure ulcer care?
Occlusive dressings create a barrier to moisture loss and a seal with normal skin around the ulcer. A moist environment results, with (semiocclusive) or without (occlusive) oxygen exchange. This moist milieu promotes formation of granulation tissue. The concern that an occluded environment brings about infection has not been substantiated for ulcers that do not appear clinically infected. The choice to use one or the other is more a matter of personal preference than influence on wound-healing kinetics. Occlusive dressings form a better seal with skin outside the ulcer margin and thus resist contamination more effectively. Examples of occlusive dressings include polyurethane film (e.g., Tegaderm, OpSite), hydrocolloid (e.g., Duoderm) and

hydrocolloid gel (e.g., Vigilon). The following treatment examples must be confirmed by experienced practitioners for specific cases:

Stage I: Cover with an occlusive dressing to prevent continued shear. Change weekly, when the dressing becomes dislodged, or when the ulcer seal is broken.

Stage II, III or IV: Treatment depends on appearance of ulcer base.

- Clean ulcers have beefy red granulation tissue without fibrinous material.
- Use wet-to-wet dressings. Examples are saline-soaked gauze and calcium alginate (e.g., Sorbsain) or hydrocolloid gel (both covered by polyurethane film). The surrounding skin should be kept dry, if possible, to avoid maceration.
- Ulcers with a white to yellow film (i.e., fibrinous exudate) require debridement (see question 7).
- Black, hard eschar (most often found on the heel), according to the Pressure Ulcer Advisory Panel, should be covered with dry gauze for protection and not debrided if "clean and dry."

7. What types of debridement are used for ulcer care? What are their indications?

Devitalized tissue promotes infection and is a barrier to reepithelialization. Therefore, it should be debrided by mechanical, enzymatic, or autolytic means. Examples of **mechanical methods** include (1) manual (i.e., surgical or "sharps" debridement), (2) wet-to-dry dressings, and (3) irrigation. Sharps debridement is usually reserved for thick or adherent eschar or infected ulcers. Eschar (and, unfortunately, viable tissue) adheres to wet-to-dry dressings during removal; hence, the method is slower to work. Prepare by soaking gauze pads in saline, wringing out the liquid, completely unraveling, loosely packing all cavities of the ulcer, covering with dry gauze, and securing with paper tape. Hydrotherapy is usually performed by physical therapists for fibrinous stage III or IV ulcers (or locally infected ulcers; see question 11). Irrigation can also be done at the bedside with, for instance, a 50-ml syringe, 19-gauge Angiocath, and normal saline. **Enzymatic debridement** (e.g., Elase) uses collagenase and other protease to break down eschar. It works slowly and is therefore used mostly in institutional or home settings. **Autolytic debridement** depends on proteolytic enzymes in ulcer fluid and is the slowest acting.

8. Should topical antiseptics, such as betadine, peroxide, or sodium hypochlorite (i.e., Daken's) solution, be used routinely?

No, according to current guidelines. Overall, these agents retard epithelialization in animal models and are toxic to fibroblasts in vitro. However, this point is controversial. Some researchers point to animal studies suggesting that short-term, low-dose treatment may not delay healing. Some of the discrepancy may lie in how the agent is applied to the wound and the definition of healing. Animal studies that use daily application of topical agents and measure the time to 50% healing demonstrate reductions in healing rate. Studies that apply single doses of topical agent or measure time to 100% healing show no difference.

9. What is the role of adjunctive treatment?

If the ulcer does not heal with conventional ulcer care, including dressings, debridements, and biomechanical interventions, adjunctive treatments should be considered. There is much research at present into adjunctive treatments, and clinical acceptance varies widely from hospital to hospital and region to region. The following list is not exhaustive:

- **Electrotherapy.** Both decubitus and leg ulcers reportedly heal more rapidly with electrotherapy of various signal types. However, it is still not approved by the Food and Drug Administration (FDA) for wound healing and hence is not routinely covered by Medicare. Contraindications include presence of a pacemaker or implanted drug pump and history of malignant arrhythmias.
- **Growth factor therapy.** Platelet-derived growth factor (PDGF), transforming growth factor beta (TGF-beta), and fibroblast growth factor (FGF) are undergoing double-blind FDA trials at present for various types of chronic ulcers. The data indicate trends in the

direction of healing rate improvement. A few clinical studies report statistically significant improvements in healing rates, that may or may not be "clinically significant." Growth factor therapy may be important in the future. However, it is not currently covered by Medicare, hence is not practiced outside of a few specialized centers.

10. What is the role of nutrition in the prevention and treatment of pressure ulcers?

A pressure ulcer may be a sign of malnutrition. Indicators of poor nutrition include a serum albumin of < 3.5 mg/dl, total lymphocyte count of < 1,800 mm^3 and body weight decrease of > 15%. Determining that the prealbumin is low is a sensitive measure of malnutrition, if available. Goals of nutrition therapy are correction of the above indices as well as a positive nitrogen balance (1.25–1.5 gm of protein/kg/day). Important vitamins for ulcer healing include vitamin C, vitamin A, and zinc. Supplementation of these substances is of questionable benefit if serum levels are normal.

11. How is an infected ulcer diagnosed and managed?

A foul smell, greenish or copious drainage, scant granulation, and dull whitish or pink base (rather than bright red granulation tissue) indicate local infection. Cellulitis is an invasion of organisms beyond ulcer margins, marked by erythema, warmth, swelling, or tenderness. Signs of bacteremia or systemic invasion include fever, elevated white count, change of mental status, or increasing insulin requirements in diabetics.

The surfaces of all ulcers are colonized by bacteria; therefore, ulcer cultures should not be performed routinely. The indications for culture are cellulitis and systemic signs. Surface swabs are misleading, because they do not isolate the causative organism. However, qualitative culture of tissue below the ulcer surface, collected under sterile conditions, is more definitive. It is routinely performed in hospital microbiology laboratories. Quantitative culture is most definitive, and results are described as colony-forming units (CFU) per gram of tissue. At levels above 10^5 CFU, ulcers heal poorly. However, quantitative culture may not be available in community hospitals.

Clinical infection is almost always polymicrobial, including both facultative aerobes and strict anaerobes. Aerobic organisms are usually found in surface swabs, whereas anaerobes are more often isolated from deep tissue and blood. In one study deep tissue isolates included *Proteus mirabilis,* group D streptococci, *Escherichia coli, Staphylococcus aureus, Pseudomonas aeruginosa, Bacteroides fragilis,* and *Peptostreptococcus* sp. Anaerobes are associated with ulcers having necrotic material and foul odor.

For locally infected ulcers, start a course of frequent ulcer inspection and mechanical debridement (e.g., wet-to-dry dressings and hydrotherapy). The Pressure Ulcer Advisory Panel recommends application of topical bactericidal agents only if infection does not resolve within 1 week. For systemic signs of infection, such as chills or sweats, fever or drop in body temperature, hypotension, or glucose intolerance (in diabetics), broad-spectrum coverage is recommended, because infection is usually polymicrobial. Urgent surgical debridement is required, because bacteremia doubtless will not clear without removal of necrotic material or drainage of abscess.

12. How is osteomyelitis in a pressure ulcer diagnosed and treated?

Osteomyelitis should be suspected in stage IV decubiti. However, the gold standard, a bone biopsy, is usually not done except as part of aggressive debridement. There is much controversy about the best noninvasive test for osteomyelitis. An elevated erythrocyte sedimentation rate, elevated white blood cell count, and positive plain x-ray, taken together, are 88% specific and 89% sensitive for osteomyelitis. (A plain film is positive in the presence of reactive bone formation and periosteal elevation). Technetium bone scan, computed tomography (CT), and magnetic resonance imaging (MRI) are of limited value because of the high incidence of false positives. In the presence of an infected ulcer and positive plain film, bone biopsy should be performed with needle aspiration through intact skin. The biopsy is positive if it shows a chronic inflammatory infiltrate (plasma cells, lymphocytes) and positive quantitative culture > 10^3 organisms/gm of bone.

13. When should surgical closure be contemplated?

Surgical closure should be done when the patient does not progress with optimal care, including available adjunctive care. In addition, the patient must agree to and be able to tolerate surgery, which may involve extensive blood loss, and osteomyelitis must be adequately treated. Frequently, stage IV ulcers require surgical evaluation. Musculocutaneous flaps are usually the treatment of choice. However, for the flap to be successful, pressure relief must be addressed; if inadequate pressure relief was the original cause of the ulcer, the skin is likely to break down again.

14. Should the goal of ulcer care always be complete healing?

Not all ulcers will heal, even with optimal care. Motivation of the patient and compliance with therapies are critical for a successful outcome. Factors associated with a high risk of non-healing include:

- Bacterial colonization by > 10^5 CFU/gm of tissue
- Osteomyelitis (25% of nonhealing ulcers)
- Chronic granulation for > 30 years (may indicate malignancy, with biopsies consistent with epidermoid cancer [Marjolin's ulcer]).

15. What is the differential diagnosis for pressure ulcers?

Skin conditions that cause erythema around perianal, perineal, or gluteal skin folds may be confused with stage I and stage II pressure ulcers. Examples include dermatophytosis (tenia cruris), *Candida albicans* (often associated with vaginal monilia), and intertrigo. Contact dermatitis should also be considered. Herpes zoster classically presents with vesicles and crusts and may occur around sacral dermatomes. Skin ulceration has a long differential diagnosis. However, subcutaneous and dermal ulcers at bony prominences at the ischeii, gluteal fold, or sacrum usually are caused by pressure. In contrast, ulceration of the lower extremities may be vascular, arterial, or infectious.

16. Can a pressure ulcer be a marker for abuse?

Yes. A pressure ulcer is likely to occur in a neglected, bed-bound patient. Unintentional abuse may result from inexperience, excessive caregiver burden, or lack of motivation. Elder abuse should be considered in the following settings:

- The caregiver has a history of mental illness, alcohol or drug abuse, is socially isolated, or has undergone recent stressful life events.
- The dependent patient presents with signs of dehydration, malnutrition, or poor personal hygiene in addition to the ulcer.

BIBLIOGRAPHY

1. Clinical Practice Guideline: Treatment of Pressure Ulcers, U.S. Department of Health and Human Services, Agency for Health Care Policy and Research, Rockville, MD, AHCPR Publ No. 950652, 1994.
2. Harding KG: Methods for assessing change in ulcer status. Adv Wound Care 8:37–42, 1995.
3. Kertesz C, Chow AW: Infected pressure and diabetic ulcers. Clin Geriatr Med 8:835–852, 1992.
4. Kosiak M: Etiology and pathology of ischemic ulcers. Arch Phys Med Rehabil 40:62–68, 1959.
5. Makleburst J: Pressure ulcer staging systems. Adv Wound Care 8:11–13, 1995.
6. Margolis DJ: Definition of a pressure ulcer. Adv Wound Care 8:8–10, 1995.
7. Yarkony GM: Pressure ulcers: A review. Arch Phys Med Rehabil 75:908–917, 1994.

40. CARE OF THE ELDERLY CANCER PATIENT

Richard H. Greenberg, M.D., and David J. Vaughn, M.D.

1. Is loss of immune surveillance the reason cancers are more common in older patients?

The question of how the loss of immune surveillance in the elderly contributes to their higher incidence of cancer is quite complicated. Theories suggest that tumor cells express specific antigens that lead to their recognition and removal by the intact immune system. Support comes from the greater incidence of neoplasia in the AIDS or organ transplant populations. Dissenters argue that the narrow range of tumor types (lymphoma, Kaposi's sarcoma) seen in these latter populations does not support the applicability of immune surveillance as a general mechanism in the control of cancer. With lymphoid and plasma cell dyscrasias, evidence suggests that loss of normal cellular regulation of the growth of these specific cell types has more to do with their malignant transformation than the absence of adequate immune surveillance. The mild loss of cellular immunity seen in the elderly may actually lead to more indolent behavior of tumors due to lower levels of nonspecific growth or angiogenesis factors in the cellular milieu.

2. What are the principal modalities for the treatment of cancer in the elderly? What are the goals?

The three main modalities of cancer treatment—chemotherapy (including biologic, hormonal, and immune therapies), radiotherapy, and surgery—may be used singly or in combination. The underlying intent of treatment can be cure, palliation, or comfort-care/symptom control. The goals of therapy typically dictate the aggressiveness of treatment and the acceptable level of toxicity.

3. Should the physician approach the management of cancer differently in the elderly than in the young?

Elderly men and women have the same right to participate fully in the planning and implementation of their cancer care and to be informed fully of their therapeutic options. Assumptions based solely on age and treatment nihilism have no place in the ethical and compassionate development of the therapeutic relationship. Appropriate clinical judgment should be used in dealing with patients with poor functional status and known limited life expectancy. Treatment options with their respective advantages and disadvantages should be presented, along with an analysis of the expected length and quality of survival compared with the level of risk to the patient. The option of focusing on symptom management in lieu of antitumor treatments also needs to be presented. An important component of the personal database for any patient, particularly the elderly, is the inclusion of the patient's wishes regarding advanced directives, living wills, durable power of attorney for health care, and preferences regarding levels of resuscitation and artificial life support. (See also Chapter 41.)

4. How does the hematopoietic reserve of the elderly patient influence management?

Aging reduces the amount of active bone marrow, as the proportion of marrow fat increases. Under steady-state conditions, there is little impact on peripheral blood counts. However, with the toxicity of radiotherapy and chemotherapy, myelosuppression occurs, and the recovery of the bone marrow is delayed and diminished. An increase in severe hematopoietic toxicity observed in Phase II clinical cancer therapy trials in patients of age > 65 as compared to their younger counterparts has been demonstrated. Modern blood-banking techniques and the use of recombinant hematopoietic growth factors (e.g., granulocyte–colony-stimulating factor) have made it easier to utilize myelosuppressive chemotherapy at higher doses and on schedule in the elderly with demonstrated decreases in neutropenia. Alternately, dose modification or the selection of less myelosuppressive drugs can avoid much of the bone marrow toxicity.

5. How does renal function influence their care?

Differences in renal function between elderly patients and their younger counterparts are the most significant determinants of alterations in cancer chemotherapy pharmacokinetics (see also Chapter 28). Changes with aging include:

- Reduced renal blood flow
- Reduced glomerular filtration

Renal impairment leads to decreased clearance and therefore the increased risk of toxicity from drugs that are renally eliminated (esp. methotrexate, bleomycin, streptozocin, and the platin-complex agents). Careful determination of renal function (creatinine clearance) as part of treatment planning is more important than assumptions based solely on age. Nephrotoxic supportive agents, such as aminoglycoside antibiotics and amphotericin, must also be approached with care in the setting of renal insufficiency.

6. Does hepatic function influence their care?

- Age-related decreases in hepatic mass, hepatic blood flow, and microsomal oxidation and reduction have been noted.
- Metabolism of chemotherapeutic agents occurs principally by hepatic phase I oxidative and reductive modification to active or inactive compounds.
- No accepted biologic marker of hepatic function exists, but appropriate clinical judgment should be exercised in the setting of significant hepatic compromise.
- The conjugating (phase II) functions of the liver do not appear to change significantly in the elderly, because alterations of metabolism at this level are typically seen only in severe hepatic dysfunction.

7. What pharmacologic issues influence the cancer care of the elderly?

Intact hepatic and renal functions are critical to the normal metabolism and excretion of cancer chemotherapeutic agents. Poor drug tolerance in the elderly is largely a product of the narrow therapeutic index of most anticancer drugs superimposed on a tendency of declining organ function reserve. Chronologic age alone should not be used as the determinant of dose modifications in chemotherapy. Adjustments in treatment intensity should rather be made based on the presence of comorbid conditions that could affect the disposition or toxicity of the intended drug. Although allowing avoidable toxicity can lead to treatment delays that compromise dose intensity, undue fear of first-line chemotherapy drugs at optimal doses is likely a major source of the observed worse response to cancer treatment seen in the elderly.

- Elderly cancer patients may have clinically relevant impairment in many pharmacokinetic processes.
- Absorption of oral drugs may be affected by the higher gastric pH, delayed gastric emptying, and altered membrane transport typical of the elderly. (However, these effects have not proved to be of significant clinical relevance.)
- Changes in body composition in the elderly (decreased body water, decreased lean body mass, increased body fat, and decreased plasma-binding proteins) can affect the volume of distribution, elimination half-life, and peak or steady-state concentrations of drugs used in anticancer therapy.

Additionally, persons aged > 65 years take an average of 4 daily medications for preexisting chronic illnesses. Evidence suggests that older adults exhibit some degree of noncompliance when required to take > 4 medications/day, as is often required by the chemotherapeutic regimen. Noncompliance stands to be exacerbated further by the multiple therapeutic and symptom control drugs, as well as their potential interactions, prescribed in the course of cancer care.

8. How does the cardiovascular function of the elderly patient influence their care?

- The use of radiotherapy to the left chest or cardiotoxic chemotherapy (anthracyclines such as doxorubicin, high-dose alkylators) may require careful pre-evaluation and treatment planning.

- Cardioprotectant agents, such as dexrazoxane (ICRF-187, Zinecard), are now available that may help in extending the safe use of cardiotoxic chemotherapeutic drugs.
- The aggressive hydration associated with the standard use of many chemotherapeutic agents must be approached with caution to avoid fluid overload.

9. How does pulmonary function influence their care?

The presence of comorbid pulmonary disease is of greater significance than age alone in determining a patient's tolerance of surgical procedures or pulmonary-toxic chemotherapy (e.g., bleomycin). However, in the well-conditioned elderly individual without significant pulmonary disease, surgical and chemotherapeutic management of malignancy should not be precluded.

10. Mucosal integrity?

- Decreased cellular proliferation, skin/subcutaneous tissue thickness, and collagen production/remodeling in the elderly lead to poorer wound healing that may complicate surgical procedures and increase the likelihood of mucositis from chemotherapy or ionizing radiation.
- Potential for decreased mobility following surgery further increases the risk of skin breakdown/ulceration and infection.
- Enhancing nutrition, increasing mobility, and careful planning of radiation or chemotherapy dosing can help alleviate the potential loss of mucosal integrity.
- Cryotherapy (sucking on ice chips) during treatment with such agents as 5-fluorouracil decreases local perfusion and can significantly reduce the incidence of the associated mucositis.

11. And neurologic function?

- Sensory and cognitive impairments are more common in the elderly, leading to a much higher incidence of treatment- and disease-related delirium.
- Losses in taste and olfaction can intensify the decreased appetite associated with chemotherapy, head/neck radiotherapy, and malignancy.
- Great care (dose modification, aggressive laxative regimen) must be exercised in the use of agents such as vincristine due to the potentially severe adynamic ileus that can result.
- The cumulative fatigue experienced with the use of cisplatin is enhanced in the elderly.

12. What factors can contribute to delirium in the elderly cancer patient?

Cancer patients are at risk for delirium due to a large number of potentially reversible causes: direct tumor invasion of the CNS, sensory overload or deprivation (e.g., removal of glasses or hearing aid), isolated or unfamiliar environment, sleep deprivation, fluid/electrolyte and nutritional imbalances, organ failure or encephalopathy, disordered bowel function, infection, fever, hypoxia. Drugs associated with cancer management, such as chemotherapy, corticosteroids, biologic response modifiers, antiemetics, antihistamines, anticholinergics, and antispasmodics, can commonly contribute to delirium.

13. How well do the elderly tolerate cancer surgery?

Despite their higher incidence of comorbid medical illness, with appropriate preparation, most elderly cancer patients tolerate surgery well. Endoscopic surgical approaches can be particularly well tolerated. Despite multi-year life expectancies that persist into their 90s, the elderly are far more likely to be denied attempts at curative resections of their tumors than younger persons. Older cancer patients are just as likely to suffer local recurrence of their disease if surgical margins are inadequate.

14. How well do the elderly tolerate radiotherapy?

Any patient with poor nutritional, hydration, or functional status is likely to experience increased radiotherapy-induced toxicity. However, studies of elderly cancer patients with good performance status demonstrate that these patients tolerate radiotherapy with significant clinical benefit. One exception was radiation for malignant CNS gliomas, in which the elderly fared poorly. Despite this, radiation for metastases to the brain is tolerated just as well by the elderly as by younger patients.

15. Do the elderly with cancer suffer more?

Studies comparing cancer patients by age, but controlling for stage of disease and life expectancy, reveal that the elderly report very similar symptoms referable to their illness and treatment. All groups, regardless of age, tend to have progressively more complaints of greater intensity at diagnosis and at recurrence, with the peak occurring as they enter the terminal phases of their disease. Other studies have suggested that increasing age is associated with less sensitivity to pain. At present, it should not be assumed that the elderly are tolerant of pain or that their analgesic program need not be as aggressive. (See also Chapter 34.)

16. Are there special considerations regarding breast cancer in the elderly?

Breast cancer continues to rise in incidence as women age. Comorbid medical illness should be a greater influence on the aggressiveness of care than age alone. Evidence suggests that breast cancer is not less aggressive in the elderly. Studies demonstrate that healthy elderly women tolerate the same treatment that would be proposed for their younger counterparts including surgery, cytotoxic chemotherapy, and radiotherapy; enjoy equivalent benefits from such therapy; and suffer poorer outcomes if their treatment is compromised. Older women should be offered breast-conserving treatments. In light of the high proportion of estrogen and progesterone receptor-positive breast cancers in the elderly, the appropriate use of tamoxifen is important in both the adjuvant and metastatic settings. Some studies even suggest that tamoxifen can be used as a primary treatment modality in certain circumstances with acceptable response rates and good quality survival. Due to its weak estrogen agonist activity, tamoxifen offers the potential of lowered serum cholesterol, decreased risk of cardiovascular death, and possibly conservation of bone density to postmenopausal women. Education of older women and their physicians is crucial to encourage greater participation in screening and breast self-examination in an attempt to increase the chance of diagnosing earlier-stage disease.

17. Are there special considerations regarding colorectal cancer in the elderly?

In the treatment of colorectal cancer, surgery, radiotherapy, and chemotherapy are considered standard in their appropriate settings. The resultant benefits to the elderly in terms of cure and palliation are comparable to those enjoyed by younger patients. Colorectal surgery in the elderly is well tolerated with appropriate preparation and the control of comorbid medical conditions. Poor outcome is associated with emergent surgeries (e.g., perforation or obstruction), so efforts should be made to react quickly to symptoms and screen for earlier detection.

The difficult adjustment associated with the creation of a colostomy in the elderly should encourage creation of primary anastamoses and sphincter-sparing procedures whenever possible. Transanal excision with radiotherapy may be considered for early-stage rectal tumors. Adjuvant chemosensitized radiotherapy is beneficial for transmural, node-positive, or locally advanced lesions. Care to avoid small bowel exposure is particularly important in the elderly. Adjuvant chemotherapy with a 5-fluorouracil-containing regimen is considered standard for node-positive colon cancers. Some care in dosing should be exercised in patients older than 75 years due to a higher incidence of chemotherapy-related toxicity.

18. Discuss special considerations for the management of prostate cancer in the elderly.

Prostate cancer is largely a disease of older men. Despite its epidemiology, screening, diagnostics, and treatment of prostate cancer often discriminates against the elderly. Radiotherapy for prostate cancer in the elderly has equivalent efficacy and toxicity when compared with its use in younger men, and it should be used as clinically indicated without age bias. For localized disease in patients with estimated survival < 10 years, surgery and radiotherapy are equivalent. Such lesions, if biologically indolent, could even be followed without active treatment in some patients. Surgery is superior if survival is not limited. In locally advanced disease, radiotherapy has less morbidity than surgery. Metastatic disease requires antiandrogen therapy. Surgical castration is fully effective, safe, economical, and ensures compliance but is personally unacceptable in 50% of patients. Gonadotropin-releasing hormone analogs are safe and effective but are costly and require long-term compliance. Cytotoxic chemotherapy has been of limited benefit in the metastatic setting. Strontium-89 is of some value in the palliation of painful bony disease.

19. Are there special considerations regarding lung cancer in the elderly?

Non-small cell lung cancer in the elderly tends to present more often as localized disease, due in part to the higher proportion of squamous cell histology. Despite more limited disease, the elderly, particularly those with comorbid cardiopulmonary disease, are often denied curative surgical approaches. Newer surgical techniques, including thoracoscopic lung resections, could make definitive surgical management more applicable to the elderly. Radiotherapy of non-small cell lung cancer can offer effective palliation, but chemotherapy outside a clinical study probably cannot be justified in this population. Small cell lung cancer in limited stage is curable in the elderly at the same rates as younger patients as long as their renal and cardiac function allow use of standard chemotherapies.

20. What about gynecologic cancer in the elderly?

Gynecologic cancers, regardless of cell type (cervical, uterine, ovarian), present at later stages of disease in older women. Tolerance of standard surgical and chemotherapeutic treatment approaches is similar irrespective of age when adjusted for comorbid illness. Studies conclude that elderly women should not be denied definitive treatment for gynecologic cancer based solely on their age. Ovarian cancer particularly results in suboptimal surgical debulking and poorer ultimate survival. Studies are presently examining the role of more-aggressive surgical debulking followed by optimal chemotherapy in the management of local ovarian cancer in elderly women.

21. Lymphoma?

The epidemiology of Hodgkin's disease predicts for a bimodal age-related incidence, with the second increase occurring in late adulthood. Age itself represents an independent prognostic variable, with age > 60 years at presentation predicting a more advanced initial stage, lower response rate, decreased survival, and increased toxicity from therapy.

Non-Hodgkin's lymphoma is also highly prevalent in the elderly with 25–35% of patients being of age > 70 years. Low-grade subtypes of non-Hodgkin's lymphoma are more common in the elderly. While not considered curable, these tumors can behave indolently over many years. Such lymphomas do not respond better to earlier treatment. Thus treatment is often reserved for patients with symptoms, compromised organs, or transformation into higher-grade histologies. Overall incidence of intermediate and high-grade histologies of non-Hodgkin's lymphoma do not vary significantly with age among adults, but the elderly consistently have worse survival independent of death from other causes. Evidence suggests that significantly improved response to treatment and survival could be attained with the use of fuller doses of chemotherapy than those typically used in the elderly. Alternate treatment regimens and improved supportive measures may prove helpful in maximizing treatment tolerance in such individuals.

22. Acute myelogenous leukemia (AML)?

AML occurs with a median age of 60 years. Despite successes in the treatment of younger patients, the elderly have lower rates of response, remission, and cure. Poor prognostic factors occur at a higher rate in the elderly and include unfavorable chromosomal aberrations, greater proportions of less-favorable subtypes, antecedent myelodysplastic syndromes, and comorbid medical conditions. Therapy is based on an anthracycline combined with cytarabine. High-dose chemotherapy approaches are particularly poorly tolerated. Despite the use of optimal regimens, efficacy of treatment in the elderly is substantially worse than that in comparable younger patients. Optimal consolidative approaches are still the subject of investigation.

23. What are some issues concerning sexuality in the elderly cancer patient?

The diagnosis of cancer brings potential threats to the sexual function of the elderly. Four of the principal issues are loss and grief, distressing symptoms, body image changes, and changes in self-esteem and self-control. Physical and sensory dysfunction may come as a result of drug side effects and sedation, hormonal blockade or ablation, psychogenic impairment/depression, and treatment-related nerve or vascular damage and fibrosis. A disruptive loss of privacy is associated with progressive physical disability, presence of outside caregivers, and the typical nursing-home living environment (semiprivate rooms, single beds, unlocked doors, lack of staff comfort with sexual issues).

The elderly patient or couple needs the assistance of the health care provider to recognize and validate these changes and to assist in the process of re-establishing sexuality and a sense of normalcy. Physical rehabilitation should include attention to sexual issues. A program of exercise gives general benefits in terms of endurance, mobility, self-image, and mood. Nutritional support and counseling improve healing, energy level, and general sense of well-being. The physical approach to sexuality may require alterations to accommodate changes in function or comfort level. Attention to rest and normalcy of sleep patterns aids energy level and concentration. Sedatives should be kept to a minimum. Counseling concerning appearance and grooming can help offset some of the changes in appearance associated with surgeries and the effects of chemotherapy or radiation. Medical interventions, such as lubricants, hormonal supplements, penile implants or injections, and vacuum erection aid devices, may have applicability to specific situations. Psychiatric referral should also be considered, when appropriate. Even in the absence of sexual intercourse, the validation of the patient's concerns and the encouragement of closeness and intimacy can provide security when the outside world threatens with hazards and losses.

24. What social needs are prominent in elderly cancer patients?

Cancer death rates are higher among the socioeconomically disadvantaged. A growing number of elderly find themselves enduring worsening financial constraints as old age advances. Almost one-third of Americans aged > 65 live alone, and approximately 30% of these have no children. Such issues impact directly on the safety and effectiveness of oncologic care, patient compliance, home-based care, and access to medical facilities for evaluation, treatment, and follow-up. A complete and understandable educational process for the elderly is important to dispel potential misconceptions about their disease and treatment. Attention must be paid to potential sensory and cognitive deficits when medical information is communicated. Rehabilitation (physical, occupational, psychological, prosthetics) is an essential component of any cancer treatment plan for the elderly and often benefits from a multidisciplinary approach.

25. How does the caregiver of the elderly cancer patient cope with the illness?

Studies have compared the experience (depression, lifestyle change, change in health, level of care provided to the patient, level of assistance provided to caregiver by friends and family) of the caregiver based on the age of the patient and the stage of the illness. When the patient is younger, the caregivers tend to be more depressed and experience greater impact on their lifestyle. These same caregivers tend to derive more support from their family and friends. As the patients' disease progresses to its terminal phases, all caregivers, regardless of age, experience higher levels of depression, greater health and lifestyle impact, and increased demands to provide care to the patient. Early phases of the patients' illness tend to place largely emotional stresses on the caregivers, while the burden of providing care to the patient dominates the late phases of the disease. Caregiver strain develops as increasing difficulty arises in the fulfillment of the caregiver's perceived responsibilities. Additionally, the level of practical and social support provided by friends and family tended to remain constant or decrease in the late stages of the illness, leaving the patient and caregiver increasingly isolated.

Physicians and social workers can intervene in this situation to provide caregivers with:

    Home care support (home health aids)

    Financial analysis/assessment of eligibility for resources

Referral to "wellness community" (community-based psychological support groups)
Treatment-center based support groups

BIBLIOGRAPHY

1. Byrne A, Carney DN: Cancer in the elderly. Curr Probl in Cancer 17:147–218, 1993.
2. Cohen HJ: Biology of aging as related to cancer. Cancer 74:2092–2100, 1994.
3. Feldman EJ: Acute myelogenous leukemia in the older patient. Semin Oncol 22(suppl 1):21–24, 1995.
4. Fleming RA, Capizzi RL: General aspects of cancer chemotherapy in the aged. Adv Exp Med Biol 330:271–286, 1993.
5. McKenna RJ Sr: Clinical aspects of cancer in the elderly: Treatment decisions, treatment choices, and follow-up. Cancer 74:2107–2117, 1994.
6. Shell JA, Smith CK: Sexuality and the older person with cancer. Oncol Nurs Forum 21:553–558, 1994.
7. Weinrich S, Sarna L: Delirium in the older person with cancer. Cancer 74:2079–2091, 1994.

41. ADVANCE DIRECTIVES

Joel E. Streim, M.D.

1. What is an advance directive?

A written document, completed by a competent person, that aims to guide health care decisions in the event that the person should become unable to communicate medical preferences or participate in medical decision-making.

2. What are the three different types of advance directives?

Instruction directives indicate the types of treatment or treatment approaches that the person would want in various clinical situations. These typically focus on lifesustaining treatments, though they may also concern less critical treatments. This type of directive may be made informally, through oral instructions given to family members, friends, or caregivers, or formally in a written "living will."

Proxy directives designate someone whom the person wants to make health care decisions on his or her behalf if he or she becomes unable to do so. This is sometimes referred to as a durable power of attorney for health care decisions.

A **values history** may also contain advance directives. This may be a written, audiotaped, or videotaped personal discussion of the person's values and goals. It provides an opportunity to make known one's specific values, beliefs and attitudes regarding life, longevity, quality of life, suffering, the dying process, and death.

3. Explain what is meant by "durable" power of attorney.

When a patient who is still competent designates a proxy decision-maker for health care matters, the patient continues to make autonomous decisions (i.e., without involvement of the proxy) as long as he or she remains competent. Decisions are not made by proxy until the patient becomes incapacitated, at which time the power of attorney "springs" into effect. (For this reason, "durable" power of attorney is sometimes called "springing" power of attorney.) From that point forward, the incapacitated person (whose judgment may now be impaired) cannot rescind the proxy appointment; hence, the power of attorney is said to be durable.

4. What does federal law require of patients regarding advance directives?

The Patient Self-Determination Act was passed by Congress as part of the Omnibus Budget Reconciliation Act of 1990 and became federal law in December 1991 (U.S. Public Law 101-508). Under this law, at the time of admission to an acute care hospital or nursing home that participates in Medicare or Medicaid programs, the admitting facility is required:

1. To ask patients if they have executed an advance directive
2. To furnish them with information about advance directives
3. To inform them of their rights under the law to execute such directives if they wish
4. To inform them of their rights to accept or refuse any form of medical treatment

All patients are thereby given the opportunity to make their preferences for future treatment known to their health care providers. However, patients are not required to draft directives or state their treatment preferences, and their eligibility for admission or treatment is not affected by their having or not having an advance directive.

5. Who should be responsible for discussing advance directives with elderly patients?

Although the staff in a hospital or nursing home admissions office may ask patients about their advance directives to comply with federal law, discussions regarding patient values and treatment preferences are probably best accomplished in the context of an ongoing primary care practitioner–patient relationship, as well as between the patient and trusted family members or friends who might later serve as proxy decision-makers.

6. Are patients who are old and frail likely to become upset when a health care provider asks them to consider hopeless situations or terminal illness?

Most patients who are in the late stages of life, including those who are near death, are relieved when someone asks about their concerns regarding the end of life. Most of them also appreciate the opportunity to express their preferences for how their health care is to be managed. The relatively few patients who are anxious about such matters will decline to discuss them or may be so highly defended that they deny such discussions are applicable to them personally.

7. How should the discussion about advance directives be focused?

While there are no established standards for these discussions, some attempts to develop guidelines in recent years have emphasized the need for patients to communicate a set of life values, even more than choices about specific treatments. This is because it is impossible for patients to anticipate all of the possible future illness and treatment situations, coupled with the presumption that a surrogate or proxy decision-maker will be better able to make a decision that reflects what the patient would have chosen for him or herself if that surrogate is well-informed about the patient's overall values. It is not expected that such discussions will be completed in one session. Getting to know a patient's values is a process that occurs over a series of visits and ideally in the context of an ongoing relationship.

Health care providers must appreciate the ways in which religious beliefs, ethnic background, and family values influence health care directives and decisions. It is important to inquire about the patient's cultural and family background and belief system, so that resultant health care choices can be respected and supported even when based on values that differ from those of the provider. Inclusion of close family members or friends in discussions of values and health care preferences is especially helpful, because they are often in the best position to appreciate nuances of the patient's culture and beliefs, to accept those important factors that serve as the foundation for the patient's directives, and to support the patient's choices regarding future health care.

8. Are health care providers and facilities legally bound to follow all advance directives contained in living wills?

No. Not all states have laws that recognize living wills. For those states that now have living will statutes, most only recognize directives that apply to situations in which a person becomes hopelessly or terminally ill; these states stipulate that patients' directives can be implemented only in conformity with existing laws, including those dealing with suicide and euthanasia. When a patient's living will anticipates clinical conditions that are not hopeless or imminently terminal, or when their directives call for health care options that would violate state or federal law, health care providers and facilities are not bound to follow the directives.

Even in situations that do not entail conflict with the law, health care providers sometimes find that a patient's advance directive is in conflict with the provider's personal or professional values. When this occurs, the health care provider or facility has the option of transferring the patient to the care of a provider or facility that can better abide by the patient's wishes.

9. Is there a legal standard for competency to execute an advance directive?

No. While there are legal standards for testamentary capacity and competency to manage one's affairs, there are no specific guidelines for competency to execute an advance directive. All adults are presumed competent to state their treatment preferences and execute an advance directive under the Patient Self-Determination Act, unless a plenary guardian of the person has been appointed under state law.

10. What happens if cognitive impairment prevents an older adult from establishing an advance directive?

Only a small minority of elderly patients with cognitive impairment are ever brought to court and adjudicated incompetent. After a person has been adjudicated incapacitated or incompetent, under most state laws he or she cannot execute valid advance directives in his or her own behalf. The court-appointed guardian of the person then is empowered to make subsequent health care decisions in the patient's behalf. However, if the patient established a power of attorney for health care matters *before* becoming incapacitated, that power of attorney springs into effect at the time the patient is found on *clinical* grounds to be incapacitated. In such cases, a legal determination of incapacity is usually not necessary.

The remainder of cognitively impaired elders retain their full legal rights to issue advance directives in their own behalf. In some cases, they continue to establish advance directives with insufficient comprehension of what they are choosing, or at the other extreme, clinicians or family members may prematurely usurp their right to make their own decisions. In other cases, when clinicians and family members believe that a patient is losing the cognitive capacity to make such decisions, they informally begin to assist in the decision-making process. Patients with some preserved cognitive function may be allowed to continue to participate in that decision-making process, expressing values and preferences that are then taken into consideration as health care providers and family members make final decisions. As cognitive impairment worsens to the point where the patient is no longer able to understand, deliberate, or communicate anything meaningful about future health care choices, an informal decision-maker is designated. Thus, even in the absence of a legally appointed decision-maker, decisions regarding future health care choices are still made, with the patient fully autonomous, partially included, or fully excluded from the process. The law does not dictate how this should be properly accomplished when patients have less than full decision-making capacity.

11. How should the clinician determine a patient's cognitive capacity to create an advance directive?

In the case of clear and total incapacity (e.g., a persistent vegetative state or coma), it is obvious that the patient cannot formulate advance directives, and there is even no legal obligation to inform the patient of their right to do so. However, in all other cases, on admission to hospitals and nursing homes, patients are required by law to be informed of their right to formulate advance directives and are presumed legally competent to establish such directives. This stands in contrast to epidemiologic estimates that approximately 6 million people in the United States have significant cognitive impairment that renders them clinically incapable of making their own health care decisions. However, no formal clinical standards exist for determining when a patient's cognitive impairment precludes them from being capable of formulating an advance directive or, conversely, when the situation safely permits a cognitively impaired patient to participate in this process.

Nevertheless, during discussions regarding the patient's rights and options in formulating advance directives, clinicians have opportunities to appraise the capacity of patients to:

1. Maintain a stable set of values and goals
2. Comprehend the relevant information
3. Reason and deliberate about their choices
4. Appreciate the situation and its possible outcomes
5. Communicate their choices

When the patient's responses during the informing process give the clinician reason to question the patient's decision-making capacity, it is still left to the clinician to judge how best to balance preservation of the patient's right to make autonomous decisions with the obligation of the clinician to protect a vulnerable patient from making flawed decisions that do not truly reflect the patient's values and goals. Many ethicists and legal scholars have suggested that in determining capacity to formulate advance directives, it is preferable for the clinician to err on the side of promoting patient autonomy. However, this debate is not yet resolved.

12. What is the role of ethics committees in disputes about the patient's ability to participate in the formulation of advance directives?

In many situations, clinicians and family members are able to reach a consensus or agreement regarding the extent to which a patient can participate in the formulation of advance directives. However, when a disagreement cannot be resolved among those who share responsibility for the care of the patient, an ethics committee may play a helpful role, and this approach is generally preferable to resorting to remedies through the legal system. Most hospital ethics committees do not render binding decisions but rather serve in a consultative capacity. They focus the goals of the deliberation, clarify the facts of the case, identify values in conflict, and make recommendations for dealing with conflicts to facilitate decision-making. Unfortunately, for patients residing in the community or in long-term care facilities, the availability of ethics committees is limited.

13. Should elderly patients with mild to moderate cognitive impairment be advised to formulate a durable power of attorney even if they are incapable of making a living will?

Yes. Some elderly patients who are already cognitively impaired at the time they choose to formulate an advance directive may not have the capacity to make a living will, but they may still be capable of appointing a health care proxy and should be given the opportunity to do so for legal, ethical, and pragmatic reasons. This important step can avert the need to petition for legal guardianship at a later date when the patient is totally incapacitated. In most states, appointment of a health care proxy is much simpler, less costly, and less time-consuming than establishing a guardianship.

14. What standards or guidelines exist for surrogate decision-making by persons appointed as proxies or guardians?

There are two main ethical standards by which surrogates can make health care decisions on behalf of incapacitated patients. The preferred standard is **substituted judgment**. This directs the surrogate to choose what he or she believes the patient would have chosen. If the surrogate decision-maker has no knowledge of what the patient would want in a given situation, then the surrogate can follow the **best interest principle**. This directs the surrogate to make the choice that is most likely to serve the best interests of the patient. When surrogates are faced with difficult decisions and unclear parameters on which to base their decisions, they can appeal for advice from health care professionals, attorneys, and hospital ethics committees. In some communities, guardianship advisory services have recently been developed.

BIBLIOGRAPHY

1. Diamond EL, Jernigan JA, Moseley RA, et al: Decision-making ability and advance directive preferences in nursing home patients and proxies. Gerontologist 29:622–626, 1989.
2. Gerety MB, Chiodo LK, Kanten DN, et al: Medical treatment preferences of nursing home residents: Relationship to function and concordance with surrogate decision-makers. J Am Geriatr Soc 41:953–960, 1993.
3. Kern SR: Issues of competency in the aged. Psychiatr Ann 17:336–339, 1987.
4. Omnibus Budget Reconciliation Act, 1990. U.S. Public Law 101-508, sect 4206 and 4751.
5. President's Commission for the Study of Ethical Problems in Medicine and Biomedical and Behavioral Research: Making Health Care Decisions, vol 1. Washington, D.C., Government Printing Office, 1982.
6. Singer PA, Siegler M: Advancing the cause of advance directives. Arch Intern Med 152:22–24, 1992.

42. ASSESSING FUNCTION

Keith M. Robinson, M.D.

1. What is functional assessment?

Functional assessment is the measurement of a patient's performance of the survival skills required to negotiate everyday life. Traditionally, it has focused on those skills that relate to basic physical and cognitive functions:

Self-care
    Activities of daily living
    Instrumental activities of daily living
Mobility/balance
Comprehension/communication

These skills generally can be thought of as those required to function safely within one's household and effectively in the local community.

Functional Survival Skills

	SELF-CARE	MOBILITY	COMMUNICATION

Household	Eating/drinking
	Bathing/grooming
	Dressing
	Toileting
	Bowel/bladder control
	Sexuality
	Cooking
	Laundry
	Housekeeping
	Taking medications
		Bed mobility
		Transfers, e.g., bed to chair,
		  chair to toilet, chair to shower
		  seat
		Ambulation with or without
		  an assistive device, level vs.
		  nonlevel surfaces (e.g., stairs)
		Balance
		Wheelchair ambulation and
		  parts management
			Hearing
			Vision
			Orientation
			Attention
			Memory
			Language (talking,
			  gesturing)
			Spatial perception
			Organization
			Problem-solving

Community	Prevocational and
	  vocational skills
	Shopping
	Banking
	Managing financial
	  and legal affairs
		Nonlevel surface ambulation,
		  with or without an assistive
		  device, (e.g., curbs, ramps,
		  uneven terrain)
		Community wheelchair ambu-
		  lation (manual vs. motorized)
		Driving
		Using public transportation,
		  e.g., bus, taxi, wheelchair, van
			Using telephones
			Writing/typing/word
			  processing
			Supervising others in
			  self-care and
			  mobility needs

2. Is functional assessment different in older people?

More functional disability is observed during normal aging. Community surveys of older Americans have documented that:

- 25% have difficulty performing heavy housework
- 20% have difficulty walking
- 10% have difficulty bathing, managing money, and using the telephone
- 5% have difficulty dressing, using the toilet, and eating

The elderly residing in long-term care institutions suffer with even more disabilities:

- 70% require assistance with toileting and transfers from bed to chair
- 50% have bowel or bladder incontinence
- 40% require assistance when eating

3. How is functional ability assessed?

The individual must be observed in relation to his or her environment. A comprehensive survey includes essential physical and cognitive functioning, the physical environment of the patient, the socioeconomic situation of the patient, and the patient's wishes concerning quality of life.

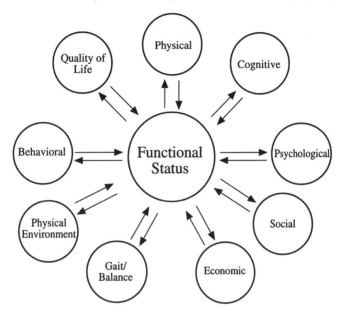

Comprehensive geriatric functional assessment.

The use of **measurement tools** to assess function has advantages and disadvantages. These tools attempt to quantify behavior and can be useful in documenting changes that occur with progressive illness or treatment, yet there are limitations to a quantitative approach. If the instrument relies on self-reports, validity is often in question. When behaviors are reduced to a numerical score, nuances that may be crucial to performance may be missed. These behaviors often are important to observe since they can be the target of specific rehabilitation interventions aimed toward optimizing function.

In **clinical practice**, functional assessment measurement tools can be used to guide a more qualitative approach for assessing function in the outpatient office or at the bedside. A quick survey of the major aspects of comprehensive functional assessment can be integrated into the traditional medical history and physical examination. Patients typically present to clinicians with **functional complaints** (e.g., falling, forgetting). The differential diagnostic approach to medical problem-solving is also quite effective in organizing functional complaints into a hierarchy of etiologies regarding impaired anatomy and physiology. The clinician must come full circle and consider the identified disease(s) and anatomic or physiologic impairment(s) more explicitly within the context of the patient's everyday life and his or her physical and socioeconomic environment. Practical solutions then may emerge for enhancing patient function with such an approach.

4. Who should do what parts in a comprehensive assessment of an older adult?

Comprehensive functional assessment is time- and labor-intensive. The physician usually is neither trained nor expected to perform such an evaluation alone or at one point in time. However, the physician is expected to be familiar with critical areas of everyday life and the contextual forces that define the lives of older patients. The physician must orchestrate the assessment by involving specific key personnel who can assist in providing this information. Further, the physician must synthesize this information so that medical decisions can be based on it. The table presents a possible division of labor among specialists who can be consulted to participate in the comprehensive functional assessment of the older adult. Many of these consultants are nonmedical rehabilitation specialists. Often, consultation with one of them or a physiatrist, who is an expert in functional assessment and functionally oriented treatments, can be useful for facilitating the functional assessment and appropriate treatment interventions aimed to enhance or stabilize function of their older patients.

Nonmedical Specialists Who Participate in Geriatric Functional Assessment

Physical therapist—Basic mobility skills including bed mobility, transfers, wheelchair mobility; ambulation, assistive devices for ambulation including canes, walkers, and wheelchairs; spasticity management with therapeutic exercises; sensory facilitation of motor control; gait training, including training with orthotic and prosthetic devices of the lower limb.

Occupational therapist—Daily living skills including feeding, grooming, toileting, dressing, and homemaking; fine motor skills of the hand and upper limbs, including splinting (orthotics) and wheelchair accessories; cognitive remediation, especially memory and visuoperception; driving evaluation.

Speech/swallowing therapist—Cognitive remediation related to communication, especially in attention, memory, language comprehension, conceptual organization, language production (including nonverbal technologies); swallowing as it relates to oral-motor and pharyngeal function, aspiration precaution, and oral feeding with different food consistencies

Neuropsychologist—Formal, in-depth, and quantitative evaluation of cognitive and intellectual function; translation of the cognitive profile of intellectual strengths and weaknesses into a behaviorally based set of strategies subsequently used by therapists, nurses, family members, and other care providers.

Behavioral psychologist—Explicit design of behavioral management strategies and programs (often in concert with medications) aimed at optimizing communication for patients having difficulty with self-monitoring, aggression, poor initiation, and other behaviors that disrupt rehabilitation treatments and social interactions.

Counseling psychologist—Psychotherapeutic treatment (often in concert with medications) of loss reactions, depression, and other affective disorders observed during recovery and sometimes disruptive to participation in therapeutic programs.

Recreation therapist—Evaluation and remediation of motor and cognitive function in both individual and group nondidactic settings while focusing on participation in leisure activities.

Case manager—Orchestrates appropriate medical, surgical, rehabilitation, and social services depending on the recovery trajectory, treatment priorities, and health insurance financial resources.

Social worker—Clarifies social support system, its ability to provide safe and stable emotional support, residential sites, personal care, and transportation; clarifies eligibility and coverage of health and welfare services and health insurance plans; mobilizes resources for coverage of essential health and rehabilitation services with informal and formal care providers acting in complementary roles; often defines the discharge plan; provides emotional support for patients and their social support system members.

Nurse—Assists and supervises the patient in using cognitive and functional skills learned in therapies; patient education of medication schedules and self-monitoring of medical problems, such as diabetes, seizure disorders, skin care, bowel and bladder training programs; facilitates coping to loss and adaptation to illness.

Nutritionist—Collaborates with physicians, nurses and therapists to establish caloric and nutritional needs during recovery; makes recommendations for nutritional support depending on the most reliable means of entry of food (oral, enteral, parenteral) and dietary advancement.

Prosthetist/orthotist—Assesses need for, and fabricates body part replacements in, amputees (prosthesis); assesses need for and fabricates devices that facilitate motor control and conserve energy consumption during mobility (orthotics), especially of lower limbs.

5. Can the traditional physical exam be changed to include a better assessment of functional status?

The traditional medical approach to data collection (history and physical examination) and differential diagnosis deconstructs the individual into a conglomeration of impaired anatomic and physiologic functions and organ systems. The power of this approach must be appreciated for making causal connections that may help to understand an individual patient's disability and handicap. Further, these organ-specific indicators become essential for measuring efficacy of medical and surgical treatments. Yet, these provide incomplete measurements of function.

The World Health Organization model becomes useful for considering function at several levels and then directs us how to extend medical data collection and problem-solving to enhance measurement of function. **Impairment** defines function at the organ system level and is measured by such indicators as pulmonary function tests and cardiac ejection fraction. **Disability** defines function of the individual in the form described under Question 1. **Handicap** defines function of the individual in relation to social roles, such as work and interpersonal aspects of living. This conceptual approach seems intuitive and common-sensical, but data collection beyond the level of impairment too often is forgotten during evaluation of older adults.

As defined in Question 1, a survey of survival skill performance is recommended to improve traditional medical history-taking. Similarly, the traditional physical exam provides limited data from which the clinician can extrapolate the functioning of the person in his or her immediate environment. For example, the presence of spastic and paretic limbs during the elementary neurologic exam provides limited data for predicting ability to transfer and walk. But direct observation of the patient performing these activities in the office or at the bedside may again provide further data to predict his or her abilities. By asking care providers and key members of a patient's social support system in the home, community, or work environments to verify the patient's self-reports and your observations of the patient's functional performance, you can gain a broader view of the functional status within his or her larger community.

6. How does mental status affect the evaluation of functional abilities?

The successful performance of most functional activities requires that basic cognitive domains (attention, memory) and higher-level cognitive domains (language, visuoperception, executive functioning) be relatively intact. The Mini-Mental Status Examination (MMSE) is a widely used screening tool. It is, however, a poor predictor of function. When comprehensive evaluation of functional abilities is required and the MMSE is abnormal, formal cognitive testing should be requested. (See Chapter 26.)

7. How are gait, balance, and falling risk evaluated in the older adult?

Risk Factors for Falling

Lower limb impairment	Generalized weakness
Visual impairment	Environmental hazards
Previous stroke	Orthostatic hypotension
Parkinson's disease	Benzodiazepine use
Barbiturate use	Antihypertensive agents/diuretics

The basic cardiopulmonary and elementary neurologic examinations provide limited information for assessing gait, balance, and falling risk. Observing the simulated or actual performance of transfers and ambulation during the physical assessment becomes essential. A baseline heart rate, blood pressure, and respiratory rate should always be compared to their response immediately after a transfer and/or ambulation trial, and then during the recovery period after the activity in the office or at the bedside. This informal clinical exercise-tolerance test can provide input regarding overall level of endurance and ability to conserve energy during movement.

A directed gait evaluation as well must be performed. To do this, a basic understanding of the normal gait cycle is necessary. Additionally, observation of the patient transferring between different surfaces that are at different heights (e.g., soft mattress to low bedside chair or commode) can be useful to assess falling risk during this aspect of basic mobility. (See Chapter 23.)

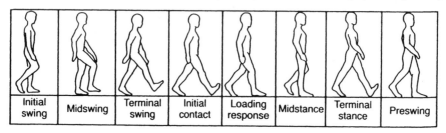

| Initial swing | Midswing | Terminal swing | Initial contact | Loading response | Midstance | Terminal stance | Preswing |

The gait cycle.

8. Describe a simple test for evaluating mobility and falling risk.

A useful instrument for assessing mobility and falling risk in the elderly is the modified **"Get Up and Go" test**. This test is done in ambulatory patients only. One practice run is allowed. The physician makes qualitative observations about each aspect of the mobility trial:

1. The patient should sit comfortably in a straight-backed, high-seat chair with arm rests.
2. Ask the patient to rise from the chair (with or without an assistive device, as is his or her usual manner of ambulation).
3. Ask the patient to stand still momentarily (10 sec) with eyes open (with or without an assistive device, as is his/her usual manner).
4. Ask the patient to stand still momentarily (10 sec) with eyes closed (again with or without an assistive device). You may need to guard them from falling.
5. Ask the patient to walk approximately 50 ft forward (with or without a device and/or assistance as appropriate, preferably toward a wall).
6. Ask the patient to turn around at the end of 50 ft.
7. Ask the patient to walk back to the chair, another 50 ft, to the original destination.
8. Ask the patient to sit down when he/she reaches the chair.

9. When are assistive devices such as canes or wheelchairs useful?

Before you recommend a specific assistive device, the weight-bearing status of the legs must be established (e.g., by the orthopedic surgeon in a patient recovering from joint replacement surgery or by the vascular surgeon in someone recovering from a vascular bypass procedure in the legs).

- Ambulation in parallel bars in physical therapy, with a walker or crutches, requires full weight-bearing by both arms and at least 50% to full weight-bearing by one leg. Use of crutches requires better dynamic standing balance than use of a walker.
- Use of a walker with wheels is appropriate when weight-bearing by all four extremities is permitted and when dynamic standing balance is compromised (e.g., in a patient with a parkinsonian gait with retropulsion).
- Ambulation with a hemi-cane, quad cane, or straight cane requires full weight-bearing by the arm in which the cane is held and in the leg on the same side, and at least 50% to full weight-bearing on the other leg that is to be unloaded. Ambulation with a cane requires good dynamic standing balance. The patient should hold the cane in the hand/arm opposite the impaired leg.

In all assistive devices, the level of hand placement (i.e., cane/walker height from the floor) is generally at the level of the greater trochanter of the hip. This position allows for approximately 20–30° of elbow flexion and the most efficient length-tension cocontraction relationship of the elbow flexors and extensors.

10. Why is an environmental evaluation important during the functional assessment of an older adult?

The environment in which a person lives should be evaluated to reduce physical barriers that prevent the elderly patient from living in his or her home. The presence of stairs on entry or inside the household may limit someone with ambulatory dysfunction to a homebound status or to one floor of their household, temporarily or permanently. If a patient ultimately proves unable to ambulate on stairs, ramping for community access, motorized wheelchairs or scooters for longer-distance ambulation, and stair-lifts or stair-glides may be considered. These are expensive and often not reimbursable by health insurance payers. Older adults with limited incomes usually cannot afford such items.

Setting up a safe, convenient, limited environment becomes acceptable to some disabled older adults when they are confined to one floor of their households:

1. Placement of essential items within reach in the kitchen can facilitate control and energy conservation during meal preparation.

2. In homes without accessible bathrooms, kitchen sinks can be adapted and bedside commodes can be used for bathing and toileting.

3. In homes with accessible bathrooms, inexpensive insurance-reimbursable equipment, such as long-handled reachers and sponges, hand-held showers, tub/shower seats, toilet/shower bars, and raised toilet seats, can be easily installed.

4. Expensive equipment, such as hydraulically controlled tub chair lifts, will require fastidious medical documentation to justify for insurance reimbursement.

5. Hospital beds with electrical controls to raise the head of the bed may help with out-of-bed transfers and re-positioning while in bed to prevent skin breakdown.

6. Lifeline systems (not insurance reimbursable) may be useful to those who live alone and are at high risk for falling.

7. Memory cueing systems in the form of signs and log books can help the forgetful person in performing specific activities, such as turning off the stove or lights.

Homecare agencies provide physical and occupational therapist who can perform home-environment assessments and make recommendations for medically necessary equipment to reduce physical barriers and optimize functional control in one's home.

11. Why is an evaluation of the social and economic context important during the functional assessment of the older adult?

The social support system surrounding the elderly patient is the major determinant for whether an elderly person can live at home again after hospitalization. Medicare reimbursement for skilled nursing or therapy services is generous but incomplete, typically limiting home health care/homemaker sessions to 9 hours over a 7-day week. This may be satisfactory for some patients, but many older people require ongoing supervision to compensate for cognitive deficits, physical assistance to perform regular toilet or commode transfers, and community-based transportation to attend outpatient visits, shop, and bank.

All possible resources must be explored in the informal care network surrounding older patients to maintain them in their own homes. The economic resources of the patient, including personal income and health insurance benefits, determine the consuming power of the older adult who requires purchase of formal services and durable medical equipment to be maintained in his/her own home. Yet, many middle-class American elderly, who are beneficiaries of Social Security and Medicare as well as secondary forms of health insurance, and who have good pension plans, cannot afford to live at home and pay for part-time or full-time home care services when necessary.

12. Is relocation to a planned community for the elderly a reliable option?

Many planned communities are being developed in this country that promise lifetime supervision and care regardless of intensity of need. However, these are expensive to buy into and are considered either risky investments or a compromise in control for some elderly people who have experienced immigration, a major economic depression, and several world wars. Some local communities have active, government-supported Agencies on Aging (AOA) that can subsidize the purchase of home-care services for income-limited disabled older adults, but medical and functional justification must be argued and waiting-lists can be long. Consultation with the social work department of the hospital or of a long-term case facility is the best strategy for implementing these recommendations.

13. What is deconditioning?

Deconditioning is a syndrome of negative anatomic and physiologic effects resulting from inactivity, bedrest, and sedentary lifestyles. With therapeutic exercise programs which primarily aim to increase cardiopulmonary endurance and muscle strength and endurance, these effects are reversible. Bedrest and inactivity can be viewed as sometimes necessary treatments in acutely ill people, but with undesirable side effects, i.e., the deconditioning syndrome.

The Deconditioning Syndrome: Effects of Inactivity and Bedrest

Musculoskeletal	**Genitourinary**
Joint contractures	Increased incidence of bladder/renal stones,
Arthrogenic	UTI, and difficulty in voiding
Soft tissue contracture	Incomplete bladder emptying
Myogenic contracture	**Respiratory**
Muscle weakness and atrophy	Diminished tidal volumes, minute volumes,
Decreased coordination	and maximal breathing capacity
Osteoporosis	Reduction in vital capacity and functional
Integument	reserve capacity
Skin atrophy	Increased respiratory rate
Pressure sores	Uneven distribution of secretions, difficulty
Cardiovascular	in clearance of secretions
Orthostatic hypotension	Impaired coughing mechanism/reduced
Increased resting heart rate	bronchial ciliary activity
Elevated systolic blood pressure	**Gastrointestinal**
Reduced stroke volume	Loss of appetite
Decline in cardiac output	Atrophy of intestinal mucosa and glands
Stasis of blood flow	Slower rate of absorption
Increased coagulability	Distaste for protein-rich foods
Endocrine/Metabolic	Constipation
Carbohydrate intolerance	Inhibition of peristalsis
Increase in serum parathyroid hormone	**Neural**
Decreased androgen level and	Sensory deprivation
spermatogenesis	Impaired balance and coordination
Increased daily nitrogen loss	Confusion and disorientation
Negative calcium balance	Anxiety and depression
Decreased Na, K	Decreased intellectual capacity

14. How are the functional consequences of deconditioning evaluated?

The assessment of the functional consequences of deconditioning focuses on cardiopulmonary endurance and on muscle strength and endurance. The length of time of required bedrest should be established, as well as the level of activity prior to bedrest. The less active a person is before forced bedrest, and the longer the period of inactivity, the more deconditioned and the longer it will take for this person to remobilize to an acceptable activity level during recovery.

The **cardiopulmonary effects** of deconditioning are fairly evident on physical examination during informal exercise tolerance testing as the reversal of cardiopulmonary conditioning or training effects: orthostatic hypotension, resting tachycardia (at least 90 bpm), abrupt increase in heart rate and respiratory rate (and sometimes systolic blood pressure) in response to minimal activity, and prolonged time to re-achieve baseline heart rate and blood pressure after discontinuing exercise. During one-trial manual **muscle testing**, strength and active range of motion may be interpreted as normal. Poor muscle endurance will be observed, however, only during repetitive (e.g., 10-trial) antigravity movements. Soft-tissue contractures (especially shoulders and heel cords) may be evident only at end-range.

Poor cardiopulmonary fitness, muscle endurance, and weakness from inactivity may not necessarily be manifest without observing the patient trying to rise from a supine position, arising from a chair, reaching overhead, or standing/weight-shifting in place for 20–30 seconds. A pattern of proximal weakness often is observed during deconditioning, since the larger muscle groups of the shoulder and hip girdles are more demanding of oxygen during antigravity movements.

15. Can deconditioning be avoided in these severely ill patients?

The effects of deconditioning can be disastrous for an older adult. Simple bedside therapeutic exercises, initiated even in the intensive care unit during the acute phase of illness and recovery, can alleviate inactivity effects:

Clearance out of bed to a chair for upright (not reclined or semireclined) sitting and progressive sitting protocols

Bathroom privileges to a bedside commode

Progressive gentle strengthening, endurance, and range of motion exercises and ventilatory muscle exercises

Ankle pumps to facilitate lower limb venous return

Bedside sitting, standing and weight-shifting activities

Progressive daily ambulation trials

Many of these therapeutic exercises can be supervised by nursing staff after consultation with physical and occupational therapists.

16. What aging-related factors influence a person's driving ability?

The ability to drive defines independence for many older adults. When you suggest to older adults that it is unsafe for them to drive, this represents a major threat to their sense of control in everyday life.

Driving is a highly integrative cognitive and motor task requiring sustained visual attention, adequate speed of mental processing and motor reaction time, and cardiopulmonary endurance. There is a growing literature that defines which older adults are at risk for being in driving accidents or having traffic violations. For example, diabetics who have frequent hypoglycemic episodes or people with heart disease with poor cardiopulmonary endurance and conduction abnormalities causing syncopal episodes are especially at risk. Visual impairments, hearing deficits, diminished proprioceptive sense (to appreciate foot movements across the pedals), and diminished proximal muscle control (to control foot pedals and the steering wheel) are aging-related changes that influence driving skills.

17. How is driving safety evaluated?

Given the limitations of making a decision about an older patient's driving safety based on a bedside or office-based examination, observing the older patient while driving is simulated or while actually driving is recommended. During history-taking, driving performance can be indirectly verified or disputed through questioning a significant other who frequently rides (or refuses to ride) with the patient.

Referral to an occupational therapist (usually insurance-reimbursable) for a formal driving screening should be made. Driving screenings at best simulate driving using video and at least probe those specific cognitive and motor skills required during driving, which are then compared to age-appropriate norms. Poor performance on a driving screen may be enough to convince an unsafe driver to stop. If not, then referral via occupational therapy to a regional driving evaluation and training center for a performance-based evaluation and driver's training is necessary. If the patient fails this, then he or she will have to forfeit his or her driver's license.

Many states have legislation requiring physicians to report disabled patients to their registry of motor vehicles, even if they are unable to drive only temporarily. If reported by a physician, a patient must participate in a more complete medical evaluation.

Driving Risk Factors

DISEASES/MEDICATIONS	IMPAIRMENTS

Heart disease with arrhythmias or compromised cardiac output causing syncope and poor ambulatory endurance	Sensory-motor
	  Visual impairment
	    Acuity
	    Fields
	    Scanning
	    Binocular vision
	    Night/twilight vision adaptation
	    Light sensitivity

Alcoholism	Poor cardiopulmonary endurance during community ambulation
Depression	Feet abnormalities
Diabetes mellitus, esp. if insulin-dependent and with retinopathy	Slow reaction time
Glaucoma	Vestibular dysfunction
Cataracts	Proprioceptive deficits
Macular degeneration	Proximal weakness

Psychotropic medications, esp. benzodiazepines and tricyclic antidepressants	Cognitive/behavioral
	  Low MMSE score
	  Sustained visual inattention or poor attentional vigilance
	  Slow speed of information or mental processing
	  Visuospatial-perceptual deficits
	  Executive dysfunction (including poor motor initiation and poor motor planning)
	  Distractibility

BIBLIOGRAPHY

1. Applegate WB, Blass JP, Williams TF: Instruments for the functional assessment of older patients. N Engl J Med 322:1201–1214, 1990.
2. Dawson D, Hendershot G, Fulton J: Aging in the eighties: Functional limitations of individuals 65 years and over. Adv Data 133:1–12, 1987. [National Center for Health Statistics, publication no. (PHS) 87-1250.]
3. Fleming KC, Evans JM, Weber DC, Chutka DS: Practical functional assessment of elderly persons: A primary-care approach. Mayo Clinic Proc 70:890–910, 1995.
4. Heaton RK, Pendleton MG: Use of neuropsychological tests to predict adult patients' everyday functioning. J Consult Clin Psychol 49:807–821, 1981.
5. Mathias S, Nayak US, Isaacs B: Balance in elderly patients: The "get-up and go" test. Arch Phys Med Rehabil 67:387–389, 1986.
6. Siebens H: Deconditioning. In Kemp B, Brummel-Smith K, Rarnsdell JW (eds): Geriatric Rehabilitation. Boston, Little, Brown, 1990, pp 177–191.
7. Tinetti ME, Williams TF, Mayewski R: Fall risk index for elderly patients based on number of chronic disabilities. Am J Med 80:429–434, 1986.

43. CORONARY ARTERY DISEASE

Joseph R. McClellan, M.D.

1. Is coronary atherosclerosis a universal consequence of aging?

The incidence of significant coronary atherosclerosis progressively increases with age, but the disease is not a universal accompaniment of the aging process. All coronary events, including angina, unstable angina, and acute myocardial infarction (MI), increase in frequency with aging. Epidemiologic studies demonstrate that approximately 30% of patients over the age of 75 have evidence of symptomatic coronary artery disease. At necropsy, approximately 60% of octogenarians and 90+% of nonagenarians have one or more coronary arteries with a 75% or greater reduction in luminal cross-sectional area caused by an atherosclerotic plaque. In addition, in older patients coronary disease is often extensive and diffuse, with generalized coronary calcification and a higher proportion of multivessel and left main disease.

2. Are the symptoms of coronary artery disease different in the elderly?

Acute and chronic coronary syndromes are less frequently recognized in the elderly. There appears to be a reduced sensitivity to pain, which results in a high incidence of silent myocardial ischemia and unrecognized acute MI. The Framingham study found that in patients aged 75–84, 42% of MIs in men and 36% of MIs in women were clinically unrecognized. This impairment in pain perception may lead to delays in seeking treatment as well as prolong the time to accurate diagnosis and institution of effective treatment strategies. The presenting features of acute MI are also different in the elderly. The incidence of typical chest pain decreases, and neurologic symptoms, including syncope, confusion, and dyspnea, predominate, especially in octogenarians. According to Bayer,[1] the most common symptom in patients over 85 years old is dyspnea; chest pain is second in frequency. Among patients younger than 75, however, the majority have chest pain. In patients over 85, MI, syncope, and confusion are much more frequent than in patients under 75. The development of angina in elderly patients strongly correlates with the presence of coronary disease. In addition, patients over 75 years old with chronic angina have a high likelihood of severe, multivessel coronary disease.

3. Should the diagnostic approach to coronary artery disease in the elderly be altered?

Cardiac catheterization remains the gold standard for the diagnosis of coronary disease and is required prior to coronary revascularization procedures. However, catheterization in the elderly has a higher complication rate, including increased vascular and dye-related complications as well as thromboembolic events. Noninvasive strategies are often preferable for initial diagnosis.

Routine exercise testing has an important role in the diagnosis of coronary disease in older patients. Because of the increased prevalence of coronary disease, the diagnostic accuracy of an abnormal stress EKG is increased in elderly patients. However, elderly patients often have additional medical problems, such as vascular or musculoskeletal disease, that limit exercise capacity and the use of treadmill testing for the diagnosis of coronary disease. Also, the baseline electrocardiogram is more likely to be abnormal as a result of coexisting conditions such as hypertension or valvular heart disease, which reduce the reliability of stress EKG interpretation. In such situations, pharmacologic stress testing with associated myocardial perfusion imaging is especially useful. Dipyridamole and dobutamine stress testing with either thallium or Tc-99m sestamibi provides accurate diagnostic and prognostic information equal to maximal exercise testing. Similarly, dobutamine two-dimensional echocardiography is a highly sensitive and specific method for the diagnosis of coronary artery disease.

4. Is modification of coronary risk factors less important in the elderly?

The importance of the well-known coronary risk factors persists in the elderly and attempts at modification should remain vigorous.

- Hypertension, including isolated elevation of systolic pressure, is a major risk factor in older patients for the development of coronary artery events as well as stroke (see chapters 20 and 36). Treatment of isolated systolic hypertension in the elderly results in a substantial reduction in stroke, cardiac death, nonfatal MI, and all cardiovascular events.
- Cigarette smoking in patients over the age of 65 is associated with a 50% increase in coronary mortality compared with nonsmokers. Cessation of smoking probably lowers this risk substantially.
- Hypercholesterolemia is also a significant independent predictor of increased coronary events in the elderly. However, less information is available about the value of treatment in older patients. Recent secondary and primary prevention trials from Scandinavia and West Scotland, respectively, demonstrated a striking reduction in cardiac mortality and nonfatal MI in patients with elevated cholesterol who were treated with HMG CoA reductase inhibitors. Of importance, significant risk reduction was seen in the first 6 months of treatment. Although, these results may not be totally reproducible in the elderly, the early benefit of therapy suggests that improvement of hypercholesterolemia with these agents will also be valuable in older patients.
- Other well-recognized risk factors, including elevated blood sugar and left ventricular hypertrophy, are also associated with increased coronary risk in older populations.

5. Is age an important risk factor in patients with an acute MI?

Age is a significant independent risk factor for mortality and serious morbidity in patients with an acute MI. Various clinical trials have documented the important effect of age on in-hospital mortality. In the first cooperative Italian streptokinase trial (GISSI), the mortality in the control group was 7.7% in patients under 65 and 33.1% in patients over 75. Similarly, the Worcester Heart Attack Study reported that mortality progressively increased with advancing age. Other major complications, including stroke, heart block, cardiogenic shock, congestive heart failure, pulmonary edema, cardiac rupture, and other mechanical complications, also increase in frequency with advanced age. This significant increase in mortality and complication rates makes the administration of prompt, effective therapy most important in elderly patients with an acute MI.

6. Are elderly patients candidates for thrombolytic therapy?

Many trials of thrombolytic therapy for acute MI excluded patients over the age of 70. However, data from GISSI, the second International Study of Infarct Survival (ISIS-II), and the recent International Trial Comparing Four Thrombolytic Strategies for Acute Myocardial Infarction (GUSTO trial) have demonstrated or suggested significant benefit of thrombolytic therapy in patients older than 65 years. The GISSI and ISIS-II trials compared streptokinase with placebo. In GISSI the mortality in patients over 75 treated with thrombolytic therapy decreased from 33.1% to 28.9%, and in ISIS-II the mortality in patients over 69 decreased from 21.6% to 18.2%. Because of the relatively high mortality, the greatest absolute benefit of thrombolysis was obtained in the older age groups. The combined mortality in the GUSTO trial of patients over 75, treated with either tissue plasminogen activator (TPA) or streptokinase, was 20%, which suggests a significant benefit from thrombolytic agents compared with historical, infarct-related mortality rates in this age group. Caution must temper the use of thrombolytics in the elderly. The incidence of stroke after thrombolytic therapy is increased in elderly patients, and other contraindications may also be more common. However, the benefit of thrombolytic therapy persists despite the increased risk of stroke. When contraindications prevent the use of thrombolytics, primary coronary angioplasty may be an effective alternative approach.

7. Should other medical therapies be altered in elderly patients with coronary artery disease?

In general, effective treatment strategies and beneficial therapies have a similar impact on morbidity and mortality in elderly and younger patients. Aspirin and beta-blockers maintain a central role in treatment of coronary artery disease and prevention of recurrent cardiac events. However, in elderly patients various alterations in drug absorption, distribution, and metabolism may affect both physiologic responses and toxicity. Both hepatic metabolism and renal excretion diminish with age. Extracellular volume diminishes, and the volume of distribution of hydrophilic drugs also decreases. In addition, end-organ responsiveness may be altered. For example, the decrease in responsiveness to adrenergic stimulation with aging may affect the cardiovascular response to beta blockade. The incidence of significant bradycardia and congestive failure after beta-blockade therapy increases with advancing age. Elderly patients may be more prone to digitalis toxicity because of reduced volume of distribution and renal clearance.

Another important physiologic alteration in older patients is a reduction in the sensitivity of the carotid baroreceptors, which blunts the cardiovascular responses to vasodilation and positional changes. Altered baroreceptor function and decreased extracellular volume increase the likelihood of orthostatic hypotension and adverse reactions to vasodilating drugs such as nitrates. In addition, significant volume reduction with diuretics may have magnified effects on posture-related changes in blood pressure. Overall, careful individualization of drug therapy is especially important in elderly patients.

8. How useful is coronary artery bypass surgery in older patients?

A randomized prospective trial comparing the impact on survival of coronary artery bypass surgery and medical therapy in elderly patients has not been performed. Older patients were excluded from the major randomized trials, including the Veterans' Administration Cooperative Trial, the Coronary Artery Surgical Study, and the European Cooperative Trial. However, many investigators have reported their experiences with bypass surgery in patients over 65, including a significant number of octogenarians. In general, elderly patients have significant symptomatic improvement after revascularization. However, operative mortality rates are increased (reported at 9–30% in octogenarians). Surgical morbidity remains a significant problem in all patients who undergo coronary bypass surgery. Perioperative delirium and mental confusion, stroke, MI, postoperative infection, and length of mechanical ventilation and hospitalization increase with advancing age. A number of factors may contribute to the higher morbidity and mortality. Elderly patients undergoing surgery have more frequent unstable symptoms, greater impairment in ventricular function, and a higher incidence of diabetes and other comorbid illness that contribute to the increased surgical risk. Surgery is usually reserved for elderly patients with extremely high-risk anatomy, such as left main or high-grade proximal three-vessel disease, extensive myocardial ischemia, or persistent symptoms despite optimal medical management.

9. Are catheter-based interventions such as percutaneous transluminal coronary angioplasty (PTCA) useful alternatives to surgery in older patients?

Coronary angioplasty has been successfully used in elderly patients for relief of symptoms and improvement in functional status. In addition, "culprit" angioplasty, which focuses on the vessel most likely accounting for ischemia and symptoms, may obviate the need for surgery in patients with multivessel coronary disease. However, PTCA in elderly patients has a lower initial success rate and higher rates of morbidity, mortality, and clinical restenosis compared with younger patients. A report from the clinical PTCA registry maintained by the National Heart, Lung and Blood Institute (NHLBI) compared results in 486 patients over age 65 and 1315 patients under age 65 for the years 1985–1986. Patients over 65 had a higher in-hospital mortality rate (3.1% vs. 0.2%) and more frequent needs for emergent (5.4% vs. 2.8%) and elective (3.9% vs. 1.6%) bypass surgery. Enhanced interventional techniques and the use of coronary stents and new anticoagulation agents and strategies are likely to improve the results of these procedures.

Coronary angioplasty is also successfully used in patients with acute MI as an alternative to thrombolysis. Primary angioplasty has a success rate similar to thrombolysis in restoring arterial patency and reducing mortality without the risk of increased hemorrhagic complications. Because of the high mortality rates of acute MI, especially in the anterior wall, elderly patients with a contraindication to thrombolytics may be an important target group for primary angioplasty. Further studies are necessary to define precisely the optimal role of PTCA in elderly patients.

BIBLIOGRAPHY

1. Bayer AJ, Chadha JS, Farag RR, Pahy MS: Changing presentations of myocardial infarction with increasing old age. J Am Geriatr Soc 34:263–266, 1986.
2. Goldberg RJ, Gore JM, Gurwitz JH, et al: The impact of age on the incidence and prognosis of initial acute myocardial infarction: The Worcester Heart Attack Study. Am Heart J 117:543–548, 1989.
3. Gruppo Italiano per lo Studio della Streptochinasi nell'Infarto Miocardio (GISSI): Effectiveness of intravenous thrombolytic treatment in acute myocardial infarction. Lancet i:397–401, 1986.
4. GUSTO investigators: An international randomized trial comparing four thrombolytic strategies for acute myocardial infarction. N Engl J Med 329:673–682, 1993.
5. ISIS-II (Second International Study of Infarct Survival) Collaborative Group: Randomized trial of intravenous streptokinase, oral aspirin, both or neither among 17,187 cases of suspected acute myocardial infarction: ISIS-II. Lancet ii:348–359, 1988.
6. Kelsey SF, Miller DP, Holubkov R, et al: Results of percutaneous transluminal coronary angioplasty in patients over 65 years of age. Am J Cardiol 66:1033–1038, 1990.
7. Scandanavian Simvastatin Survival Study Group: Randomized trial of cholesterol lowering in 4444 patients with coronary heart disease: The Scandanavian Simvastatin Survival Study (4S). Lancet 344:1383–1389, 1994.
8. Shirani J, Yousefi J, Roberts WC: Major cardiac findings at necropsy in 366 American octogenarians. Am J Cardiol 75:151–156, 1995.

44. HEART FAILURE IN THE ELDERLY

Iris Reyes, M.D., and Jerry Johnson, M.D.

1. Why is heart failure considered a relevant medical condition especially in the elderly?

More than 2 million Americans have heart failure, with approximately 400,000 new cases developing each year. The total treatment costs for heart failure, including drugs, physician costs, and nursing home stays, are estimated to consume > $10 billion in health care expenditures yearly. Heart failure shortens life expectancy, resulting in 5-year mortality rates of 50%. The incidence of this condition rises markedly above age 65, and its prevalence approaches 10% in individuals over age 80. As the elderly population encompasses a higher percentage of the general population, the importance of properly managing this condition and decreasing morbidity and mortality grows.

2. What causes heart failure?

- Coronary artery disease is the most common cause of heart failure, accounting for 50–75% of patients with heart failure.
- Hypertension is the second most frequent cause of heart failure, and in African-American elderly, it holds particular significance because of relative undertreatment.
- Cardiomyopathy is the next most common cause of heart failure. This includes all of the various causes of cardiomyopathy (alcoholic, viral, asymmetric hypertrophic cardiomyopathy, idiopathic, and others).
- Valvular heart disease causes heart failure less commonly. The two most common forms of valvular heart disease in the elderly are mitral regurgitation (usually secondary to left ventricular dilatation but may also be due to degenerative or rheumatic disease) and aortic stenosis (most commonly due to degenerative disease).

3. What are the major pathophysiologic abnormalities leading to heart failure?

Although multiple diseases can lead to heart failure, the pathophysiologic abnormalities fall in two categories: (1) left-ventricular (LV) systolic dysfunction with an ejection fraction < 35–40%, in which cardiac contractility is reduced; and (2) LV diastolic dysfunction in which LV filling is impaired because of stiffness or abnormal relaxation. The prevalence in the community of heart failure due to diastolic dysfunction is unknown, but data from clinical studies suggest 20–40%. In the elderly, this figure may be higher because of increased LV stiffness due to age and the increased prevalence of hypertension. Interestingly, the most common causes of heart failure, ischemia and hypertension, may result in systolic *or* diastolic dysfunction. Knowledge of the pathophysiologic mechanism is necessary to plan an effective and safe management strategy.

4. Which symptoms are suggestive of heart failure?

Patients who complain of dyspnea at rest or on exertion, paroxysmal nocturnal dyspnea, or orthopnea should be evaluated for heart failure unless the history and physical examination point toward a noncardiac cause. Dyspnea on exertion is probably the most sensitive symptom among patients with heart failure. Decreased exercise tolerance, due to dyspnea or generalized weakness, may be a nonspecific symptom of heart failure. The interpretation of leg edema may be complicated; if found along with symptoms such as dyspnea, it may indicate heart failure, but if found alone, it is more often caused by venous insufficiency. In the demented elderly patient, nonspecific symptoms such as worsening cognitive function, fatigue, and decreased food intake may be due to heart failure.

5. Can physical findings suggest the diagnosis of heart failure?

In patients with suspicious symptoms, finding an elevated jugular venous pressure, hepatojugular reflux, laterally displaced apical pulse, and a third heart sound may indicate heart failure.

The presence of rales with this complex of signs and symptoms is indicative of heart failure. It is important to note that some patients with mild to moderate LV systolic or diastolic dysfunction have none of these signs of heart failure. In these patients, the physician must rely on diagnostic studies. The finding of wheezing, especially in someone with no prior history of lung disease, should alert one to the possible presence of heart failure.

6. What diagnostic studies should be performed once heart failure is suspected?
The diagnostic studies chosen should provide information regarding the possible precipitating, complicating, or primary causes of heart failure. However, no test should be ordered unless the result will influence a management decision. Even a seemingly benign test can tax a frail elder.

Chest x-ray: In symptomatic patients, cardiomegaly is highly suggestive of heart failure, especially when accompanied by evidence of pulmonary vascular congestion. Although a normal chest x-ray makes the diagnosis of heart failure unlikely, it does not rule it out.

EKG: While there is no specific EKG finding for heart failure, the tracing may reveal possible precipitating factors. These include acute ischemia, prior myocardial infarction, arrhythmias, LV hypertrophy, and conduction abnormalities.

CBC: Anemia may aggravate underlying heart failure by decreasing O_2 carrying capacity. Anemia may trigger signs and symptoms of heart failure, even in patients with no underlying cardiac abnormalities.

Serum electrolytes: These may be helpful in the decision regarding drug selection.

Creatinine: An elevated serum creatinine may indicate renal insufficiency, requiring adjustments of drug selection or dosage.

Albumin: Hypoalbuminemia may lead to increased extravascular fluid.

Urinalysis: The finding of proteinuria or hematuria may indicate renal causes as precipitants of heart failure.

T4/TSH: Thyroid studies, including thyroxine (TH) and thyroid-stimulating hormone (TSH) levels, should be obtained in all elderly patients with heart failure with or without atrial fibrillation, as hyper- or hypothyroidism may present with heart failure as its initial manifestation in patients over age 65.

7. List the general criteria for admitting a geriatric patient with heart failure.
Patients in whom heart failure is present or suspected should be admitted if there is:
• Evidence of acute myocardial ischemia
• Pulmonary edema or severe respiratory distress
• Oxygen saturation < 90%
• Other severe complicating medical illness such as syncope, hypotension, and anasarca
• Heart failure unresponsive to outpatient therapy
• Inadequate outpatient social support to manage the condition safely
Some patients with these findings may be managed as outpatients if adequate monitoring and follow-up care can be arranged. Home visits by physicians, nurse practitioners, or registered nurses have demonstrated effectiveness in outpatient management of heart failure.

8. Do echocardiography and radionuclide imaging have roles in the evaluation of patients with heart failure?
Because clinical symptoms and signs do not reliably distinguish patients with heart failure due to systolic versus diastolic dysfunction, it is essential to measure LV function in patients with suspected heart failure. Noninvasive studies, radionuclide scanning or echocardiography, can reliably distinguish between systolic and diastolic dysfunction, a necessary step in planning therapy. Echocardiography also adds the ability to determine the presence of vascular and pericardial disease. The distinction between diastolic and systolic dysfunction is particularly relevant in the elderly population. While the elderly may tolerate mild diuretic therapy, the use of ACE inhibitors, digoxin, or nitrates may carry significant risks and should be used only if

specifically indicated. Patients with heart failure secondary to LV diastolic dysfunction may experience hypotension and its attendant sequelae when given these medications.

9. When should diuretics be started in older patients with heart failure?

Diuretics are useful in patients with heart failure with evidence of volume overload whether due to systolic or diastolic dysfunction. Patients with heart failure and signs and symptoms of volume overload, such as peripheral edema and pulmonary congestion, should be started on diuretics immediately. Those with evidence of mild heart failure can be managed with thiazide diuretics. Those with findings indicating severe heart failure require loop diuretics. The dosage used is severity- and patient-dependent. It is important, however, to consider starting elderly patients on low dosages (e.g., 25 mg of hydrochlorothiazide or 20–40 mg of furosemide) and titrating up as needed. The timing of diuretic administration is also relevant, especially in those with urinary urgency or incontinence. Patients managed with diuretics need to be monitored for possible volume depletion, hypokalemia, hyponatremia, hypomagnesemia, and azotemia.

10. What is the role of the ACE inhibitors in the management of heart failure?

Angiotensin-converting enzyme (ACE) inhibitors should be started in all patients with heart failure due to LV systolic dysfunction unless a specific contraindication exists. Several studies provide strong evidence that ACE inhibitors reduce mortality in patients with LV ejection fraction below 35–40% and symptoms of mild to advanced heart failure. Asymptomatic patients with low ejection fractions due to coronary artery disease have also been shown to have a prolonged survival. ACE inhibitors have been shown to improve cardiac hemodynamics and functional status. Contraindications include:

- Serum potassium greater than 5.5 mEq/l
- History of adverse drug reaction to these agents
- Symptomatic hypotension

ACE inhibitors should be used with caution in patients with serum creatinine > 3.0 mg/dl or creatinine clearance < 30 ml/min.

Although the largest randomized clinical trials have employed captopril or enalapril, the reduction in mortality in patients with heart failure due to systolic dysfunction is probably a class effect. In using any of these drugs in the elderly, the physician should start with a low dose equivalent to 2.5–5 mg of enalapril or 12.5 mg of captopril while monitoring the patient's blood pressure and electrolytes. If tolerated, titrate up to the equivalent of 20 mg of enalapril.

11. What are the side effects of ACE inhibitors?

Hypotension is a possible side effect of ACE inhibitors, especially when starting or titrating the dose upward. Therefore, patients should be euvolemic, not hypovolemic, when initiating therapy with an ACE inhibitor. Increases in serum creatinine and potassium have also been noted in some patients. ACE inhibitors should be used with caution in patients with renal insufficiency. However, chronic renal insufficiency is not an absolute contraindication. Potassium supplements and potassium-sparing diuretics should be discontinued before starting ACE inhibitors. Cough is a common complaint in patients on this medication. As cough is also a symptom of heart failure, these patients should be evaluated for possible pulmonary vascular congestion. Angioedema has been reported in some patients and, when involving the oropharynx, is an absolute contraindication to continuing ACE inhibitors.

12. When are direct vasodilators indicated in the management of heart failure?

Vasodilators such as isosorbide dinitrate and hydralazine are appropriate alternatives for afterload reduction in patients who are intolerant of ACE inhibitors. This combination has been shown to decrease mortality from 19–12% at 1 year and from 47–36% at 3 years in one trial when compared to placebo. Side effects including palpitations, headache, and nasal congestion are somewhat more likely with these agents. Anti-ischemic agents are also indicated when transient episodes of ischemia are suspected.

13. What is the role of digoxin in the management of heart failure?

While digoxin is routinely used in patients with heart failure with atrial fibrillation and a rapid ventricular response, its use remains controversial in those with sinus rhythm. Evidence suggests that digoxin improves functional status and can prevent clinical deterioration in some patients with LV systolic dysfunction. Its effect on mortality is unknown. Based on these findings, it may be beneficial to start digoxin in patients with severe heart failure due to LV systolic dysfunction who remain symptomatic despite treatment with ACE inhibitors and diuretics. Digoxin should be avoided in patients with diastolic dysfunction and in patients with COPD unless a rapid supraventricular arrhythmia is present.

When initiating treatment with digoxin, lower dosages should be used in elderly patients, those with renal insufficiency, and in patients with baseline conduction abnormalities. Patients should be aware of signs of toxicity which include confusion, nausea, visual disturbances, and anorexia. The clinician should be aware that digoxin levels may be raised by medications such as quinidine, verapamil, amiodarone, antibiotics, and anticholinergic agents. Therefore, digoxin levels should be checked approximately 1 week after starting any of these medications. Digoxin's narrow therapeutic window means that it must be used with care in older patients. More frequent monitoring than in younger patients is warranted.

14. How should diastolic dysfunction be treated?

The survival of older patients with heart failure due to diastolic dysfunction, although not as poor as in systolic dysfunction, is still reduced with an annual mortality of 8–22%. However, randomized clinical trials to determine the efficacy of alternative pharmacologic approaches in treating patients with diastolic dysfunction have not been conducted. Pharmacologic therapy should be directed at:

Decreasing central blood volume with diuretics

Controlling heart rate with calcium channel blockers or beta blockers as tachycardia further decreases ventricular filling in these patients

Enhancing the rate of relaxation with calcium channel blockers

Decreasing left ventricular wall thickness with antihypertensive agents such as calcium channel blockers

ACE inhibitors theoretically should benefit patients with diastolic dysfunction.

15. How should patients be monitored and educated to prevent hospitalizations?

Readmission to the hospital for heart failure is common. It has been reported that heart failure patients over age 70 have a readmission rate as high as 57% within 90 days of discharge. Factors associated with readmission include inadequate follow-up, poor social situations, noncompliance with a low-salt diet, and noncompliance with medication. It is essential that these issues be addressed as soon as heart failure is diagnosed, whether as an inpatient or outpatient. Patients should be taught the symptoms of worsening heart failure, particularly dyspnea on exertion and weight gain, and advised to notify the physician if these symptoms arise.

The physician should arrange for follow-up contact by phone or in person within 1 week of instituting new medications or after discharge from the hospital. During this contact, the proper use of medication and compliance with diet should be addressed. Because weight gain is a crucial objective sign of fluid overload, patients should be instructed to weigh themselves almost daily and to report a weight gain of 3–5 lbs. Laboratory studies including electrolytes, BUN, and creatinine should be checked during this visit, and medications adjusted as needed. Repeat imaging studies of the heart offer little value in monitoring the progress of heart failure once its pathophysiology has been characterized.

BIBLIOGRAPHY

1. Heart failure: Evaluation and Care of Patients with Left Ventricular Dysfunction. Rockville, MD, Agency for Health Care Policy and Research. June 1994. [AHCPR Guideline no ll; DHHS publ no 94-0612.]
2. Stevenson LW, Perloff JK: The limited reliability of physical signs for estimating hemodynamics in chronic heart failure. JAMA 261:884–888, 1989.
3. Wong WF, Gold S, Fukuyama O, et al: Diastolic dysfunction in elderly patients with congestive heart failure. Am J Cardiol 63:1526–1528, 1989.
4. SOLVD Investigators: Effect of enalapril on survival in patients with reduced left ventricular ejection fractions and congestive heart failure. N Engl J Med 325:293–302, 1991.
5. O'Neill CJ, Bowes SG, Sullens CM, et al: Evaluation of the safety of enalapril in the treatment of heart failure in the very old. Eur J Clin Pharmacol 35:143–150, 1988.
6. Vinson JM, Rich MW, Sperry JC, et al: Early readmission of elderly patients with congestive heart failure. J Am Geriatr Soc 38:1290–1295, 1990.
7. Tresch DD, McGough MF: Heart failure with normal systolic function: A common disorder in older people. J Am Geriatr Soc 43:1035–1042, 1995.

45. DIABETES MELLITUS

Cheng-An Mao, M.D., M.P.H.

1. How prevalent is diabetes mellitus in the elderly?

The prevalence of diabetes mellitus is 7–10% in people over age 65 years and increases with age. The rate can be as high as 15% in nursing home populations. Possible factors contributing to the increased prevalence are:

Weight gain
Reduced physical activity
Postreceptor defects
Impairment of insulin-mediated glucose uptake

2. Is diabetes mellitus different in older people?

An increasing ratio of adipose tissue to lean body mass leads to a decrease in insulin sensitivity. Studies have shown that the number of insulin receptors is unchanged by age, but the impairment of insulin-mediated glucose uptake could be due to postreceptor defects. Older persons also have elevated insulin levels. This change could be explained by insulin resistance and/or decreased insulin degradation. Impairment of beta-cell function may play a role, but autopsies have indicated that islet cell morphology does not change with aging. Glucose tolerance declines with age. It is controversial whether the glucose intolerance of aging is a normal aging process or an abnormality that needs to be corrected.

Diabetes mellitus is commonly seen in the elderly. The classic symptoms such as polydipsia, polyuria, and hunger may not present at the time of diagnosis. The most common type in older persons is non-insulin-dependent diabetes mellitus (NIDDM), so-called type II diabetes.

3. What are the criteria for diagnosing diabetes mellitus in older patients?

The National Diabetes Data Group's criteria for diagnosing diabetes are based on fasting plasma glucose levels, which are relatively unchanged by age. Studies have shown fasting plasma glucose level increases by 1–2 mg/dl/decade after the age of 50 years. Useful criteria for diagnosis are:

1. Fasting plasma glucose level > 140 mg/dl on > 1 occasion, or
2. Random plasma glucose level > 200 mg/dI, accompanied by symptoms

In patients without symptoms, random plasma glucose levels of > 200 mg/dl should be followed by determination of fasting plasma glucose levels. An oral glucose tolerance test (OGTT) is only performed if the patient does not fit the above criteria and diabetes mellitus is highly suspected. Older persons have higher rates of impaired OGTT, which may result in inconclusive results. Interpretation of glycosylated hemoglobin (HbA1c) levels in the elderly is also problematic. HbA1c levels are elevated with aging and some medical conditions, such as chronic renal failure and hypoxia. Using HbA1c to diagnose diabetes may result in a higher false-positive rate. Persons who are very obese, have a family history of diabetes, or have a history of gestational diabetes are considered at high risk. These groups should be carefully evaluated, and their random plasma glucose levels should be measured as part of periodic health examinations.

4. Which conditions other than diabetes mellitus raise plasma glucose levels?

Because acute physical stress can produce transient hyperglycemia, the diagnosis of diabetes mellitus in acutely ill patients is always difficult. Even though patients may need blood sugar control during hospitalization, they may not require diabetic treatment after being discharged. Diseases or conditions affecting plasma glucose levels include:

Stress	Hyperparathyroidism
Pancreatic disease	Hyperthyroidism
Glucagonoma	Acromegaly
Cushing's syndrome	Hemochromatosis
Primary aldosteronism	Infections
Pheochromocytoma	

5. Which drugs might increase plasma glucose levels?

Clinicians also need to be aware of those medications that induce high plasma glucose levels. Hyperglycemia is a complication of medications used to treat hypertension, heart failure, hyper-cholesterolemia, seizures, bipolar disorder, and asthma. Over-the-counter medications with a sugar-content such as cough syrups, can raise plasma glucose levels, too.

Thiazide, furosemide, diuretics	Lithium
Glucocorticoid, estrogen, growth hormone	Phenytoin
	Isoniazid
Diazoxide	Sympathomimetic agents
Niacin	Sugar-containing medications (e.g., cough syrups)
Phenothiazine, chlorpromazine	Alcohol

6. What complications can arise in diabetes mellitus in the elderly?

Vascular diseases—myocardial infarction, stroke, peripheral vascular disease
Ophthalmologic disease—diabetic retinopathy
Renal disease
Nervous system disorders—polyneuropathy, autonomic neuropathy, diabetic amyotrophy, cognitive impairment
Hypoglycemia
Hyperglycemia—hyperosmolar hyperglycemic nonketotic coma

7. Discuss the vascular complications of diabetes mellitus.

Diabetic patients have a 2–3-fold higher risk of myocardial infarction and stroke than nondiabetic persons. In NIDDM, 60% of mortality is from vascular diseases. Hyperglycemia, hyperinsulinemia, and hyperlipidemia are all associated with vascular disease and are commonly seen in older diabetics. In addition, diabetic patients are prone to hypertension and obesity, which are also risk factors for coronary artery diseases.

When choosing medications for hypertension control in diabetic patients, angiotensin-converting enzymes (ACE) inhibitors are preferred because they decrease the rate of proteinuria and preserve renal function. Hydrochlorothiazide and furosemide may induce hyperglycemia and may worsen glycemic control. Beta-blockers should be used carefully, as they may mask tachycardia induced by hypoglycemia.

Peripheral vascular disease can be caused by both macro- and microvascular angiopathy. When peripheral vascular disease combines with neuropathy, there is a high rate of diabetic foot ulcers.

8. Which ophthalmologic complications occur in diabetes?

Vision impairment is a common problem in patients with NIDDM. One-third of the blindness in these patients is due to diabetic retinopathy. Diabetic patients are also prone to cataract formation and macular edema.

The prevalence of retinopathy tends to increase with the duration of disease. Although studies have demonstrated that intensive glycemic control could reduce the incidence of retinopathy in patients with insulin-dependent diabetes mellitus (IDDM), the same correlation has not been shown in patients with NIDDM.

Intensive treatment always brings the worry of possible hypoglycemia in older patients. Early detection and photocoagulation therapy seem to be the best strategies to manage this complication. Regular eye examinations by ophthalmologists are recommended.

9. Which sign offers an early indication of diabetic nephropathy?

About 5% of deaths in patients with NIDDM are from renal disease. Diabetic patients have higher renal mortality rate than nondiabetic patients. **Microalbuminuria** (30–300 mg of urinary albumin excretion per day) is an early sign of nephropathy. The subsequent development of renal insufficiency is correlated with the appearance of microalbuminuria in patients with IDDM, but not always in NIDDM. Urinalysis can be used as a follow-up test to detect urinary albumin.

10. Describe the diabetic complications affecting the nervous system.

Nerve damage in diabetes mellitus may be due to either ischemic changes or exposure of the neurons to high glucose concentration or to abnormal glucose metabolites (e.g., sorbitol and fructose). The prevalence of **polyneuropathy** in NIDDM patients increases with the disease duration. Again, studies have shown intensive glycemic control decreases the incidence of neuropathy in IDDM patients, but there are no well-controlled trials to prove this decrease in NIDDM patients. Peripheral polyneuropathy usually presents with numbness and paresthesia. Tricyclic antidepressant drugs, phenytoin, carbamazepine, and topical capsaicin have been used to treat painful peripheral neuropathy.

Autonomic neuropathy has multiple presentations and is difficult to treat. Postural hypotension can result in falls; nausea and vomiting can be from gastroparesis; urinary tract infections may be secondary to urinary retention caused by dysfunction of bladder contractions. Other complaints, such as constipation, diarrhea, and impotence, are not uncommon. Treatment is mainly for symptom relief. Erythromycin and metoclopramide can be tried in cases of gastroparesis. Tetracycline may be helpful in diabetic diarrhea. Increased salt intake, elastic stockings, position modification, and mineralcorticoids have been used in treating postural hypotension.

Diabetic **amyotrophy** is an unusual syndrome of atrophy and weakness of pelvic girdle and upper leg muscles accompanied by anorexia and depression. The muscular problem is asymmetric and associated with severe pain. The syndrome usually resolves spontaneously within 1 year.

Cognitive impairment is noted more frequently in diabetic patients than nondiabetic patients. This impairment can be due to ischemic strokes, recurrent hypoglycemic episodes, and osmolarity changes. Mental status evaluation and follow-up are necessary.

11. How are the complications of glycemic control managed?

Hypoglycemia: Older patients are at a higher risk for hypoglycemia when undergoing treatment with hypoglycemic agents. The elderly have decreased abilities to compensate for hypoglycemic episodes, so prevention is the key to managing this complication. The most common cause of hypoglycemia is mistakes in dosages of hypoglycemic agents, with visual impairment being one of the major reasons for these mistakes. Decreased renal function prolongs the half-life of insulin and some hypoglycemics, thereby causing hypoglycemia. Reduced calorie intake can be caused by depression, infections, or disabilities in the elderly. Unless medication dosages are decreased as food intake falls, hypoglycemia may develop. When hypoglycemia happens, the patient's dietary habits, renal functions, and medication dosages should be carefully evaluated.

Hyperglycemia: In older patients, hyperosmolar hyperglycemic nonketotic coma occurs more frequently than ketoacidosis. Demented patients with uncontrolled diabetes mellitus should be carefully treated, especially when they become dehydrated or infected. Early diagnosis and aggressive treatment are the best practices to deal with these situations.

12. What are the principles of treating diabetes mellitus in geriatric patients?

Although there is no strong evidence to prove that good glycemic control reduces complications in geriatric patients, strict metabolic control can prevent dehydration, obesity, and polyuria. Treatment plans should be carefully reviewed with patients and caregivers. Many factors, such as vision acuity, renal function, cognitive status, functional condition, and support systems, should be considered when creating a treatment plan. To avoid hypoglycemia, plasma glucose levels are usually maintained just under 200 mg/dl in older patients.

Because older people may have multiple medical problems, the care of diabetes mellitus in the elderly can be challenging. Regular medical examinations and cooperation of patients and caregivers ensure successful management. Prevention of complications and functional preservation are the two main goals of diabetic treatment in the elderly.

Wearing appropriate shoes and avoiding bare feet prevent unnecessary injuries. Good foot care avoids amputations, saves medical expenses, and maintains life quality. Podiatry referral is useful in almost all elderly patients with diabetes.

Because ACE inhibitors preserve renal function in both IDDM and NIDDM, they can be used in diabetic patients for renal protection. Protein restriction has been advocated by the American Diabetes Association, but may not be suitable in older patients because of the possibility of malnutrition. Even though tricyclic antidepressants can be used for pain control, nortriptyline may be a better choice because it has fewer side effects. An EKG should be performed before starting tricyclic antidepressants to rule out heart blocks, which are contraindications. Nortriptyline can be started with a low dose, 10 mg, at bedtime. Capsaicin cream 0.075% is an over-the-counter topical that has been demonstrated to alleviate peripheral nerve pain. The cream is applied topically 3 or 4 times a day and takes at least 1 week to show effects.

Diet and lifestyle modifications, such as exercise and weight reduction, may control plasma glucose levels well for about one-third of older NIDDM patients. If plasma glucose levels are not under good control after a 3–6-month trial of dietary therapy, medications often can be the next step in therapy. Although oral agents are simple to use and highly acceptable, some patients may require insulin therapy.

13. How is dietary control used in managing diabetes mellitus?

Dietary therapy has few side effects, but dietary habits are not easily changed, especially in older persons. A good diet for diabetics should be a balanced diet, with restricted saturated fat. The requirement of daily calories varies but should be around 30–35 kcal/kg of ideal body weight, depending on the patient's situation. Acutely ill patients may need higher daily calories. Obese patients can have caloric restrictions for weight reduction, but minerals and vitamins supplements may be required if daily caloric intake is restricted too low. The diet can contain 50–60% of the calories from carbohydrates. Because many older diabetic patients are not obese when they are diagnosed, caloric restriction may not be indicated. Malnutrition is a potential risk for older patients and should be carefully evaluated when prescribing a restricted calorie diet.

Clinicians often suggest that patients avoid simple sugars, though there is no evidence to demonstrate that sugar can cause more adverse effects than other carbohydrates. Fructose only slightly elevates plasma glucose, and thus patients should not avoid fruits or vegetables. Alternative sweeteners, such as saccharin and aspartame, can be used safely to increase flavor, if the daily consumed doses of alternative sweeteners are below the acceptable dose recommended by FDA. Alcohol is relatively contraindicated in diabetic patients because alcohol can induce hypoglycemia, especially in patients treated with hypoglycemic agents.

Poor dietary compliance is the main reason of treatment failure. Allowing diverse options of food can encourage patients to adhere to the dietary program. Educating both patients and family members is important because some patients rely on families to prepare food for them.

14. Can older patients benefit from exercise?

Many studies demonstrate the benefits of exercise for older patients. Exercise improves obesity, glucose tolerance, lipid profiles, and physical abilities and may also reduce cardiovascular risk. Noncompetitive, low-impact, aerobic exercise is favored. Walking is a simple and inexpensive exercise. Swimming is nonweight-bearing and good for patients with arthritic disorders. Tai chi and stretching exercises are other good examples. Wearing appropriate shoes and socks, monitoring orthostatic hypotension, and warming-up before exercise can prevent unnecessary injuries (see also Chapter 15).

Diabetic patients should have a complete physical examination before starting exercise. For those beginning energetic exercise programs, an exercise stress test should be performed to disclose coronary artery disease. Patients should attempt to reach their targeted heart rate slowly because sudden cardiac death may occur during vigorous exercise. Patients with proliferative retinopathy need to avoid isometric exercise, such as lifting, that increases intraocular pressure and can cause further damage.

15. What treatment adjustments are warranted for exercising patients?

Exercise expends more glucose than ordinary activities and therefore can be associated with hypoglycemia if treatment adjustments are not made. In normal persons, hypoglycemia is avoided by production of glucose through hepatic glycogenolysis and gluconeogenesis. In patients treated with insulin, the high insulin concentration suppresses hepatic glucose production and causes hypoglycemia. Oral hypoglycemic agents may also increase the chance of hypoglycemia during exercise. Several strategies can be used to prevent this hypoglycemia:

Eat 15–30 gm carbohydrates before exercise
Reduce the regular dosage of hypoglycemic agents before exercise
Avoid drinking alcohol
Keep insulin injection sites away from exercising muscles
Never skip meals
Take medications after morning exercise

16. Which oral hypoglycemic agents are preferred to treat older diabetics?

When controlling hypoglycemia by diet and exercise fail, oral hypoglycemic agents are often the next therapy because they are painless and easy to use. **Sulfonylureas** have been the most commonly prescribed oral hypoglycemic agents. Their mechanisms are related to enhanced insulin secretion and tissue sensitivity. Compared to second-generation agents, first-generation agents have higher risks of hypoglycemia. Hypoglycemia can also be induced by drug interactions when first-generation agents are combined with salicylates, nonsteroidal anti-inflammatory drugs (NSAIDs), warfarin, sulfonamide, beta-blockers, and monoamine oxidase inhibitors.

Chlorpropamide, a first-generation agent, is not safe in the elderly due to its longer half-life and the possibility of hyponatremia. Second-generation agents, such as **glyburide** and **glipizide**, may be the better choice when treating the elderly. Patients should be started on a low dosage. Side effects are equal in both agents. Glyburide has mildly active metabolites that are not supposed to increase the risk of hypoglycemia. Some clinicians suggest glyburide may have less chance to develop hypoglycemia in renal failure patients because glyburide is metabolized by both kidney and liver. However, all of the hypoglycemic agents should be carefully prescribed in patients with renal insufficiency because of the prolonged half-lives.

Metformin, a biguanide, has been used in other countries for a long time and recently has been approved by the FDA. Its mechanisms are considered to involve inhibition of hepatic glucose production and intestinal glucose absorption. Sulfonylureas can result in hyperinsulinemia and weight gain, but metformin does not induce hypoglycemia and achieves blood sugar control without increasing body weight or hyperinsulinemia. The side effects include GI discomfort and lactic acidosis. From the recent studies, the incidence of lactic acidosis is very low. Renal and hepatic diseases are contraindications.

17. When does insulin become necessary?

Patients may need insulin treatment if oral agents fail to maintain carbohydrate metabolism. Insulin regimens can be either single or mixed. **NPH**, an intermediate insulin, is the most commonly used single agent. **Regular insulin** may be added for better glucose control. Premixed regimen (e.g., insulin 70/30) is convenient for some geriatric patients who have difficulties in mixing the regimens.

Patients or caregivers should be taught how to prepare and how to give insulin injections. Treatment failure can be from the lack of education. The service from visiting nurses is very helpful and should be frequently used. A home glucose monitoring machine can be offered to appropriate candidates.

Insulin plus sulfonylureas have proved to be effective in the middle-aged population, but there is no sufficient evidence indicating that the combined regimen produces better results in treating the elderly. Actually, this regimen should be avoided in the geriatric population because of the high risk of hypoglycemia.

Pharmacokinetics of Hypoglycemic Agents

	ONSET (HRS)	PEAK (HRS)	DURATION (HRS)
Glipizide	0.25–0.5	1–3	0–16
Glyburide	0.25–1	2–4	24
Metformin	0.9–2.6	2	12
Regular insulin	0.5–1	2.5–5	8
NPH	1–1.5	4–12	24

18. What are follow-up plans for geriatric patients?

- Regular medical examinations as recommended for general diabetic patients.
- Mental status evaluation and functional assessment.
- Use blood samples to follow-up glucose control. Testing glycosuria is a less accurate method to monitor diabetes mellitus in older patients because renal function is frequently impaired and renal glucose threshold increases with aging.
- Periodic HbA1c levels to monitor glucose control. Chronic renal failure, hypoxia, and drugs such as high-dose salicylates and opiates may alter HbA1c levels.
- Yearly influenza vaccinations administered before the the winter season. Pneumococcal vaccine appears effective for life after a single immunization.

When treatment fails, examine the patient to rule out the possibility of acute infections or physical stresses. Drug side effects or interactions should be considered. Noncompliance is the most common reason of treatment failure. To improve the compliance, a concerted effort from patients, caregivers, visiting nurses, and family members is needed. Team work is important in ensuring successful treatment.

BIBLIOGRAPHY

1. Bailey CJ: Biguanides and NIDDM. Diabetes Care 15:755–772, 1992.
2. Betts EF, et al: Pharmacologic management of hyperglycemia in diabetes mellitus: Implications for physical therapy. Physical Therapy 75:84–94, 1995.
3. Clark M, Lee DA: Prevention and treatment of the complications of diabetes mellitus. N Engl J Med 332:1210–1227, 1995.
4. Diabetes mellitus in elderly people. Diabetes Care 13(Suppl 2):1990.
5. Franz MJ, et al: Nutrition principles for the management of diabetes and related complications. Diabetes Care 17:490–518, 1994.
6. Hazzard WR, et al (eds): Principles of Geriatric Medicine and Gerontology, 3rd ed. New York, McGraw Hill, 1994.
7. Reikel W: Care of the Elderly: Clinical Aspects of Aging, 4th ed, Baltimore, Williams & Wilkins, 1995.

INDEX

Page numbers in **boldface type** indicate complete chapters.